Occupational Health Services

T0174156

Injured workers and their families, employers, and society as a whole benefit when providers deliver the best quality of care and when they know how to provide effective services for both prevention and fitness for duty, and understand why, instead of just following regulations.

Designed for professionals who deliver, manage, and hold oversight responsibility for occupational health in an organization or in the community, *Occupational Health Services* guides the busy practitioner and clinic manager in setting up, running, and improving health care services for the prevention, diagnosis, treatment, and occupational management of work-related health issues. The text covers:

- an overview of occupational health care in the USA and Canada: how it is organized, who pays for what, how it is regulated and how workers' compensation works;
- how occupational health services are managed in practice, whether within a company, as a global network, in a hospital or medical group practice, as a free-standing clinic, or following other models;
- management of core services, including record-keeping, marketing, service delivery options, staff recruitment and evaluation, and program evaluation;
- depth and detail on specific services, including clinical service delivery for injured workers, periodic health surveillance, impairment assessment, fitness for duty, alcohol and drug testing, employee assistance, mental health, health promotion, emergency management, global health management, and medicolegal services.

This highly focused and relevant combined handbook and textbook is aimed at improving the provision of care and health protection for workers and will be of use to both managers and health practitioners from a range of backgrounds, including but not limited to medicine, nursing, health services administration, and physical therapy.

Occupational Health Services

A practical approach

Second edition

Tee L. Guidotti, M. Suzanne Arnold,
David G. Lukcso, Judith Green-McKenzie,
Joel Bender, Mark A. Rothstein,
Frank H. Leone, Karen O'Hara,
and Marion Stecklow

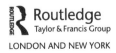

Routledge
Taylor & Francis Group

LONDON AND NEW YORK

First edition published 1989
by American Medical Association

This edition published 2013
by Routledge
2 Park Square, Milton Park, Abingdon, Oxon, OX14 4RN

Simultaneously published in the USA and Canada
by Routledge
711 Third Avenue, New York, NY 10017

Routledge is an imprint of the Taylor & Francis Group, an informa business

© 2013 Tee L. Guidotti, M. Suzanne Arnold, David G. Lukcso,
Judith Green-McKenzie, Joel Bender, Mark A. Rothstein, Frank H.
Leone, Karen O'Hara and Marion Stecklow

British Library Cataloguing in Publication Data
A catalogue record for this book is available from the British
Library

Library of Congress Cataloging-in-Publication Data
Occupational health services : a practical approach / [edited by]
Tee L. Guidotti ... [et al.]. – 2nd ed.
    p. ; cm.
    Rev. ed. of: Occupational health services / Tee L. Guidotti,
    John W.F. Cowell, Geoffrey G. Jamieson ; with the assistance and
    contribution of Alan L. Engelberg. c1989.
    Includes bibliographical references.
    I. Guidotti, Tee L. II. Guidotti, Tee L. Occupational health
    services.
    [DNLM: 1. Occupational Health Services. 2. Accidents,
    Occupational–prevention & control. 3. Occupational Diseases–
    prevention & control. WA 412]
    LC classification not assigned
    363.11–dc23   2012010800

ISBN13: 978-0-415-50281-8 (hbk)
ISBN13: 978-0-415-50282-5 (pbk)
ISBN13: 978-0-203-09574-4 (ebk)

Typeset in Baskerville
by HWA Text and Data Management, London

This book is dedicated to the workers who will be protected, treated, cared for, and, on occasion, saved by occupational health professionals, and to their families.

Contents

Figures

Tables

Boxes

Exhibits

Contributors

Authors

M. Suzanne Arnold, RN, PhD
Assistant Professor, Occupational Health Program,
McGill University, Faculty of Medicine
Montreal, Quebec, Canada
627 Kochar Dr.
Ottawa, Ontario
Canada, K2C 4H2
Suzanne.Arnold@McGill.ca and msarnold@istar.ca

Joel Bender, MD, PhD, FACOEM
Global Medical Director
U.S. Preventive Medicine, Inc.
47970 Ravello Ct.
Northville, MI 48167
JBender.MD@uspm.com and jbender@twmi.rr.com

Judith Green-McKenzie, MD, MPH, FACOEM, FACP
Associate Professor
Residency Program Director
Division of Occupational Medicine
Department of Emergency Medicine
University of Pennsylvania Medical Center
Ground Silverstein
3400 Spruce Street
Philadelphia, PA 19104
judith.mckenzie@uphs.upenn.edu

Tee L. Guidotti, MD, MPH, FRCPC, FCBOM, FFOM, FACOEM, FACP, DABT, QEP
Vice President for Health/Safety/Environment & Sustainability
Medical Advisory Services
1700 Research Blvd., Ste. 240
Rockville, MD 20850
tguidotti@nmas.com

Frank H. Leone, MBA, MPH
President and CEO, RYAN Associates, and
Executive Director, National Association of Occupational Health Professionals (NAOHP)
c/o RYAN Associates
226 East Cañon Perdido, Suite M
Santa Barbara, CA 93101
fleone@naohp.com

David G. Lukcso, MD, MPH, FACOEM
Medical Director
Medical Advisory Services
1700 Research Blvd., Ste. 240
Rockville, MD 20850
dlukcso@nmas.com

Karen O'Hara, BA
Managing Editor
UL PureSafety
730 Cool Springs Blvd, Suite 400
Franklin, TN 37067
karen.ohara@puresafety.com

Mark A. Rothstein, JD
Herbert F. Boehl Chair of Law and Medicine
Director, Institute for Bioethics, Health Policy and Law
University of Louisville School of Medicine
501 East Broadway #310
Louisville, KY 40202
mark.rothstein@louisville.edu

Marion Stecklow, MLT, CHCM
Environmental Health Consultant
12901 Prosperity Drive # 250
Silver Spring, MD 20904
Masstecklow@aol.com

Contributing Coauthors

Ian M. F. Arnold, MD, MSc, DOHS, FRCPC, CRSP, CEA, CSPQ
Consultant in Occupational and Environmental Health and Safety
627 Kochar Dr.
Ottawa, Ontario
Canada, K2C 4H2
imfarnold@ca.inter.net

Sami A. Bég, MD, MPA, MPH
Associate Medical Director
U.S. Preventive Medicine, Inc.
12740 Gran Bay Parkway, Suite 2400
Jacksonville, FL 32258
sbeg@uspm.com

David J. D'Souza, MD, MPH, FACOEM, FAAFP
Chief, Division of Occupational Medicine
Medical Director, Business Health Services
Beth Israel Medical Center
317 East 17th Street, 2nd floor
New York, NY 10003
davedsouza@pol.net

Raymond J. Fabius, MD, FAAP, FACPE
Chief Medical Officer
TRUVEN Health Analytics
1500 Spring Garden St.
4th Floor / C.701
Philadelphia, PA 19130
raymond.fabius@truvenhealth.com

Donna Lee Gardner, MSc
President
Gardner & Associates, Inc.
958 Aaron Branc Road
Bakersville, NC 28705
donnaleegardner@msn.com.

Paul Joos-Vandewalle, MBBCh
Occupational Health & Wellness Consultant
Shi Bisset & Associates
Strategic Partner of CHALLY Group Worldwide
Suite 1102, Block 10
Lane 460 Jinhui Lu
Shanghai 201103
People's Republic of China
paul.vandewalle@gmail.com

Craig Karpilow, MD, MPH, FACOEM, FRSTM&H, MRO, DME
Medical Director, Occupational Medicine Division
Workplace Medical Corp
130 Wilson St.
Hamilton,
Ontario L8R 1E2
Canada
craig.karpilow@workplacemedical.com

Ronda Brewer McCarthy, MD, MPH
OSHA and Regulatory Medical Expert Panel
Concentra
Medical Director, City of Waco Employee Health Services
1415 N. 4th Street
Waco, TX 76702-2570
ronda.b.mccarthy@gmail.com

Preface

Occupational health is the provision of care and health protection for workers, primarily through three core activities: (1) preventing, identifying, treating, and managing the consequences of injury and illness arising out of work; (2) evaluating fitness to work at a job; and (3) protecting and promoting personal health and productivity. These services are primarily provided by health care providers such as physicians and occupational health nurses in facilities or programs operated by employers or in community-based institutions, such as hospitals. Many providers and managers of institutions that sponsor occupational health services do not take the time to study occupational health services and never appreciate how it differs from conventional personal health care. Their half-baked initiatives may perform with disappointing results as a business and fail to meet their potential in providing health care. Careless managers then write off the potential of occupational health care when it was their model that failed. However, occupational health care can certainly be profitable and good occupational health services can and do provide excellent medicine and nursing care. This book is intended to show how.

This is a practical book intended as guidance on managing occupational health services, for professionals who deliver, manage, and hold oversight responsibility for them in an organization. It is not a handbook to clinical practice, a detailed evaluation of occupational health within the health care system, or a comprehensive textbook on occupational medicine or nursing. It is focused on the delivery of occupational health care, which is certainly enough for one book. The authors are writing for providers, managers, and health workers in any occupational health setting: corporate health departments, on-site medical centers, hospital or medical group-based occupational health services, free-standing occupational health medicine centers, and the many other forms that occupational health services take. Not every chapter pertains to every type of service, but there is enough overlap and similarity among them that it made sense to organize the book primarily by function. Still, there are dedicated chapters devoted to the special issues of corporate, hospital-based, and occupational medical centers and much in each of those chapters is of value in the other settings.

The current authorship team has deep experience in the practical delivery of occupational health care. Their backgrounds span academic life, corporate practice, and community-based services. The current authors were each assigned chapters or parts of the book to revise from the first edition, rewrite, or to write from the beginning. In several cases they invited coauthors for their chapters, who are designated "contributing authors." Several chapters had material moved around among them. Mark Rothstein kindly reviewed the legal content of several chapters to ensure accuracy. This interaction has made this a stronger, interdisciplinary, and more useful book. All chapters were edited extensively in order to achieve consistency, a helpful and accessible tone, and ease of use when readers look up a specific topic. Because this was a group effort but individuals took responsibility for a topical area, the specific views expressed in any passage are not necessarily held by every author and each author reserves the right to a personal opinion or interpretation of any given passage.

Some authors moved while the book was in preparation. In the case of RYAN Associates, which was assigned several chapters, individual chapters were delegated to contributing authors. Karen O'Hara, who had been Senior Vice President and Editor-in-Chief of RYAN Associates and the National Association of Occupational Health Professionals, left those related positions for the position of Managing Editor at UL PureSafety.

The work began as revision of a book first published in 1989 and subsequently reissued in facsimile as a "classic" in occupational medicine. The first edition of *Occupational Health Services: A Practical Approach* was published in hardcover by the American Medical Association (AMA) in 1989 in an edition of 4000, all of which sold, mostly through OEM Health Information (Beverly Farms, Massachusetts). Tee Guidotti, Geoffrey Jamieson, and John W.F. Cowell were the original authors, with Alan Engelberg participating on behalf of the AMA.

How this happened is a convoluted story. To simplify, the original three authors, who were based in Canada, had planned a work for the Canadian market but soon realized that it would have a greater and more positive influence on practice, wider distribution, and more impact if it covered both the US and Canada. They discovered that the AMA had previously published a five-booklet series based on a series of articles published in 1975 in the *Journal of Occupational Medicine* (now the *Journal of Occupational and Environmental Medicine*) by Henry Forbush Howe, an official in the AMA responsible for occupational medicine and environmental health. The series was itself a revision of earlier articles constituting a guide to occupational health practice, taken from various sources. Although the earlier articles were an inspiration, and excellent for their time, the booklets were greatly in need of revision. The authors offered to develop a new and much more comprehensive work, to be published by the AMA and sold rather than given away. Thus it happened that a book that was noted for carrying more Canadian content than any previous work on occupational health services happened to be published by the *American* Medical Association. The current team of authors continues the tradition of Canadian and American cooperation.

The first edition went out of print around 1997, as all available copies from the AMA printing were sold. In 2000, the book was recognized as a "classic in occupational medicine" by Blackburn Press, a small publisher that specializes in reissues of books that are out of print but of historical interest. In 2001, Blackburn printed a facsimile reissue of the 1989 first edition in paperback format. Meanwhile, used copies circulated and some institutions photocopied the entire work (with and without permission) for use in classes on occupational health.

By 2011, the time was long overdue for a new edition. It became clear that although the basic format and structure was sound, and that some things had not changed over 22 years, the new work would require more than just updating. Occupational health care would need to be rethought for a new generation and a new time. A new authorship team was then chosen with broad perspective, relevant experience, and compatible visions of the field, so that their individual contributions to the mosaic would fit seamlessly into a complete picture of occupational health practice in the 21st century. The challenge was to do this in a relatively compact book.

This book specifically addresses practice in the US and Canada. Although there are significant differences in the constitutional level of occupational health legislation and regulations, health care financing system, and workers' compensation systems in the two countries, the practicalities of occupational health practice are sufficiently similar to be covered adequately in one work, which is convenient for the many employers that operate in both countries. There are certain topics, such as hospital-based occupational health services for employers in the community, obstacles in strategic planning, and "hard-sell" marketing that are unique to the US and scarcely apply at all to Canada, which is hardly mentioned in those chapters. There are others, such as psychological safety and health, in which the Canadian experience is more advanced and is presented in detail. There is one topic, absence, that is best developed in the UK, from which both countries can learn.

We refer at times to "North America" as the US and Canada. We are aware that "North America" as a geographic term includes Mexico, and sometimes the islands of the Caribbean and western Atlantic, but we are using the term as it is commonly used by Americans and Canadians and as implied in the Spanish "norteamericano," referring to residents of the two countries. Occupational health services in Mexico and the rest of Latin America are organized differently and, while of great interest, are outside the scope of this book. Readers who are interested in comparative international systems are referred to references at the end of Chapter 7, "Global Occupational Health."

The authors supported their participation in this project through their own resources and effort. Medical Advisory Services, of Rockville, Maryland, provided support in kind for production of the book. Ms. Sam Motyka, a fine artist based in Edmonton, Alberta (Canada), prepared the drawn figures in her characteristic clean line, which is easy to read and results in clear photocopies. Dr. Joos-Vandewalle supplied the photographs of health institutions in Chapter 6. Praeger ABC-Clio gave permission for the reproduction of figures in Chapters 1 and 8, from *The Praeger Handbook of Occupational Health*.

1 The Occupational Health Care System

Tee L. Guidotti

Occupational health services are those health care services primarily concerned with managing injuries and illnesses that arise from work and maintaining the health of people at work or those who were at one time injured or exposed to a hazard while on the job. There are four essential elements to the mission of occupational health services:

- Prompt and effective care for injuries and illness arising out of work.
- Documentation of the cause of the injury or illness and its relationship to work, for purposes of compensation and future prevention.
- Management of chronic conditions that are aggravated or affected by the work environment.
- Management to promote health, productivity, and well-being.

The value added by occupational health professionals is not limited to the management of work-related disorders, as important as that is. It also comes from preventive programs, guidance to the employer on health affairs, problem-solving, risk management, careful documentation as the foundation for fair and equitable compensation, and productivity gains for the employer. From the point of view of the worker, this translates to better health, better and more sustainable benefits, fewer risks, better outcomes, better protection from hazards, and income security.

Box 1.1 summarizes issues that face virtually all employers in North America and that define the core mission of the occupational health service.

Occupational Health Care is a Separate System

In the US and Canada, as in many countries, occupational health services are provided by a separate and parallel health care system that shares many of the same providers with the general health care system but has a different payment mechanism and managers. The occupational health care system is driven by workers' compensation and management issues and is self-contained and more or less insulated from broader health care financing issues, except as they affect the price of clinical services in the market.

Most health professionals think of occupational health care as a subset of the general health care system or an alternate payer system. However, this is not accurate because the occupational health care system is not only separately financed but is driven by different factors (chiefly economic and technology trends), and organized around different principles than general health care, principally prevention and compensation. If occupational health

Box 1.1 Occupational Health Issues Faced by Most Employers

- Health care for employees, insurance being the obvious expense and wellness and health promotion being a proactive strategy
- Health care for employees injured on the job (in some states employers have the right to specify which doctor sees the employee first)
- Preventing work-related injury and illness by identifying and controlling hazards in the workplace
- Preventing work-related injury and illness by monitoring the experience of workers over time
- Preplacement medical evaluation for new hires
- Accommodation for health problems and impairment (compliance with Americans with Disabilities Act)
- Communication with health care providers to ensure an early and safe return to work for injured employees, whether the injury was work-related or personal
- Evaluating workers' compensation claims and tracking experience with work-related injuries and disease
- Certification of "serious" illness in an employee or dependent (under the Family and Medical Leave Act)
- Return to work and fitness for duty
- Certifying sickness absence
- Managing "presenteeism" (when an employee comes to work but is not functioning effectively due to health problems)
- Health promotion and wellness, for the employees' benefit and to improve sustainable productivity
- Drug screening and how to manage it without disrupting the workplace and risking ethical, legal, and privacy problems
- Product safety and liability and the due diligence required of a producer
- Protecting the health of employees in company-run facilities, such as cafeterias and canteens
- Defending against "toxic tort" lawsuits and third-party legal actions
- Environmental hazards and managing the risk and liability beyond simple compliance with EPA regulations
- Compliance with federal and state regulations for occupational health (not all of which are OSHA).

services are compared to other payers and organized systems in health care in the US, it would be about the third or fourth largest health care sector, after private health care, Medicare, the US Military Health System, and possibly the Veteran's Administration. The uncertainty comes from the absence of data on employers' direct payment for services. Expenditures by employers are not publicly disclosed and so are invisible to the rest of the health care system. The workers' compensation component of the occupational health care system looks smaller than it really is because service provision is fragmented by state and province and large parts of it, such as the appeals mechanism, are invisible to the average health professional. On the other side, the cost of occupational health and safety management effort within the plant and the aggregate total of payment from employers for direct health services are business expenses not routinely reported or tracked and therefore not publicly visible. Provision of occupational health services in the community is fragmented among different providers, most of which do not identify themselves as specializing in occupational health, and is often informally provided (such as fitness for duty evaluations) or casual, as a small part of a private practice, and so providers typically have a low profile in their community.

Occupational health services are paid for by either workers' compensation (universally called "workers' comp") carriers or directly by employers. Some companies are self-insured and so pay directly either way. However, there is a hidden subsidy from the general health care system to workers' compensation because costs for many disorders arising from work are absorbed in the general health care system. This happens most often because patients do not declare that the disorder is work-related, because the occupational association is not recognized, or because the effort made to file a claim is not attractive to the injured worker (particularly after retirement or for noise-induced hearing loss claims). Major insurers and managed care organizations search diligently for cases that might be work-related, because their expenses for those cases can be pushed over to workers' compensation. This issue becomes particularly acute in long-term disability, when the workers' compensation carrier and the long-term disability (LTD) carrier sometimes come to a standoff over whether a case is or is not work-related. On the other hand, there is an offset in the other direction, probably much smaller, in that personal health problems may be misclassified as work-related, often unintentionally but sometimes intentionally. The most often-cited example is weekend sports injuries that are declared on Monday morning as work-related, although how often that really happens is unclear. The latter offset is a source of continuing controversy, particular in low back pain and musculoskeletal disorders associated with repetitive strain.

Workers' compensation typically pays for medical care and income replacement for injuries and illnesses arising on the job, using funds derived from insurance premiums paid by employers (see Chapter 2). Workers' compensation is state-based in the US (with systems for federal employees, the District of Columbia, and US possessions, and special systems for interstate and maritime workers, there are 60 workers' compensation systems in total) and province-based in Canada (13, counting the territories and federal employees). Some disorders that arise from activities off the job, such as sports injuries, are misclassified as work-related, sometimes by intent, but the evidence is clear that far more disorders, especially illnesses, are not recognized as work-related, especially when they arise after retirement.

Employers pay directly for preventive services, fitness-for-duty evaluations (see Chapter 22), health promotion and wellness programs (see Chapter 30), and specialized services, such as consulting and medicolegal expert work (see Chapter 32). Much of this is directed at managing and mitigating costs in the workers' compensation system but increasingly employers are making what they consider a strategic investment in a healthy and productive workforce.

In the US and Canada (but not in some countries), the same medical providers generally attend to both occupational and nonoccupational cases. For most practitioners, nonoccupational cases constitute the great majority of their practice. The needs of the occupational health care system are very specific, particularly with respect to documentation, but it reimburses at a rate roughly equal to or only slightly higher than Medicare (US) or general health care (called "Medicare" in Canada). This means that few practitioners make an effort to become accomplished at managing the occupational dimensions of cases. Those few who do have usually developed streamlined, high-volume, well-integrated practices that manage workers' compensation documentation efficiently and manage individual cases intensively through rehabilitation and return to work.

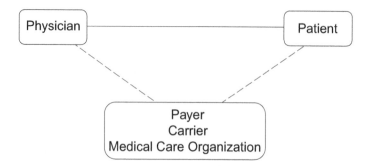

Figure 1.1 Relationship between the patient and the physician in the general health care system is modified by the third-party payer but remains primary in personal health care. (From *The Praeger Handbook of Occupational and Environmental Medicine* © Tee L. Guidotti. Reproduced with permission of ABC-Clio, LLC, all rights reserved.)

The path followed by the US and Canada is not the only way that occupational health services can be organized. In France, occupational health care is provided by well-organized specialized medical groups. In Finland, the occupational medicine physician is the primary care provider for working-age adults, performing a role much like the general or primary care internist in North America. In many developing countries, occupational health services have been the foundation for general health care in newly urbanized or settled areas of industrial development, as was true in North America in times past. For example, railroads and large employers such as Kaiser Permanente built much of the American health system and many of its most important institutions. Much of the health care system in the Middle East, Mexico, and Venezuela was built on the employee and dependent services infrastructure of the oil industry. Occupational health services sponsored by government have also been provided as part of a centrally-managed health care system in Quebec and Kuwait and in the socialist era in Eastern Europe and China.

The occupational health care system is built on different assumptions than the general or personal health care system. In a traditional fee-for-service setting, the primary relationship is that between physician and patient (the traditional "physician–patient relationship"), with the managed care organization, insurance carrier or other third-party payers influencing that traditional role (Figure 1.1). The degree to which third parties affect the physician–patient relationship has been very controversial and much debated but there is no real debate that the traditionally exclusive one-on-one physician–patient relationship of the past is over, at least in North America.

In occupational health care in North America, the number of players with a legitimate interest in the case and with influence on its management includes, at a minimum, the physician, the patient, the employer, a government regulatory agency (such as the Occupational Safety and Health Administration, OSHA), and the workers' compensation carrier (Figure 1.2). The physician's relationship to the patient is fundamentally the same but modified by other relationships and is governed by very explicit rules and procedures within the system which are designed to protect the legitimate interests of the employer and the carrier and by government regulation. The physician often acts outside the physician–patient relationship (see Chapter 3), reporting to the employer or to the carrier rather than on behalf of the individual patient. Among these agencies, information circulates subject to legal requirements, with accepted rules of confidentiality and authority for decisions and responsibility for compensation according to the role of each player.

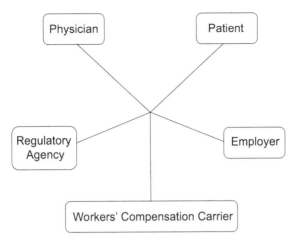

Figure 1.2 In the occupational health care system, the treating physician is essential but only one element in a network in which information about the specific injury, responsibility, and authority is shared with others, including the employer, the workers' compensation carrier, regulatory agencies (such as OSHA), and often workers' advocates. (From *The Praeger Handbook of Occupational and Environmental Medicine* © Tee L. Guidotti. Reproduced with permission of ABC-Clio, LLC, all rights reserved.)

Organization of Occupational Health Services

Occupational health services can be divided into "on site" and "off-site" facilities and services. For a century, in-plant services dominated the delivery of occupational health care. Then, in the 1980s, major corporations more or less in unison adopted a set of congruent management policies that were applied to functions outside the company's core business:

- *Outsourcing.* Corporate medical departments were closed and the services were contracted out to practitioners outside the employer's organization. This trend had the paradoxical effect of increasing the total number of occupational health professionals and the proportion based in the community. However, the trend resulted in a reduction of influence within companies, less engagement in the employer's specific needs, and loss of familiarity with the workplace. Some employers are now recruiting again because they have found that they need sufficient in-house capacity to manage contractors and to deal with internal matters.

- *Delayering.* Probably the most significant trend of all, delayering reduced or eliminated the upper- and middle-management layers of the company in order to streamline the organization, shorten the communications link, improve accountability, and increase efficiency. This trend was particularly important because these organizations lost the senior level of management that had been most familiar with occupational health services and its value proposition. Since outsourcing removed occupational health services from view and since the value of occupational health is rarely taught in business schools, new Master of Business Administration (MBA)-level managers almost never know how to manage occupational health services or how they contribute, unless they happen to have prior experience.

- *Downsizing.* Downsizing was the trend toward drastic reduction in the size of organizations, to the minimum required to conduct business. The objective was to boost profitability, force gains in productivity, and to streamline operations. Later, this was modified to "right-sizing," reducing the workforce to the optimum required to do business. With a much smaller workforce, many employers saw no need to maintain in-house occupational health services.

- *Devolution.* Some employers substituted occupational health nurses for physicians or assigned reporting accountability for contract physicians to non-physicians, for functions that did not require a medical license. Many physicians were alarmed at the time and believed that nurses were taking their jobs, which led to some friction between the professions. However, neither the salaries nor the decision-making authority of nurses who took on these responsibilities rose commensurate with the reassignment of professional accountability. The trend did not lead to the advancement at the corporate level that many nurses expected. In retrospect it seems clear that the trend was motivated simply by cost containment. Had there not been a substitution of lower-paid individuals for physicians, the positions would probably have been outsourced or cut.

Although the outsourcing trend, in particular, shook the field of occupational health services at the time, many positive outcomes resulted from these trends, as well as negative consequences. The number of practitioners in the field actually increased (as indicated by measures such as membership in professional organizations), and more practitioners became available in the community, making occupational health services more accessible to medium-sized employers and even small enterprises.

Providing Occupational Health Care

Occupational health care has a different emphasis than general health care, where the overriding objective is to treat the acute condition and the priorities are diagnosis and treatment. In occupational health care, diagnosis and treatment takes priority in an emergency or when the injured worker is in pain but otherwise accurate documentation is of equal importance. This is because the occupational health care system rests on different pillars than the general health care system:

- *Causation.* For purposes of workers' compensation, establishing the relationship of the injury or illness to work is critical, more important even than the exact diagnosis.
- *Compensation.* Workers' compensation is driven by the cost of care and replacement of lost wages. The prevention of disability ("tertiary prevention") and the assessment of impairment are therefore pivotal in occupational health care.
- *Fitness for duty.* For most physicians, an evaluation undertaken before a patient takes a job or certification for return to work is peripheral to care and is often performed in a perfunctory (and sometimes unprofessional) manner. In occupational health practice, it is central to the mission of providing care and quality is critical.
- *Exposure assessment.* For almost any complicated occupational health problem, assessing or estimating exposure to the hazard in question is a critical part of the evaluation. In general health care, it is rarely even attempted, except for taking the history of cigarette smoking.
- *Prevention.* In general health care, prevention and individualized health promotion are primarily about changing personal behavior with respect to health-related behaviors. In occupational health, prevention is primarily about compliance with regulation and training and the appropriate use of protective technology and personal protective equipment that, properly used, are independent of individual behavior.

- *Population health.* In general health care, the individual is the central concern. Except in cases of extreme risk, such as serious communicable diseases, issues of public health generally take a second priority to the patient's own interests and well-being. In occupational health, the practitioner of course manages individual health problems but also manages programs designed for protecting health at the level of populations, in this case the workforce.

In practice, most workrelated disorders are injuries on the job. Occupational injuries constitute the great majority of disorders related to work and include sprains, strains, burns, lacerations, occasionally fractures, and, rarely, severe multiple trauma; the emphasis, however, is on soft-tissue injuries, rehabilitation, functional assessment, and the management and prevention of chronic problems such as back pain and repetitive strain injuries. In the terminology of workers' compensation, injuries are single acute traumatic events, which may include burns and poisonings, and diseases are disorders that arise from repetitive or cumulative exposure. As a result, in the world of occupational health, many musculoskeletal disorders are classified as diseases, including repetitive strain injuries of the upper extremity and sometimes low back pain (more often considered an injury because there is assumed to be a precipitating event).

Occupational diseases typically encountered by the occupational physician include dermatological problems, eye conditions, acute respiratory disorders, and noise-induced hearing loss. Although important, poisonings due to hazardous chemicals, cancer related to work exposure, neuropathies, and other chronic conditions are relatively uncommon in a primary care-level occupational health service and are usually handled by referral to consultants or specialists. Cardiovascular disease is typically treated as a personal health and wellness problem, although there is new attention to occupational risk factors for heart disease. Psychological ("mental") stress at work (see Chapter 29) resulting in mental health issues (called "mental–mental" in the jargon of workers' compensation) presents a difficult management problem that is generally dealt with poorly, because it involves deeper issues of workplace culture and control. These disorders may be caused by conditions in the workplace but they may also arise from factors outside the workplace, presenting a dilemma of causation.

In addition to disorders caused by occupational exposures, there are many conditions related to work by exacerbation (temporary worsening of a pre-existing general condition) or aggravation (worsening of a pre-existing occupational condition), such as pre-existing asthma made worse by workplace exposure ("work-exacerbated asthma"). Neck pain may result from a vehicular collision where degenerative joint disease already exists in the cervical spine. Psychological safety and health at work may aggravate substance abuse issues, which are usually considered to be personal health problems in the domain of employee assistance programs (see Chapter 28). Such issues require the occupational health service to address the personal health of the worker and sometimes even to intervene in the primary care provided. These situations characterized by work factors interacting with personal health are very common, probably much more common than purely work-caused disease.

Much of the day-to-day work of occupational health services involves assessing the implications of personal health for capacity to work. For example, an important function of an occupational health service is fitness-for-duty evaluation, determining whether a candidate otherwise suitable for a specific job and who has been offered the position contingent on medical evaluation has the capacity to do the work required safely, and whether accommodation is required.

Although clinical aspects of occupational health care are similar to practice in general health care, administration and communications are more obviously part of day-to-day practice in occupational medicine and occupational health nursing. A real opportunity exists to prevent injury and disease and to promote good health.

Prompt and effective treatment of the injured worker can save that individual from unnecessary disability. An early return to work, when medically indicated, can also assist in rehabilitation. Acute care of an occupational injury, however, is more than a simple health care service function, as it might be in a hospital emergency room. It creates an opportunity to use the lessons learned from each injury, either singly or as aggregate statistical data, to prevent future injuries. The ultimate goal of an occupational health intervention, of course, is to control the hazard that led to the problem in the first place.

Communication is an essential aspect of occupational health care. The physician never acts alone in an occupationally-related case. Each action is reviewed and discussed behind the scenes and often generates multiple decisions and communications in the form of telephone authorizations, claims, chart reviews, and requests for clarification. Maintaining confidentiality can be particularly tricky, as some parties to the case are entitled to full information and others may not be.

Many physicians who do not understand the logic and structure of the process balk at the amount of paperwork involved in workers' compensation cases, in particular. However, the forms are usually simple and straightforward and require little more effort than a dictated progress note or a brief hospital discharge summary and physicians can bill for the time spent preparing them. Refusal to complete them, delay in filing them, or lack of attention to their content may severely harm the patient, distort health care costs, mislead regulatory activities, and result in health services not being covered by the carrier. To assist in the process and to expedite billing, it is important to train clerical staff to be skilled and to become experienced in workers' compensation. A brief telephone call by the physician or nurse to the employer to report on the patient's fitness for duty (see Chapter 22) should be considered a routine part of most patient visits, not an additional, onerous task.

There are some legitimate differences in medical practice between occupational and personal health services. For example, clinical practice guidelines generally work quite well for injured workers. Workers, because they are sufficiently well to hold down a job and seldom of advanced age, are on average healthier and more fit as a group than the general population or patients in primary care generally, and much healthier than patients in most specialty practices and geriatrics. (This principle is called "the healthy worker effect.") Practice guidelines can therefore be followed more consistently, with fewer exceptions because of co-morbidities, and outcomes are more predictable.

A basic difference between the occupational and the general health care systems is the level of utilization considered appropriate. The interests of the employer, insurance carrier, and the patient usually favor a speedy return to work which may be facilitated by a more intensive level of services in occupational cases. A day or two earlier return to work, because fitness for duty is determined sooner or more accurately, outweighs the cost of an additional clinic visit or physical therapy session for an injured worker receiving workers' compensation benefits. Careful monitoring for fitness for duty and extra therapy sessions, when they are justified, cost far less than a second injury, leaving aside the personal setback for the injured worker a premature return to work may represent.

More intensive use of services such as physical therapy may be required, to a degree that would seem over-utilization in general health care but which may be quite appropriate to the objective of returning the patient to work as soon as the patient is able. The intensity of care is intended to further the interests of all parties: to return the patient to work promptly, to reduce losses to the employer from absence, to promote prompt settlement of claims, and to reduce long-term expense on the part of the carrier. Physical or rehabilitation therapists may also monitor the progress of an injured worker's recovery more frequently and at less cost than through medical appointments.

In the setting of workers' compensation services, the physician is compensated on a fee-for-service basis according to a state-determined or contractual fixed fee schedule. In a predominantly fee-for-service setting, incentives built into the system tend to favor over-utilization of services because the profit margin increases (or the losses are diminished) when more services bring in more revenue. This tendency to raise the intensity of care is somewhat offset by adherence to practice guidelines and by the relative health (with many exceptions) of the workforce. However, there remains a potential systemic incentive to over-utilize services, especially when occupational health services offer physical therapy on site. This has led third-party carriers to institute utilization review (UR) procedures. UR is required to keep the balance and to prevent the compensation system from being abused. Unfortunately, UR is also often used by payers to prevent or delay delivery of care in an effort to reduce costs.

In the vast majority of cases, representing straightforward injuries, the occupational health care system works more or less automatically and reasonably well. In a tiny fraction of disputed or unclear cases, particularly for occupational disease, the system tends to jam and creates horrific complications and delays. For this reason, documentation is paramount and must be accurate and complete. An important motivating factor in the system is to reduce the number of appeals and expensive litigation.

Another distinct aspect of delivering occupational health care is the importance of correct handling of medical records. These records are subject to review not only by the patient, but also by the insurance carrier, the employer, or outside consultants when a claim is appealed, and may be subpoenaed in some circumstances. Occupational health records for employees must be maintained separately from their personal health record in order to prevent inadvertently breaking confidentiality. Some information, such as the family history, should not be kept in occupational health records because of legal implications and the risk of disclosure. Occupational health records must be retained for 30 years under the OSHA Records Retention Standard (see Chapter 13).

Occupational Health Professionals

This text is written primarily for physicians and nurses and secondarily for health services managers. Some physicians are board certified in occupational medicine and have been specially trained for this work, but most physicians working in this field of practice have not. Some nurses are certified occupational health nurses (COHN), specialists in their closely related field. Chapter 14 describes appropriate preparation and qualifications for health care professionals entering this field.

It must be emphasized that occupational medicine and occupational health nursing are not solitary practices. In occupational health practice, the physician and the occupational health nurse is each always a member of a team and not necessarily the team leader. There are many occupational health professionals beyond physicians and nurses. Chapter 14 also describes the various occupational health professionals and their roles, training, and credentials.

Types of Occupational Health Services

Occupational health services, like general health services, can be seen as a pyramid with three well-defined levels, illustrated in Figure 1.3.

- *Primary care.* Services that deal with acute problems of a more basic level of medical complexity. Occupational health services that specialize in this level of care are generally geared to a high-volume, low-margin operation, meaning that the number of patients is large and reimbursement for services is constrained, usually by a set fee schedule. The key to financial viability is to keep costs low, and to standardize common functions such as workers' compensation reports, and to refer anything complicated.
- *Secondary care.* Services that receive referrals for more complicated cases, conduct independent medical evaluations, or that are engaged in managing complicated problems on behalf of an employer. This specialized level of care is geared to problem-solving and is not readily standardized. It usually involves a mix of diagnoses for patient problems or consulting services for population-level program management issues.
- *Tertiary care.* Services that deal with a high-level referral or consulting function at the apex of the referral pyramid. Examples may include program design and evaluation, management consulting, quality assurance, and monitoring or managing programs for clinical screening, as opposed to the day-to-day operation of such programs.

Where these services are provided depends on the organization of occupational health services in the community and employer preference. Table 1.1 provides a classification of occupational health services, in the sense of service providers, based on whether care is

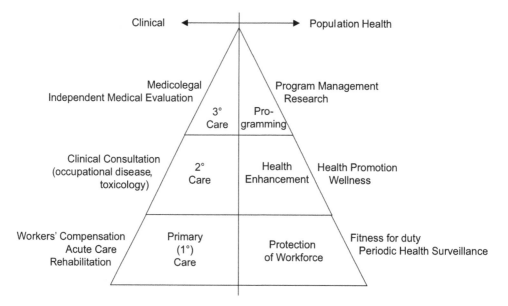

Figure 1.3 Pyramid structure of occupational health services. On the left, the clinical functions of providing occupational health services comprise primary care, secondary referral, and tertiary high-level consultant tiers, just as in general medicine. On the right, these three tiers have their counterparts in functions for the protection of the workforce and population health (See Chapter 20 for an explanation of why periodic health surveillance is a population rather than an individual health function.)

Table 1.1 Template for Organization of Occupational Health Services

Location where service provided	Serving one employer	Serving multiple employers
Employer's location: • On site (In-plant) • Employer's offices • Multiple locations	Model: clinic facility in plant or nearby, staffed by full- or part-time physician, nurse. Names: occupational health service, employee health service, health unit, occupational health service.	Model: clinic facility in an industrial park or regional center staffed by full- or part-time physician, nurse. Names: occupational health center.
Provider's location: • Office • Clinic • Group practice • Hospital • Network	Model: practitioner with a contract to serve employees of one company in a community-based facility, usually part-time. Sponsor: rare, mostly practitioners formerly employed by a company who were given a contract after services were outsourced.	Model: clinic facility based in community staffed by full- or part-time physician, nurse. Names: occupational health/ medicine clinic/center. Sponsor: free-standing medical service, hospital, multispecialty group practice, physician's private office, occupational (formerly "industrial") health center.

provided at the employer's location or in the provider's facility. This is more than an issue of real estate, because the venue of the clinical encounter largely determines access and control.

Employer's Venue ("On site")

The two levels of occupational health services under the control or in the venue of the employer are corporate health services and "on-site" services, at a particular facility or location. (The traditional term "in-plant", for on-site facilities, reflected an era of manufacturing dominance, when factories typically had an infirmary or dispensary.) Corporate policy, quality assurance, and standardized protocols, where they exist, are developed at a corporate level, usually at company headquarters but sometimes coordinated by a contract physician who is in charge locally. Corporate functions are discussed in Chapter 6; this discussion will focus on on-site services. The "corporate medical director" and his or her staff may coordinate the care of plant or on-site services and delivery of care by community-based contract physicians.

On-site services are provided within the employer's facilities, by a practitioner directly employed by the company or under contract. In a given location, the company may employ an on-site physician (traditionally called a "plant physician"), a nurse, or a nurse practitioner whose responsibility may range from simple triage and first aid to fairly comprehensive primary care, but never setting corporate policy. An on-site occupational health service under the employer's control is often called the "employee health service," particularly in hospitals. In a large company with many locations, these providers would be supervised by a corporate or regional medical director.

The mix of services rendered depends on the industry and the plant's historical experience. A shipyard or major manufacturer with a high trauma risk may maintain a full-service clinic capable of treating most primary health problems and stabilizing cases of major trauma. A financial institution with the same number of employees may contract for part-time services of a physician whose duties are mostly to conduct preplacement and fitness for duty evaluations, and to review workers' compensation claims. Many employers have their own guidelines that on-site physicians are expected to follow but most do not, beyond essential corporate policies. Most employers large enough to have in-house services have some form of wellness program in which the occupational health service is involved (see Chapter 30).

One hospital (see Chapter 9), divides in-house occupational health services into two offices, called "employee health" and "occupational medicine" or "occupational health," both of which report to human resources but sometimes through separate managers. The concept is that "employee health" manages issues that primarily relate to before-injury care, including wellness, fitness for duty and retention, while "occupational health" manages after-injury care and compensation. (This division of responsibilities is not generally accepted in the occupational health community, which holds prevention as a core value.) In this system, "employee health" therefore would deal with preplacement evaluations for applicants and fitness for duty evaluations for current employees, but also return to work, following protocols that are standardized and require minimal supervision; staffing is usually by nurses, at the Registered Nurse (RN) level. "Occupational health" would deal with management of difficult cases, impairment evaluation, and disputed workers' compensation cases; staffing is usually by nurse practitioners with physicians available as needed. Hospitals may like this divided system because it allows routine services to be performed at lower cost, reduces the need for health professionals with special training (such as certified occupational health nurses), and places the occupational health service in a close but subordinate working relationship with human resources. The disadvantages derive from lack of coordination, especially in fitness to return to work, confusion on the part of employees (since the notion of what "occupational health" really is gets lost), inconsistency, and fewer opportunities for involvement in prevention on the part of more skilled health care professionals. This system tends to work best when procedures are standardized or prescribed, as in a hospital setting where procedures are largely determined by criteria of the Joint Commission on Accreditation of Hospitals.

Some facilities serve many employers in a shared facility or area of industrial development (and so can be characterized as "on site"), often with assistance and support from a sponsor. The Slough Industrial Health Service project (now called Corporate Health Ltd.) is a famous and influential British prototype that was established in 1947 as a not-for-profit foundation, providing both medical and hygiene services integrated as a comprehensive system for employers in a large privately-owned industrial park in Berkshire, west of London, and the surrounding area. There have been attempts to initiate the full Slough model in Canada, most notably in Red Deer, Alberta, in the 1970s, but that project required a government subsidy to be sustained and ultimately was discontinued. In the US and Canada today, private providers may be co-located in an industrial area for better service but they are almost never part of an organized system in the Slough model.

Occasionally a large company will assist its vendors or contractors by providing occupational health services to their suppliers and contractors. This is increasingly rare because of liability issues, since it runs counter to the unstated purpose of many contracts, which is to remove liability from the larger company.

The most recent trend in employer-sponsored health care is the "on-site health clinic," which provides primary and urgent care on site on the grounds of large employers. The overriding purpose for an on-site health clinic is to provide services so that employees do not need to take time off work and to manage chronic disease among employees, not for delivery of occupational health services. However, these facilities have the potential to develop sophisticated and responsive occupational health services for the employers that sponsor them. Many are getting deeply involved in wellness and health promotion programs.

This is actually the return of an old idea. Employer-sponsored primary care has always been provided in remote sites, such as mining communities or in foreign operations of multinational corporations. Although perhaps not a felicitous model, "polyclinics" were also established in socialist Europe and China in large industrial operations to provide health care to workers; after the collapse of communism, many of these facilities were privatized. Employer sponsorship of medical care is an old model, used extensively in the 19th century by the railroads, in the early 20th century by employers such as John Deere, and famously in the mid-20th century by the Kaiser Company, which in the 1930s of necessity set up a health care network serving workers building the Hoover Dam and later both employees and their dependents at the Grand Coulee Dam site and later again in shipyards. This was the origin of the Kaiser Permanente system, which, as did others like it, adopted a prepayment financial plan and transformed itself into a health management organization. The few surviving examples of direct-care employer-sponsored health clinics essentially disappeared by the 1950s in the face of strenuous opposition by the American Medical Association (AMA).

On-site clinics are usually set up on a contract basis with local primary care providers, not with occupational health service providers. The objective is to have personal medical care readily available to employees to minimize time off work for medical appointments, for better management of chronic disease, and to expedite urgent but minor care. Major employers have made a commitment to this trend, including Toyota, Boeing, Intel, Pepsi Bottling Group, Credit Suisse, Sprint Nextel, and, notably, Perdue, where the clinics have become the major source of medical care for their low-wage, primarily Spanish-speaking employees in poultry production. Estimates cited in converging studies suggest that in 2010 roughly one quarter of employers with more than 1000 employees sponsored such on-site clinics, although the trend was slowing. Some employers were questioning whether an on-site clinic would encourage excessive utilization and others were deferring the capital expense during the recession.

Whether the new generation of on-site clinics will provide a high quality of occupational health services remains to be seen. They are oriented more toward personal care but at least one health care system specializing in staffing employer-sponsored health clinics, Aurora Health Systems, offers a full range of occupational health services, on-site rehabilitation, employee assistance programs, and wellness services together with the more usual urgent and primary care. During the H1N1 epidemic of 2009, some clinics were reportedly able to obtain vaccine early to protect their sponsors' employees, through the distribution system set up to give priority to clinics.

Provider's Venue

Over the past few decades, "off-site" or community-based health care facilities have displaced on-site services as the principal form of organization for providing occupational health services. They exist in many variations:

- *Primary care outreach*. Many practitioners, especially family physicians, provide such services in the course of their practice out of their own office. They often do not consider themselves occupational health providers because this is usually not a major part of their practice. Many practitioners view important occupational health functions, such as certifying fitness for duty and preplacement evaluations, solely as a service they provide for their patients' convenience, without further professional interest. Others intentionally branch out into occupational health care, usually at the primary care level only, in order to diversify their patient base.

- *Urgent care centers.* The proliferation of urgent care centers in the US has been a major trend in health services in recent years. Occupational health services are considered a major "business line" for urgent care centers. Most of these centers provide primary injury care and perform fitness for duty and preplacement evaluations but not more advanced care. Urgent care centers can be free-standing or affiliated with a hospital or medical group.

- *Occupational medicine centers (OMCs).* OMCs are free-standing, community-based occupational health centers, typically a medical group or practice primarily devoted to providing occupational health services for local employers and not affiliated with local hospitals or multispecialty practices. They have the advantage of streamlined procedures and staff trained and experienced in handling paperwork for worker's comp and important services such as the US Department of Transportation Commercial Driver Medical Examination program. The business model is based on high-volume management of common or simple problems and referring more complicated problems elsewhere. Because of their importance and rapid growth, Chapter 19 is devoted to this provider model.

- *Multispecialty group practices.* Large group practices have always provided occupational health services and many well-established groups were founded to provide such care. Some, such as the Guthrie Clinic in northeastern Pennsylvania and Scott & White Healthcare in Texas, have roots in railroad medical services and networks established in the 19th century. Others, such as Kaiser Permanente, originated from occupational health services for employees which were expanded to a broader patient base. Historically, this sector has been responsible for many innovations in health care generally.

- *Hospital-based occupational health services.* Because occupational injuries only infrequently require hospitalization and most services are delivered in outpatient settings, hospitals were relatively late in developing occupational health services beyond their own employee health services. Their entry into the market was marked by a miscalculation, which was that offering occupational health services would "lock in" large groups of employees into their health care system for personal care and drive utilization of hospital services. In fact, that rarely happens. As a result of their aggressive pursuit of this strategy, however, hospital-based services have emerged as the dominant model for occupational health care in the US within the last 20 years.

- *Union-sponsored or labor-affiliated occupational health clinics.* Only a handful of these facilities survive, principally in New York and Canada, but they were once more common. They have been very important where they exist in providing a counterweight to employer influence in the occupational health care system by providing advocacy and access to specialized expertise for workers.

- *Consultants.* By definition, consultants are health care providers who assess more difficult cases and do not provide care in the first instance. A small number of full-time private consultants in occupational medicine specialize in performing independent medical evaluations, disability evaluations, assessing causation and work-relationship for disputed workers' compensation and medicolegal cases; in other words, they function on the second and third levels of the pyramid in Figure 1.3. They are usually located in major cities and often associated with university programs. Unlike primary care practitioners, the business model for consultants usually depends on a smaller volume of cases, usually difficult or contested, that are "high-value" with respect to costs and compensation and for which higher fees are paid. Consulting practice is usually limited to individual practitioners who have extensive experience and have either earned a personal reputation in the field or have special or unusual expertise to offer. Consultants sometimes associate in consulting firms in order to share overhead and expertise.

* *Academic occupational health clinics.* Many academic medical centers sponsor referral clinics for evaluation and recommended management of suspected occupational disease, mostly associated with training programs in occupational medicine and nursing. They are valuable resources for referral but generally cannot provide acute injury management. They are represented by the Association of Occupational and Environmental Clinics (www.aoec.org).

Much occupational health care is provided outside this framework. Hospital emergency rooms deal with innumerable occupationally-related cases as a matter of routine, usually providing only acute or episodic care.

What are the Common Occupational Health Services?

Occupational health services, in the sense of functions, may be divided into two categories, ameliorative and preventive. Ameliorative services are intended to cure or limit disease or to manage existing problems. The word "ameliorative" is used here rather than curative because health care does not always cure disease or heal injury but always seeks to make the condition better. Preventive services seek to avoid exposure of the worker to hazards, detect disorders at an early and potentially curable stage, and to limit disability. Table 1.2 categorizes the principal occupational health services in this way. This is a conventional way of viewing such services but certainly not the only way it can be done, and elsewhere in this book (see Chapter 16) other taxonomies are used.

Acute care of the injured or ill worker is the most common role in occupational health performed by the primary care physician. Although most occupational injuries are straightforward to manage clinically, occupational illnesses are often overlooked or their

Table 1.2 Classification of Common Primary Care-Level Occupational Health Services

	Ameliorative[1]	*Preventive*[2]
Occupational medicine	Acute and chronic care for work-related injury and illness	Fitness for duty evaluation (Periodic health surveillance)[3] Health monitoring
Personal health care	Expedited primary care to reduce absence, monitor chronic disease (such as on-site health centers)	Preventive health services (such as influenza immunization) Case management of chronic disease (such as blood pressure checks)
Hazard control	Health hazard evaluation (Periodic health surveillance)[3] Regulatory compliance[4]	Worker education Personal protective equipment (e.g. respirator fit testing)
Wellness	Employee assistance programs Absence certification	Health promotion

1 To cure, mitigate or ameliorate a problem.
2 Always preventive, never "preventative".
3 Periodic health surveillance serves two purposes: to monitor the health of the individual worker and to ensure that hazard control is effective for the workforce.
4 Hazard control is not primarily a medical function but many regulatory standards have mandated surveillance and other medical requirements.

occupational association may not be recognized. Proper management of occupational disorders requires reporting of the case (a legal requirement of the Occupational Health and Safety Administration, on the "OSHA 300 Log") and prompt communication with the carrier and the employer if the injured worker will need time off work. Preparation of a "physician's first report" validates the case in the workers' compensation system (as the case has usually been initiated by the "employer's first report") and the physician is expected to file "supplemental" reports on the patient, concluding with a final report when the patient either is fit to return to work or has recovered as much function as is to be expected given the nature of the injury ("maximum medical improvement").

Fitness-to-work evaluations are a major responsibility of the occupational physician; these include preplacement, periodic health, "return-to-work," and disability evaluations, among other types. Preplacement evaluations, periodic health evaluations, "return-to-work evaluations" (following an injury or illness), and medical "certification" of absence due to illness are often spoken of as separate services, but they are all examples of fitness-for-duty evaluations, discussed in detail in Chapter 22.

Preplacement evaluations are medical evaluations of newly hired employees to determine whether they are able to perform safely and satisfactorily, with reasonable accommodation, the duties of the position offered. Knowledge of the precise work to be performed and the physical requirements imposed by the work is essential to a well-conducted preplacement evaluation. A preplacement evaluation is conducted after the decision has been made to hire the worker, contingent on physical capacity to do the job, if necessary with reasonable accommodation. In the past, the term "pre-employment examinations" was used, implying medical screening to perform any job, but the newer concept, and therefore the term "preplacement," is now required under the Americans with Disabilities Act (see Chapter 23).

Periodic health evaluations are usually given to employees at risk because of exposure to a known health hazard for early detection of the outcome in question; this is called "surveillance" (see Chapter 20). When required by law, such periodic screening for disease is called "mandated surveillance." Mandated surveillance is required by OSHA for workers exposed to a number of hazards, including lead, asbestos, and noise. Observance of a population without reference to an expected outcome is called "monitoring." The most common use of monitoring in industry is the "executive physical," a routine comprehensive medical evaluation for executives and key personnel whose health is thought essential to the company's future.

In impairment evaluation, the physician's role is to measure, to the extent possible, the physical capacity of the worker (who by then is usually not a patient) for purposes of assessing the level of disability for purposes of compensation (see Chapter 26). The physical assessment of impairment performed by the health care provider is only one part of disability evaluation but it is essential to the process. The suitability of the workers' skills, motivation, and aptitude for employment is evaluated by a work evaluation or rehabilitation counselor. The labor market for the workers' skills is also a critical factor in determining whether an award is made by workers' compensation.

Occupational health care providers are frequently part of teams to assess hazards or to investigate incidents. Chapter 21 provides an introduction to occupational health hazards.

Absence certification or management is a function of human resources departments, which review and certify illness requiring time away from work based on the report of a treating physician or the occupational health service, typically when the absence is longer than three days (see Chapter 24). Many, perhaps most, companies require employees to obtain certification in the form of a "note from the doctor," omitting the diagnosis and personal health information, for absence of more than three days. The note is usually presented to the human resources department or to the occupational health unit. An on-site physician reporting to the employer may review problem cases or requests for leave. Of course, the occupational physician generally has no way of knowing whether the illness was actually a valid reason for absence or even whether it occurred. The occupational physician's role is therefore to assess the plausibility of the absence, the explanation given, and the note from the treating physician, because the physician can request protected health information, including the diagnosis, but human resources cannot. Absence certification is usually combined with return-to-work evaluation but at a cursory level. As a practical matter, the occupational physician usually becomes involved only in extreme or questionable cases, which may involve employees who are absent more often than appears justified on the basis of health or who are given more time off work than appears reasonable after recovery from an illness or injury. The proper role of the physician is to identify causes for repeated or unauthorized absence, to assist the worker if possible, and to advise the personnel officer if absence will continue. This function is in contrast with the discredited practice of assigning physicians the role of "absenteeism control," tracking, investigating, and reviewing all absence in the organization. The physician must never act as policemen or timekeeper for the workforce because it erodes trust and obviates cooperation with employees on health protection.

Employee assistance programs (EAP) are organized by employers to identify employees with substance abuse, mental health, or other personal problems and to refer them for treatment, support and motivate them to complete treatment, and to assist in their rehabilitation. Most EAPs are focused on alcohol and drug abuse and mental illness, but others include family and adjustment problems, financial mismanagement (particularly overextended credit and other debt), and stress. A typical EAP operates primarily by self-referral of patients who are then triaged to local health care or counseling facilities. The employer monitors the progress of the employee and guarantees return to the same or similar work; EAPs usually do not provide direct treatment except for initial counseling. EAPs are discussed in detail in Chapter 28.

Wellness and health promotion programs are designed to keep workers well and to enhance both personal well-being and productivity as a workforce. They are discussed in detail in Chapter 30.

Recommended Reading and Resources

Guidotti TL (2010) *The Praeger Handbook of Occupational and Environmental Medicine*. Santa Barbara CA, Praeger ABC-Clio.

Guidotti TL, Kuetzing BH (1985) Competition and despecialization: an analytical study of occupational health services in San Diego, 1974–1984. *Am J Ind Med*, 8:155–165.

Harber P, Rose S, Bontemps J, Saechao K, Liu Y, Elashoff D, Wu S (2010) Occupational medicine practice: one specialty or three? *J Occup Environ Med*, 52(7):672–679.

Harber P, Rose S, Bontemps J, Saechao K, Liu Y, Elashoff D, Wu S (2010) Occupational medicine practice: activities and skills of a national sample. *J Occup Environ Med*, 52(7):1147–1153.

Moser R Jr. (2008) *Effective Management of Health and Safety Programs: A Practical Guide*. Beverly Farms MA, OEM Press, 3rd ed.

2 Workers' Compensation

Judith Green-McKenzie

Workers' compensation is the oldest form of social insurance in the United States and the third largest source of support for disabled Americans after Social Security and Medicare. Workers' compensation systems started in the US and Canada during the early part of the 20th century for the purpose of providing monetary compensation for medical and rehabilitation costs and lost wages to certain workers with work-related injuries or disabilities. Since then, a network of systems has evolved over the years to cover many more categories of workers since its inception. However, even today, a century after its inception, almost 10 percent of workers in the United States are still not covered, regardless of whether their jobs are hazardous. On the whole, however, the workers' compensation system can be credited for helping to create a more humane environment for all workers in North America, as workers covered by this system do not have to fear becoming impoverished or leaving their families destitute after a work-related injury, illness, or death.

This chapter is intended to provide an overview of workers' compensation systems, reviewing the principles and main characteristics. Workers' compensation in the US is not one unified system but is governed by different laws in the various states, federal jurisdictions, and US territories. In Canada, workers compensation systems are organized by province and show more consistency, because they were all established on a template closer to the original German model.

This chapter will address the historical roots of workers' compensation in North America, how the system is organized, what is compensable, workers' compensation insurance, how claims are handled, rehabilitation and disability management, and how disputes are resolved.

Origins

Germany, under Chancellor Otto von Bismarck, was the first country to pass laws establishing a workers' compensation system (1884). The German compensation system became a model for the industrialized world. The Austro-Hungarian Empire followed in 1887 and developed a very large insurance industry. Norway, Finland, Denmark, Italy, France, Spain, The Netherlands, Sweden, Greece, Russia, Belgium, and Switzerland all passed workers' compensation laws before 1910.

The German model was adapted by the UK in 1897 as the "Workman's Compensation Act." This adaptation became the model for the US and most industrialized Commonwealth countries (except Canada, which preferred the original German model). The UK eventually terminated its workers' compensation system when the National Health Service was phased in and insurance coverage for work-related injury became redundant.

Wisconsin passed the first US worker's compensation law on May 3, 1911, after much controversy. Prior to this event, special employer liability laws had been adopted by many states, which helped prepare the way for the workers' compensation laws that followed. Eight other states followed Wisconsin's lead that same year and passed their own workers' compensation laws. By 1920, all but eight states had passed workers' compensation laws. Mississippi (1948) and Hawaii (1963) were the last states to do so.

Workers' compensation in Canada began at about the same time when the province of Ontario organized a Royal Commission chaired by Mr. Justice William Meredith, the report of which outlined a model for workers' compensation based on five principles: no-fault compensation, collective liability of employers, security of payment, exclusive jurisdiction, and political independence. The model was closer to the original German system of public ownership than the British adaptation which influenced the US. Ontario introduced the first Canadian system in 1914, based on these "Meredith Principles." Other provinces followed suit, following the Meredith template closely.

Before workers' compensation, litigation was usually necessary for full compensation. Workers rendered injured or ill due to a work-related injury or illness bore the full brunt of medical care and lost wages unless employers voluntarily offered compensation, as many did but not always at levels adequate to support a family. Although an employee could file suit, that employee as plaintiff had to prove that the injury or illness was caused by employer negligence. The sole legal grounds for the disabled worker was the common-law principle that an employer is responsible for the injury or death of a worker if it is caused by employer negligence. Hence, in order for the worker to benefit from common law, he (injured workers who sued were almost always male) would have to bring suit against his employer, effectively cutting off all possibility of voluntary compensation if it had been offered, and making the worker effectively unemployable even if he could work, because other employers who knew of the lawsuit would not hire him. Workers who sustained a work-related injury or illness rendering them unable to return to work but who were unable to litigate successfully were left destitute. During this period in American and Canadian history there was no social safety net except for charity.

For the suit to succeed, the worker would then have to prove that the employer had been negligent and that the negligence had caused the injury. Under a common-law system, disputes are settled through an adversarial exchange of arguments and evidence where both parties present their cases before a neutral fact finder, either a judge or a jury. The judge or jury evaluates the evidence, applies the appropriate law to the facts, and renders a judgment in favor of one of the parties. Following the decision, either party may appeal the decision to a higher court. This process was invariably prolonged, difficult, and expensive. Very few workers were in a position to undertake legal action, given the prohibitive cost and the workers' low wages, and unions were usually not strong enough yet to help them. The process was also complicated by legal delays which worked strongly against workers who were not earning wages due to their disabilities.

In general, judges tended to take the side of the employer, especially when an industry was viewed as vital to the prosperity of a community. This was justified by the logic of the time because the courts did not want to interfere unnecessarily with the engine of economic growth. In the 19th century, both the US and Canada were developing their economies rapidly and with increasing linkages, but both had been beset by serious economic upheavals, especially in 1873 and 1893, and their prosperity was viewed as fragile. Judges were reluctant to impose what were seen as unreasonable burdens on employers. Juries, however, were less predictable and often sided with the worker. However, many cases did not get that far.

Employers had recourse to strong defenses under the law. One defense was the doctrine of "contributory negligence," whereby the worker would not be covered if he had in any way contributed to his own injury, regardless of the extent of employer negligence. Another was the "fellow-servant rule," whereby the worker could not collect damages if it could be shown that actions of a fellow worker had contributed to the extent of the injury. Finally, there was the "assumption of risk," whereby damages would not be recovered by the worker if the injury had been caused by inherent hazards of the job or by unusual hazards of which the worker was aware. The worker, under this doctrine, had assumed the risk by accepting the job.

The worker generally lost the case, because not only did common law protect employers but the informal constraints held workers back even if they had the resources to pursue litigation. Attorneys were expensive, the legal process was slow, and fellow workers who witnessed the injury were easily coerced not to come forward, especially if a case could be made that they contributed in some way to the injury. By the time the case was decided, the worker could be penniless or dead. Most claims were settled under terms favorable to the employer and very few illnesses were compensated, or even recognized.

As public policy, neither the employer nor the worker was satisfied with this common-law system. Employers were dissatisfied because they faced an increasingly large financial risk as juries became more restive and unpredictable and as medical costs and wages increased. Unions were gaining strength and voicing discontent with how the system was rigged against the worker. "Industrial accidents" were gaining more and more publicity during this time, resulting in increasing public pressure to improve working conditions in industrial settings, which were now felt to be more dangerous than agriculture or mercantile work. As the numbers and sizes of injury awards increased at the turn of the century, employers started to seek and accept passage of laws that would cap their liability, creating a rare moment of agreement between employers and workers which made passage of these laws possible.

No Fault System

Workers' compensation was founded on the principle of providing a compulsory "no-fault" form of insurance for workers injured in the course of employment, so that employers, through an insurance mechanism, are held responsible for compensation for work-related injuries and illnesses, regardless of findings of cause. In exchange for certain and prompt compensation (as it was seen then) through the no-fault system, the worker accepts compensation limited to the standard amount specified by each state, whether or not the payment fully covers lost wages, pain, and/or suffering. The benefits are limited and prescribed by statute and damages for "pain and suffering" are not recoverable. Employers as a group pay premiums to support compensation as a cost of doing business, although individual employers may have their premiums adjusted by an "experience rating" based on their record of claims.

If the disability is permanent (partial or total) the injured worker usually receives regular indemnity (compensatory) payments indefinitely. If both the employer and the employee agreed upon a "lump-sum" settlement, however, then this lump sum is in lieu of the indemnity payments and nothing more can be claimed in the future. There may be survivor benefits in the event of a fatality in some cases and some systems provide direct services such as retraining or rehabilitation.

When the workers' compensation statutes were first promulgated, it was expected that such laws would provide fair and equitable protection for both the injured employee and the employer. By forgoing their right of access to the courts, workers could expect to receive prompt income and medical benefits for work-related injury, and to avoid court delays, legal costs, the necessity to prove negligence, and the uncertainty of outcome. Employers, on the other hand, no longer faced the possibility of judgments by juries resulting in high settlement or restitution costs, since these costs were to be pooled and assessed outside of the personal injury litigation system. In addition, the public good would be served by relieving government and charitable organizations of the potential cost of supporting uncompensated disabled workers. Employers would also be encouraged through the incentive of insurance premium expense to minimize the occurrence of workplace accidents and injuries.

In practice, therefore, the workers' compensation system generally features compulsory, near-universal insurance coverage with income protection for work-related disability in order to provide benefits to injured workers and to protect the employer from litigation risk. Liability and compliance is enforced in the US by administrative agencies at the state level, with names such as the board of workers' compensation or industrial commission, also helping to avoid litigation. In some states and the District of Columbia and Canadian provinces, workers may seek care from any physician of their choosing (although a declaration of the employee's preferred provider usually must be made in advance); in most US states, however, the first medical encounter must be with a physician of the employer's choice (or selected from a list provided by the employer or the insurance carrier) for workers' compensation to pay for care. Workers have a basic right to refuse any recommended medical care or procedures. However, workers who do not cooperate with medical or rehabilitative care risk cancellation of their benefits.

Exclusive Remedy

Workers' compensation statutes are based on the legal principle of "exclusive remedy" whereby an injured employee can only claim compensation within the system. Workers in effect have given up the right to sue the employer at common law. In return, the injured employee receives total reimbursement for the medical costs incurred, as well as full or partial wage replacement during the period during which the employee is unable to work. Litigation is generally allowed only on issues of process and constitutionality of the workers' compensation system.

Exceptions do exist to the rule of exclusive remedy when issues in the case extend beyond the employer–employee relationship, as in the "dual capacity doctrine" discussed below. The most common is third-party liability, in which the manufacturer or distributor supplies a product that is defective, acted negligently, or fails to warn that the product is unsafe, is separately liable and can be sued by injured workers. Third-party liability is the grounds for most asbestos litigation. Another exception would be if the injury results from a deliberate, intentional act of the employer, in which case criminal charges can and have been laid.

The "dual capacity doctrine" refers a rule of law under which a defendant, who has two or more relationships with a plaintiff, may be liable under any of these relationships. For example, if the product or service that caused the injury to the worker is also produced by that employer, the employer is liable both as the employer of the injured employee and also as the producer of the product or service that caused injury to the employee. The injured employee may then either collect benefits for job-related injuries under workers' compensation, or file suit against the employer as the producer of the defective product or service. Thus the worker may still sue at common law if the injury results from the action of an employer in a relationship with the worker other than a worker–employer relationship.

As always, legal advice should be sought from a lawyer experienced in this specialized field before considering such unusual tactics.

Systems

The US does not have a unified workers' compensation law. Within the workers' compensation system, each state, three federal jurisdictions and each US territory (e.g. Guam, Puerto Rico, and the Virgin Islands) have individual systems, statutes, and regulations. As such, most workers' compensation systems are under state control. Many states protect workers from termination or retaliatory actions when a workers' compensation claim is filed. Some states have laws limited to physical injuries while some have laws which provide compensation only for specific injuries. States also differ in other aspects as well, such as the funds allotted for compensation to the claimants, in reporting procedures, in the amount of funds paid to the provider, and the administrative procedure. There are common threads, however. In general, federal and state programs provide benefits to employees who sustain a work-related injury, or to their dependents if workers are killed as a result of work, or if workers acquire an occupational disease. Significant variations do continue to exist even as the fundamental principles that underlie the many workers' compensation systems and programs have evolved over the years since inception. Six states have state-owned "monopoly" single-payer insurance carriers, as in Canada; many others have state-owned residual funds for employers who cannot afford or cannot obtain commercial insurance.

The 10 provincial Canadian "workers' compensation boards" (WCBs) are governed by appointed but autonomous boards and combine claims management, employer services, and insurance as single-payer "monopoly" systems under the oversight but not direct control of elected officials. There is also a combined territorial system for the Northwest Territories and Nunavut, a separate system for Yukon, and a system for federal employees, claims for which are administered by the provincial WCBs. As a result, Canadian WCBs tend to be larger and more often involved in providing direct services (such as rehabilitation) than the state-level businesses of commercial workers' compensation carriers in the US.

There are exceptions to coverage under workers' compensation. Although workers' compensation laws cover most wage and salary workers and the concept of workers' compensation could be made applicable to all workers, most workers' compensation legislation exclude coverage of certain types of work or renders some workers exempt for largely historical reasons. Most commonly excluded are agricultural workers, domestic (household) workers, and casual laborers. Coverage for other types of work may be limited, such as independent contractors, the self-employed, business owners and partners, workers employed by small companies with five or fewer employees, state and municipal employees, and nonprofit institutions. (Canada also excludes bank employees.) In addition, workers' compensation insurance is not compulsory for most private employment in some states (e.g. Texas). However, if the employers decline coverage they lose the legislated defense against being sued.

National Commission on State Workman's Compensation Laws

Decades after the first workers' compensation laws were passed in Wisconsin, The Occupational Safety and Health Act of 1970 was promulgated with the aim of assuring "... safe and healthful working conditions for working men and women ..." The National Commission on State Workman's Compensation Laws was also created under this Act and offered a thorough appraisal of the workers' compensation system. The Commission issued 84 recommendations, which influenced states to update their laws. The commission recommended coverage of workers who may not have been previously covered such as agricultural, domestic, and government workers. The commission also recommended coverage of all employers regardless of the number of employees and for all work related diseases. It also recommended an increase in weekly cash benefits. In general, it led to an increase in the types of workers covered under workers' compensation laws in various states, although several categories are still, today, yet to be covered.

Federal Workers' Compensation Programs

Notwithstanding the predominantly state-level organization of workers' compensation in the US, there are systems for federal employees and for workers in industries that cross state boundaries, administered mostly in the Department of Labor. In Canada, the system for federal employees is administered by provincial and territorial WCBs and is managed overall by Human Resources and Skills Development Canada (under the Minister of Labour).

The Federal Employees' Compensation Act (FECA) exists to administer the compensation for most US federal employees and provides workers' compensation coverage to three million federal and postal workers for employment-related injuries and occupational diseases. These benefits include partial wage replacement, benefits for total or partial disability, medical benefits, and vocational rehabilitation. This Act also provides survivor benefits to eligible dependents in the event that the worker dies. FECA is administered by the Office of Workers' Compensation Programs (OWCP).

The Federal Employees Liability Act of 1908 (FELA) applies to employees of interstate railroads. This is a modification of tort law, reducing the burden of proof on the plaintiff, rather than a no-fault workers' compensation statute. The injured employees may sue the railroad employer directly. The Jones Act or Merchant Marine Act of 1920 allows qualifying seamen the same protections afforded to US railroad employees under the FELA.

The Longshore and Harbor Workers' Compensation Act (LHWCA), initially passed by the US Congress in 1927, covers any person engaged in maritime employment, with the exception of seamen. LHWCA provides employment-injury and occupational-disease protection to workers who are injured or contract occupational diseases on the navigable waters of the US, or in adjoining areas, as well as for truck drivers, forklift operators, crane operators, employees on fixed oil production platforms, persons who work in shipyards building, repairing or tearing down vessels, and persons involved in building docks or other structures over the water, among others.

The Federal Coal Mine Health and Safety Act of 1969 amended by the Black Lung Benefits Act of 1972 is a social protection program for coal miners with coal workers' pneumoconiosis and related dust-induced respiratory diseases. This act regulates both the compensation system and the safety of coal miners. It allows provision of monthly payments and medical benefits to coal miners totally disabled from pneumoconiosis (black lung disease) arising from their employment in or around the nation's coal mines and provides monthly benefits to a miner's dependent survivors in the event that a miner dies from pneumoconiosis.

The Federal Veterans Compensation Program covers military personnel. It provides cash benefits and medical care to veterans disabled on duty. The Veterans Benefits Administration provides compensation for service-related and non service-related disabilities.

Adjudication

A worker qualifies for workers' compensation benefits if the injury or illness "arose out of or in the course of employment." A work injury that aggravates a pre-existing condition is also compensable. By definition, and contrary to common usage, an "injury" in workers' compensation occurs as the result of a single (although possibly complicated), discrete event. A "disease" is the result of a causal process that unfolds over time, notwithstanding that some diseases, such as infections, can result from discrete events. Therefore, when a worker falls off scaffolding and breaks his or her ankle, it is an "injury." When a worker develops a repetitive strain injury resulting in a tendonitis, it is a musculoskeletal "disease," along with occupational cancers, infections, lung disorders, etc. In order to make sense out of this, and to more easily apportion causation and disability, the concept of "cumulative injury" has evolved in workers' compensation. This idea recognizes that some work-related conditions are the result of the sum total of numerous small injuries, such as sound pressure on the ear that adds up to noise-induced hearing loss, or repetitive motions that add up to a repetitive strain injury, or low back pain that does not arise from a single event. Cumulative injuries are treated as a type of "disease" in workers' compensation. An exacerbation occurs when there is an increase in symptoms from any disorder caused by work. Aggravation refers to a change in the pre-existing condition leading to a temporary or permanent increase in disability or leading to a need for additional or different medical treatment. (These terms are generally applicable, but some workers' compensation systems and common usage use the reverse definitions.)

A common occupational example is low back injury. This type of claim, which in round numbers represents about 15 percent of all workers' compensation claims, not only tends to be disproportionately expensive, accounting for about 30 percent of all workers' compensation costs, but this disproportionate cost is driven by only about 10 percent of claims for this condition.

Occupational disease claims are also more difficult to adjudicate because of the factors of causation involved. Workers' compensation has focused mainly on injury claims. As cause and effect became clearer over the years, occupational diseases increasingly received recognition under workers' compensation. However, it was not until 1976 that occupational disease was covered in all states. Despite legislation, even today demonstrating proof for some occupational diseases is onerous.

Attributing occupational exposure to an illness may be challenging for the compensation adjudicator if the scientific evidence linking exposure with effect is weak, if it is not based on epidemiology (which the adjudication system strongly prefers to toxicological evidence), if the mechanism is not explained, or if the association has not been extensively studied. "First cases" of a newly recognized occupational disease usually have a hard time winning acceptance.

Often, causation of a disease is not unique to occupational exposure and many diseases have multiple causes. Unless the relationship between the exposure and disease is clear and evaluated with attention to the magnitude of risk conferred by each exposure and their potential interaction, it may be difficult or impossible for the worker to prove that the exposure led to the disease. For example, lung cancer may occur much more frequently in a smoker but it is also occurs in nonsmokers. It is a matter of informed judgment and interpretation of the facts in a given case to determine whether the lung cancer is due to chance, environmental causes (such as sidestream tobacco smoke or radon), other occupational carcinogens, asbestos exposure, or smoking (roughly in ascending order of potency), or some combination thereof, since interaction is known to occur and to amplify risk. In this way, lung cancer is unlike mesothelioma, which is reliably associated with asbestos exposure, even for brief periods in the remote past.

Time presents many issues. Many occupational diseases, especially cancers, have long latency periods. If there is a long latency period and much time has elapsed, the memory of events and exposure may be clouded. In addition, historical data may be difficult to obtain as written documentation of any exposure to a hazard or written documentation of records of employment may not be available at the time of disease onset. By the time some diseases develop, such as cancer, or impairment becomes severe enough to interfere with daily life, as in noise-induced hearing loss, many workers are long past retirement. It is not surprising, then, that a disproportionately low number of claims are submitted for occupational disease given their known and suspected prevalence and that disease claims are much more likely to be disputed than injury claims.

In diagnosing an occupational illness or disease, the occupational health provider must carefully review the case and all supporting materials including laboratory data, any industrial hygiene exposure data (current or historical), and medical records. A thorough history, assessing all previous workplace and environmental exposures, and a thorough physical examination are necessary. In general, an occupational disease or illness is considered compensable if an occupational exposure is the cause or one of several causes contributing to the disease, if the exposure aggravates a non-occupational condition, or if the exposure hastens the onset of a non-occupational condition. The burden of proof to demonstrate that the disease is occupational falls on the worker submitting the claim. The key elements of assessing causation and estimating impairment are similar to conducting an independent medical evaluation and are described in Chapter 25.

Simple cases, such as witnessed injuries and characteristic occupational diseases (such as mesothelioma following asbestos exposure) are almost always accepted by workers' compensation carriers without dispute. Complicated cases and most occupational diseases (such as multiple injuries or lung cancer in a smoker) are almost always denied. The system expects the injured worker to come back on appeal, providing evidence and carrying the burden of proof. As a result, whether such cases are ever accepted often depends on the availability of occupational physicians trained in recognition of these diseases and the evaluation of causality. Workers with chronic occupational illness often wait more than a year to receive compensation and they usually incur administrative and legal costs.

Apportionment

In some states (notably California), the physician may be required to make a determination not only as to whether the claim is valid but also to estimate the extent to which the exposure or purported cause contributed to the worker's condition. This is called "apportionment of causation." "Apportionment of impairment" refers to the process where a determination of what fraction of the resulting impairment was due to a particular injury or whether a portion of a worker's permanent disability is due to a cause other than the current injury, either occupational or non-occupational. Apportionment allows distribution of the financial responsibility, helping to ensure that the employer's carrier only pays for the portion of the disability putatively caused by that employer's workplace.

Insurance

Workers' compensation insurance provides coverage for work-related injuries or illnesses. It typically includes employer's liability insurance used to protect the employer if the worker is awarded damages outside the scope of workers' compensation. All states except Texas and all Canadian provinces require all businesses with employees (with few exceptions) to carry workers' compensation insurance coverage. This can be achieved through a commercial carrier, on a self-insured basis, or through a state workers' compensation insurance program. Employers are required to obtain workers' compensation liability insurance to pay for claims filed by employees. The result is a health care payment system within a legal system.

Self-insurance is preferred by large corporations (the 1 percent of US employers that employ 10–15 percent of the workforce), which have sufficient financial resources, and legal and medical staff to manage it successfully. The sheer size of the workforce allows the employer to spread risk across the large employee population. Mid-sized firms (14 percent of employers employ 70 percent of the workforce) usually purchase commercial market insurance. Small firms (85 percent of employers employ 15 percent of the workforce) are class rated and generally pay a payroll premium based on the industry's injury or illness history. High risk industries that cannot get reasonably-priced insurance on the open market may have access to state insurance funds in the US, such as California's State Compensation Insurance Fund.

Workers' compensation premium rates are set on the basis of each industry's injury/illness experience, using data such as the frequency and severity of claims, which reflect the hazardous risks of the workplace and of the employer's workers' compensation experience. The National Council on Compensation Insurance (NCCI) compiles experience data annually. Each state then sets specific experience rates for the employers operating within its borders. Some jurisdictions apply additional rate adjustment factors that relate to the industry or the specific company's accident record over a recent, defined period.

Insurers charge appropriate premiums and pay out or deny claims. Insurance carriers or self-insured employers may contest workers' compensation claims if the work relatedness of an injury is questioned or if the amount of the claim exceeds the amount a carrier is willing to pay. Contest over payment is most likely to occur for expensive claims, for example those involving permanent total disability or death.

In most states (Texas is the main exception) and provinces, having workers' compensation insurance is mandatory for covered employers. Uninsured employers may be penalized heavily in the form of fines, loss of common-law defenses, increase in the amount of benefits awarded, and payment of costs. The risk of the employee filing a civil suit is the biggest deterrent to those employers who choose to "go bare," as the cost of one expensive claim can threaten a company's financial stability. All states have "uninsured insurance" funds from which funds for compensation of workers can be drawn in such a contingency, although the company will then be expected to repay the fund and is subject to a civil suit.

"Second-injury funds" are established for the purpose of compensating workers in situations in which a previous impairment existed and impairment from the additional trauma has led to greater total or proportionate disability than the new injury would have produced alone. Compensation for the difference between the impairment apportioned to the present injury and total impairment due to the combined effects of previous impairment and the current injury is then paid to the worker from this second injury fund. The second-injury fund encourages employers to hire previously injured workers. In jurisdictions without such a system, the employer or insurance carrier is usually assessed for the total disability. This has the effect of discouraging some employers from hiring disabled workers, because they anticipate that if that employee is injured, they will be assessed for everything, including impairment that pre-existed the hire date.

Social Security Disability (SSDI)

There is usually an offset in benefits if a claimant for workers' compensation is eligible for other insurance programs, as there is in commercial insurance. Some workers may also be eligible for supplemental monthly benefits from disability from Social Security (SSDI) or Canada Pension Plan Disability Benefits. These benefits are available after a wait period (five months for SSDI) post-injury. They are calculated as if the disabled individual had reached the age for social security retirement benefits. The worker is eligible if he or she is unable to carry out substantial gainful employment, if the disability is expected to last more than one year, or if premature death will result. The combined SSDI plus workers' compensation benefit cannot be more than 80 percent of the worker's average earnings or the total family benefit under Social Security before the injury. SSDI benefits are reduced if the total benefits exceed the aforementioned. Some states will, however, reduce the workers' compensation benefits by all or part of the Social Security payments.

Disability

Disability is an inability or limitation in performing activities, roles, and tasks within a social or physical environment. Impairment refers to an anatomic or functional abnormality or loss. Workers' compensation carriers derive disability from impairment in a formula that also takes into account the job market and skills of the claimant. Disability may therefore vary among individuals with the same impairment, due to economic demand, and educational factors. Impairment is discussed in detail in Chapter 26.

There are four types of disability under workers' compensation:

- *Temporary total disability* (TTD), in which the worker is unable to work for a period of time but recovery is expected. Most injured workers fall under this category. Benefits are paid to the worker while out on disability. There is a waiting period before benefits are paid out, with the wait time depending on the state.
- *Permanent total disability* (PTD), in which the disability resulting from the work-related injury or illness is such that the worker is unable to undertake gainful employment and further treatment will not lead to recovery. These workers receive wage replacement (indemnity payments). Some states provide additional funds to dependents. Some states limit their duration of payment, while some provide compensation for life.
- *Temporary partial disability* (TPD), in which a worker sustains a work-related injury or illness such that the worker is unable to perform usual duties but is capable of working in some capacity at the same job (modified duty). The injured worker may receive the same wages. If modified duty is not available and the worker works in some other capacity, the worker may be compensated for the difference in wages earned before the injury and wages earned during the period of temporary partial disability (usually at two-thirds of the difference).
- *Permanent partial disability* (PPD), in which there is a permanent loss of one or several functions. Work is possible, but the worker may need to work at a modified duty capacity or at a different job. Payment may depend on the part of the body damaged, may be subject to a minimum and maximum limit, and may be based on the difference in the wages earned before and after the injury.

When an injured worker has recovered as much as they are likely to, and have reached a stage of permanent disability, they are said to have reached "maximum medical improvement"

(MMI) or to be "at permanency." Being at permanency does not imply that the condition will never change in the future, due to aging, co-morbidity, or second injury, nor does it mean that the worker with partial disability cannot return to any work or work at "light duty" before MMI is fully reached. However, determining whether a case is at permanency or has reached MMI is a necessary first step before impairment can be meaningfully evaluated for permanent disability of any kind.

Benefits

Workers' compensation benefits to workers and their families fall into two broad categories:

- Income replacement, which may include cash disability benefits (permanent total, temporary total, permanent partial, and temporary partial disability), survivor benefits, and vocational rehabilitation benefits, which is intended to lead to a new source of earned income on completion.
- Medical care benefits and (variably, for fatalities) funeral costs.

Payment for medical services resembles other forms of health insurance. Full medical benefits are generally provided with no time or monetary limitations involving no deductibles or co-pay. Medical benefits cover reimbursement for professional services, hospital stays, diagnostic tests, medications, wheelchairs, crutches, prostheses, and medical appliances. Most states require that all reasonable costs be covered, including transportation to and from medical care if it would otherwise be a hardship for the injured worker. Medical benefits may be restricted by fee schedules, however, to limit unnecessary costs. The employer and the insurance carrier have the right to challenge overuse of medical services administratively, a particular issue with respect to physical therapy. Independent review systems or utilization review organizations have been established to review medical treatment related to a case for medical necessity and to assist the administrative law judge or other reviewer as to necessity for the treatment.

Approximately 75 percent of all compensable claims for workers' compensation and 25 percent of cash benefits paid involve temporary total disability. For both temporary total disability and permanent total disability, workers typically receive two-thirds of their average daily wages with each state having a minimum and a maximum amount to be disbursed. These benefits are not taxed. Workers with permanent disability may be given a lump sum or paid on a monthly basis. Many jurisdictions do not adjust for cost of living. Approximately 1 percent of all compensable workers' compensation claims involve permanent total disability. In the event of a fatality, survivor benefits and funeral expenses are paid at a rate established for total disability. Benefits for surviving children typically end at age 18 or 19 but can be extended to ages 23 or 25.

The post-injury period of time before the cash benefits begin varies in each state from one to seven days. Most compensation agencies provide a retroactive adjustment to the actual date of injury if the disability continues beyond a certain threshold period.

Rehabilitation

Rehabilitation is an important aspect of workers' compensation and is included as part of workers' compensation benefit packages. Rehabilitation is the process of assisting an individual, disabled from any cause, to achieve a maintainable maximum level of functional and psychological independence in relation to self, family, home, and community. Optimally, the rehabilitation process begins as early as possible and is continued until functional independence is achieved. It benefits both the system and the worker to achieve the greatest possible degree of recovery in the shortest possible time. Vocational and psychological counseling or retraining and job placement are typical benefits provided to some degree by all states in order to return the worker to the workplace at either full duty, modified duty, or in another capacity. Some Canadian provinces, such as Alberta, have run their own rehabilitation centers for injured workers.

Vocational Rehabilitation

Vocational Rehabilitation refers to the provision of those vocational services such as vocational guidance, and vocational training. It also allows elective placement, designed to enable a disabled person to secure and retain suitable employment. Rehabilitation benefits such as physical therapy and occupational therapy are paid. Vocational rehabilitation involving retraining and counseling may also be covered.

Survivor Benefits

Dependents of employees who die as a result of a work-related injury or illness are paid death benefits under workers' compensation. States vary in the method of determining the amount of the benefit. Survivors are given a percentage of the worker's wage, usually paid to a surviving spouse until remarriage, and to children until they reach a specified age. These benefits to the survivors include burial allowances.

Adjudication and Appeals

Claims are reviewed in the first instance by the insurance carrier, which may use in-house experts to decide whether to accept or reject a claim. Most cases are straightforward and are accepted. Decisions concerning the relationship of an injury to the worksite are based on a "physician's first report," made on a form of the same name, that an injury of a certain type has been treated and that recovery requires the worker to be off work for a certain period of time. This is supported by the employer's confirmation, on a similar form, that an accident or toxic exposure affecting the worker occurred at the workplace on the date specified. The claim is then referred to a case manager, who, these days, is usually either a nurse or has some other background in clinical health care.

Although workers' compensation statutes were passed as an alternative to costly, time-consuming litigation in civil court, there have always been disputed claims. These disputes can be costly and adversarial, and the need to keep them out of the courtroom led to the formation of the first "alternative dispute resolution" mechanisms in North America.

In most states, an administrative law judge or hearing officers, rather than the court system, decides disputed cases. Some states have a workers' compensation specific judge or tribunal. In other states, workers' compensation judges are part of an administrative system of law judges that hear all kinds of administrative disputes. Appeals are possible, although generally appellate courts do not overturn findings of a judge. State administrative agencies have a variety of names, such as the Board of Workers' Compensation, the Industrial Commission, the Department of Labor and Industry, and the Industrial Accident Board. These organizations are responsible for supervising and insuring compliance with the compensation act and regulations, the investigation of worker claims, supervision of medical care and rehabilitation of workers, management of all premiums, administrative and compensation funds, and the collection and analysis of occupational injury and illness data.

In Canadian provinces, there is a level of appeal within the workers' compensation board, and if the dispute is not resolved there then it is decided by an autonomous workers' compensation appeals tribunal, which has the power to retain its own experts.

Differences in opinion which arise in workers' compensation cases are usually over either the work-relatedness of the injury or illness or the extent of impairment, and therefore final determinations of disability. The occupational health professional, usually a physician, may be requested to render an "expert" medical opinion (see Chapter 25, "Independent Medical Evaluation"). Other reasons for a dispute may involve issues of insurance coverage, provision of medical care, amounts of entitlement, the injured worker's earning capacity, and timeliness of a claim's work-relatedness. (Fault, however, can never be an issue, except in the exceedingly rare instance of alleged criminal intent.) These differences in opinion may arise among the employer, the insurance carrier, and the worker. If the disagreement persists, a hearing by the competent workers' compensation agency or court maybe requested. If resolution is unsatisfactory, parties may appeal. This administrative process eliminates the use of a jury and places the responsibility of deciding issues of fact, as well as issues of law, with an administrative judge or panel of judges.

Adjudication is the act of giving a judicial or administrative ruling, such as a judgment or decree. The assessment of a claim for compensation requires the answer to two questions: can the injury or illness be said to be caused or aggravated by workplace events, and do the facts fulfill the requirements of workers' compensation law? The first question is, in large part, medical; the second is strictly legal. For some claims of temporary disability and for all claims of permanent disability, the question is more complex. The compensation authorities must be satisfied that a claimed permanent disability is indeed permanent. As such, cases of severe disabling trauma (traumatic amputations, paralysis from falls, serious burns, etc.) may be thoroughly investigated with great reliance on medical advice.

Claims Management

The workers' compensation system has many moving parts, all centered on the injured worker. It is the worker's responsibility to initiate a claim for compensation. The employer is also expected to file a "first report," but that assumes that the employer acknowledges the claim. Standard forms are available for use in each jurisdiction for the initial claim, the most important of which to the physician is usually called the "doctor's first report." Figure 2.1 shows this form for the state of California.

There are time limits within which a worker must file a claim as well as time limits in which the worker must notify the employer about the work-related injury or illness. The time limits depend on the jurisdiction. Often, medical treatment is provided even before a claim has been submitted. (The Occupational Safety and Health Administration also has uniform requirements for employers to report injuries but these are unrelated to workers' compensation.)

Prompt filing of the claim and efficient claim investigation procedures are essential in order to allow for timely payment for medical care and payment of indemnity benefits.

STATE OF CALIFORNIA

DOCTOR'S FIRST REPORT OF OCCUPATIONAL INJURY OR ILLNESS

Within 5 days of your initial examination, for every occupational injury or illness, send two copies of this report to the employer's workers' compensation insurance carrier or the insured employer. Failure to file a timely doctor's report may result in assessment of a civil penalty. In the case of diagnosed or suspected pesticide poisoning, send a copy of the report to Division of Labor Statistics and Research, P.O. Box 420603, San Francisco, CA 94142-0603, and notify your local health officer by telephone within 24 hours.

	PLEASE DO NOT USE THIS COLUMN
1. INSURER NAME AND ADDRESS	Case No.
2. EMPLOYER NAME	
3. Address No. and Street City Zip	Industry
4. Nature of business (e.g., food manufacturing, building construction, retailer of women's clothes.)	County
5. PATIENT NAME (first name, middle initial, last name) 6. Sex □ Male □ Female 7. Date of Mo. Day Yr. Birth	Age
8. Address: No. and Street City Zip 9. Telephone number ( )	Hazard
10. Occupation (Specific job title) 11. Social Security Number - -	Disease
12. Injured at: No. and Street City County	Hospitalization
13. Date and hour of injury Mo. Day Yr. Hour or onset of illness a.m. _____ p.m. 14. Date last worked Mo. Day Yr.	Occupation
15. Date and hour of first Mo. Day Yr. Hour examination or treatment a.m. _____ p.m. 16. Have you (or your office) previously treated patient? □ Yes □ No	Return Date/Code

Patient please complete this portion, if able to do so. Otherwise, doctor please complete immediately, inability or failure of a patient to complete this portion shall not affect his/her rights to workers' compensation under the California Labor Code.

17. **DESCRIBE HOW THE ACCIDENT OR EXPOSURE HAPPENED.** (Give specific object, machinery or chemical. Use reverse side if more space is required.)

18. **SUBJECTIVE COMPLAINTS** (Describe fully. Use reverse side if more space is required.)

19. **OBJECTIVE FINDINGS** (Use reverse side if more space is required.)
   A. Physical examination

   B. X-ray and laboratory results (State if non or pending.)

20. **DIAGNOSIS** (if occupational illness specify etiologic agent and duration of exposure.) Chemical or toxic compounds involved?   □ Yes   □ No
   ICD-9 Code ____ ____ - ____

21. Are your findings and diagnosis consistent with patient's account of injury or onset of illness? □ Yes   □ No If "no", please explain.

22. Is there any other current condition that will impede or delay patient's recovery? □ Yes   □ No If "yes", please explain.

23. **TREATMENT RENDERED** (Use reverse side if more space is required.)

24. If further treatment required, specify treatment plan/estimated duration.

25. If hospitalized as inpatient, give hospital name and location   Date   Mo. Day Yr.   Estimated stay   admitted

26. WORK STATUS -- Is patient able to perform usual work?   □ Yes   □ No
   If "no", date when patient can return to: Regular work ___/___/___
   Modified work ___/___/___   Specify restrictions _____

Doctor's Signature _____   CA License Number _____

Doctor Name and Degree (please type) _____   IRS Number _____

Address _____   Telephone Number ( ) _____

FORM 5021 (Rev. 4)
1992

Any person who makes or causes to be made any knowingly false or fraudulent material statement or material representation for the purpose of obtaining or denying workers' compensation benefits or payments is guilty of a felony.

Figure 2.1 The "Doctor's First Report of Occupational Injury or Illness" form as used in California

Several stakeholders participate in the process of managing and moving the claim forward. The main parties are the treating physician, occupational health care providers advising the employer, the employer (supervisor, manager, or other representative), the insurer (claims adjuster, case manager, or other representative), and sometimes a workers' advocate (usually a union representative).

The Care Management Team

The insurance adjuster becomes involved when the claim is initially filed. Once the worker is under the care of a health care provider, the adjuster may contact the worker, the worker's supervisor, and the provider or provider's representative. The adjuster may use this time to introduce himself to the parties involved and gather information about the case. The adjuster may try to assess the severity of the injury as well as the target return-to-work date. The adjuster may use this time to inform the worker about lost wage benefits as well as about how the medical bills will be paid.

Physicians play a pivotal role in the workers' compensation system. The physician provides medical care to the injured worker and is the primary party responsible for documenting how the injury or illness was related to work, establishing the diagnosis, assessing the prognosis for recovery or permanent or temporary disability and extent of the impairment, providing or referring for rehabilitation and determining ability to work and in what capacity throughout the course of treatment, and in documenting progress and the final outcome. Fitness for duty (see Chapter 22) must be evaluated and documented as the injured worker recovers, with the most accurate possible determination of when the injured worker is fit to return to work and whether accommodation is required. Residual impairment (permanent partial or total disability) should be documented in detail.

Evaluation and documentation of the injured worker prior to the initiation of treatment should include pain level, objective physical findings, and current temporary impairment that interferes with functional capacity, both at home and at work. Subjective information should be noted but emphasis should always be given to objective findings. A clear statement regarding what objective or functional goals are to be achieved throughout the treatment period is useful, functional improvement should be tracked throughout this period, and evidence of progress towards meeting the functional goals should be sought. Examples of documentation supporting improved function would be increased physical capabilities (with a focus on job specific activities). Resolution of physical findings (such as increased muscle tone, radicular symptoms, or weakness), increased range of motion, strength, or aerobic capacity may be physical examination correlates of improved function. The physical therapy reports, if such a referral was made, document this for reference in physician-generated progress reports. The compensation authority uses these progress reports to help determine whether benefits are warranted or continue to be warranted.

Other health care providers, such as the occupational health nurse, occupational health nurse practitioners, and physician assistants, provide care to the injured or ill workers, support the process, and document the worker's progress. All health care providers in the system ought to be conversant with the laws in the state or province in which they provide workers' compensation care, in order to help ensure efficiency as well as appropriate care and counsel to the injured or ill worker.

In many settings, nurse case managers and medical assistants assist the occupational medicine provider together with other occupational health professionls, forming a team under physician leadership. Nurse case managers play a central role in the care management in that they enhance communication among all parties, that is, the specialists, physical therapists, safety personnel, workers' compensation administrators, and employer/supervisor, helping to bring the necessary information to the provider who can then integrate the information into his report.

Medical assistants play an ever-increasing role assisting the physician to ensure greater efficiency. Indeed, research supports the use of an integrated care management approach in managing the case of an injured or ill worker or a worker population, adding preventive measures to the program. This approach allows increased efficiency and reduced cost without sacrificing quality of care. Some of the elements of this integrated care approach are the use of preferred provider networks where injured workers are referred to specialists with whom the occupational health care provider has a relationship and from whom reports can be obtained in a timely fashion.

Physical therapists should be part of this team and not only provide treatment but timely and detailed reports on both progress and function, so that the occupational medicine (OM) provider receives up-to-date information on the progress of the injured worker allowing the provider to increase work restrictions as deemed appropriate based on the physician assessment and physical therapist report of progress.

Return to Work and Modified Duty

The injured worker's condition and temporary impairment should be managed with the end point being a return to work (sometimes called "return to function"), and preferably to the functional status that will allow the worker to return to the job he had been doing prior to the injury.

"Modified duty," "light duty" (an imprecise but traditional term), or "return to work with restrictions," when available, is a first step in a progressive increase in resuming duties as the injured worker's functional capacity increases. The injured worker's work restriction or modified duty parameters should match the modified job requirements. The provider may need to obtain the job description from the supervisor and base the modified duty work restrictions on this information. Sometimes a recommendation can be made for an ergonomist or another qualified professional to evaluate the work station. Modified duty allows the worker to reintegrate into the workplace or return to the workplace sooner, rather than waiting until the worker is able to carry out the full duties required. Modified duty accommodation has several advantages over waiting for recovery to fitness for full duty. It may prevent the worker from having to leave the workplace at all, so that the worker remains a part of the workplace culture while recovering; it may allow earlier reentry into the workplace; and use of modified duty leads to a reduction in indemnity costs to the employer, as there is less or even no lost time.

The supervisor is a vital part of the team in this respect, being in the best position to ensure that the work modifications are being met and that the worker is not being requested to do more than he or she is able given his or her injury and recovery status. Not observing the modifications set forth by the provider may result in a lack of progress by the injured worker or even a worsening of the condition. Regular visits to the provider are important so that progress can be monitored and interventions made as needed.

Some workplaces do not offer modified duty and will not accept an employee back to work until they have been given a release to full duty. The employer may be concerned about liability from a second injury, the risk to others, or the personnel issues that are raised when employees are not treated exactly the same. However, increasingly employers do not offer modified duty because with automated, high-production work processes there are no "light duty" tasks available and the pace of work is perceived as too intense for someone who may not be able to keep up. This problem often interferes with early and safe return to work.

The objective for the provider is not necessarily to return the worker to a state completely without pain or to wait until impairment is fully resolved before returning the worker to the job in some capacity. The goal is functional restoration. This return in function allows the worker to carry out work activities, activities of daily living, and to fulfill home and social obligations.

The optimal end point of the claim is a return to full duty. However, the nature of some injuries and workers is such that a full duty release is not possible. The provider may determine that the worker is at maximal medical improvement and has recovered to the extent possible. It is then determined that further medical care will not provide substantial improvement in function, although there may be other benefits for chronic conditions. It does not mean that the worker cannot be gainfully employed in another capacity. The worker may then have a permanent restriction reflecting permanent partial disability, or may be totally disabled. The injured worker may not be able to return to the same job or even to the same workplace. An assessment called a functional capacity evaluation may be requested at this point to determine what the worker is able to do and to help with job placement.

A "functional capacity evaluation" (FCE) is a comprehensive battery of performance-based tests used to determine an individual's ability to work and conduct activities of daily living. The FCE can be used by the provider as an aid in the determination of restrictions necessary for the worker to perform work duties safely. The FCE gives a more objective, measured assessment of what the worker can actually do, for example the quantified weight a worker is able to lift or the worker's range of motion.

Recommended Reading and Resources

Ballen DT (1994) The sleeper issue in health care reform: the threat to workers' compensation. *Cornell Law Review*, 79: 1291–1302.

Federal Coal Mine Health and Safety Act of 1969, Title IV – Black Lung Benefits Act (1969) Title 20. Employees' Benefits. Available at: http://law.justia.com/cfr/title20/20-2.0.1.1.8.html#20:2.0.1.1.8.1.283.1. Accessed September 4, 2011

Green-McKenzie J, ed. (2004) Managing workers' compensation costs. *Clin Occup Environ Med*, 4(2):1–5 (also the entire issue which was devoted to this topic.)

Green-McKenzie J, Behrman A, Emmett EA (2002) The effect of a health care management initiative on reducing workers compensation costs. *J Occup Env Med*, 44(12): 1100–1105.

Green-McKenzie J, Gershon R, Karkashian C (2002) Infection control practices among correctional healthcare workers: effect of management attitudes and availability of protective equipment. *Inf Control and Hosp Epi*, 22(9): 555–559.

Guidotti TL, Cowell JWF, eds. (1998) Workers' compensation. *Occup Med: State of the Art Rev*, 13(2): 241–450. (Entire issue devoted to topic.)

Harris J (2003) Workers' compensation. Chapter 18, in: McCunney RJ, ed. *A Practical Approach to Occupational and Environmental Medicine*. Philadelphia PA, Lippincott Williams and Wilkins, pp. 242–266.

Krohm G, Lore K, eds. (2011) *Workers' Compensation Centennial Commemorative Volume 1911–2011: Reflections on the History and Development of Workers' Compensation in the United States*. International Association of Industrial Accident Boards and Commissions, Madison WI, pp. 87–96.

Neumark D, Barth P, Victor R. (2007) The impact of provider choice on workers' compensation costs and outcomes. *Industrial and Labor Relations Review (Cornell)* 61(1): article 7. Available at: http://digitalcommons.ilr.cornell.edu/ilrreview/vol61/iss1/7. Accessed December 22, 2011.

US Department of Labor. Division of Federal Employees' Compensation (DFEC). Q&A Concerning Benefits of the Federal Employees' Co. Available at: http://www.dol.gov/owcp/dfec/regs/compliance/feca550q.htm. Accessed August 30, 2011.

Victor R, Carrubba L, eds. (2010) *Workers' Compensation: Where have we come from? Where are we going?* Cambridge MA, Workers' Compensation Research Institute.

Yang R, Liu J. (2011) *WCRI Medical Price Index for Workers' Compensation*, 3rd Edition (MPI-WC). Cambridge MA, Workers' Compensation Research Institute. Available at: http://ww1.prweb.com/prfiles/2011/11/10/8955935/wcri_med_cpi_3_final.pdf. Accessed December 22, 2011.

3 Occupational Health Law

Mark A. Rothstein

Federal and state laws enacted in the last several decades have attempted to protect occupational safety and health, prevent discrimination based on physical and mental disability, promote privacy and confidentiality of health information, and achieve other laudable goals. Many of these laws directly or indirectly affect the practice of occupational medicine. Knowledge of the legal context and implications of a medical assessment is likely to improve the practice of occupational medicine for physicians, nurse, and patients alike.

Decisions on legal actions should not be taken on the basis of general or background information such as that provided in this chapter. Always consult a lawyer experienced in occupational health law for guidance in specific cases, contracts, and in drafting binding policies.

This chapter is limited to the law of the US. Practitioners in Canada are advised to review applicable provincial or federal legislation and case law because the law differs, sometimes considerably, from American law. A particularly valuable resource for information is the Canadian Centre for Occupational Health and Safety.

Physician–Patient and Practitioner–Patient Relationships

The central legal issue surrounding occupational medicine is the nature and significance of the relationship between the physician and the individuals they examine or treat. Is there a physician–patient relationship? If not, what is the nature of the relationship and what legal duties are imposed on physicians? Although the main focus of the chapter and most of the legal cases involve physicians, the same principles apply to other health professionals, including nurses, pharmacists, and physical therapists.

In all settings, the physician–patient relationship is legally considered to be based on an implicit contract and characterized by the following: (1) the physician is selected by the patient or someone authorized by the patient (e.g. a referring physician); (2) the physician is paid by the patient or some third-party authorized by the patient (e.g. a health insurer); (3) the physician acts for the benefit of the patient; and (4) treatment may result. In the occupational setting, most, if not all, of these criteria are absent.

Rather than a traditional physician–patient relationship, therefore, occupational physicians and the individuals they examine have a "third-party" or "hybrid" relationship, which gives rise to numerous real or perceived conflicts of interest. Both salaried and independent contractor physicians owe a duty of loyalty to the entities that hire them as well as to the individuals they examine. (These issues arise almost entirely in the context of examining and evaluating workers for the purpose of making an assessment and offering recommendations to a third party, and excludes treatment; see Chapter 25.) The unusual relationship also creates a significant challenge to physicians in establishing and maintaining the trust of the examinee. The level of trust for an occupational physician by an individual employee and applicant can be envisioned on a continuum, ranging from a completely distrustful and adversarial relationship to a trusting fiduciary relationship identical to physician–patient relationships in private practice. In the former situation, complete lack of trust, the individual may engage in defensive measures, such as failing to provide or distorting key health information, thereby interfering with the physician's ability to assess accurately the individual's current health and future risks. In the latter situation, "excessive" trust, the individual may reveal confidential information without realizing that the physician is obligated to provide management with medical recommendations based on the information. If medical conclusions based on health information are revealed to management the individual may feel betrayed by a perceived breach of confidentiality. Even more troubling is the common situation where individuals forego visiting their regular health care provider because they erroneously believe they had a satisfactory checkup, even though the occupational medicine assessment they received was limited to determining their fitness for duty.

Although it is essential that occupational physicians and examinees understand the specifics of their special relationship, it should be recognized that the third-party medical relationship is not unique to occupational medicine. It exists in many other medical arrangements when examining physicians are employed for the benefit of an entity or person other than the individual whose health is being assessed. Other comparable relationships exist when there are medical examinations for insurance, workers' compensation, Social Security disability, military and prison health care, veterans' benefits, and litigation.

As further described in the following section, legal recognition of a physician–patient relationship generally has been a prerequisite to finding liability for medical malpractice. This is one of the reasons why physician groups traditionally have rejected the notion that there is a physician–patient relationship in occupational settings. In 1999, the American Medical Association (AMA) added section 10.03, Patient-Physician Relationship in the Context of Work-Related and Independent Medical Examinations, to its AMA Code of Medical Ethics. The provision states, in part, that "When a physician is responsible for performing an isolated assessment of an individual's health or disability for an employer, business, or insurer, a limited patient-physician relationship should be considered to exist …" The AMA's explicit recognition of a limited physician–patient relationship in occupational medicine contrasts with the position of the American College of Occupational and Environmental Medicine's Code of Ethics which still does not recognize even a limited physician–patient relationship and continues to refer to examinees as "individuals" rather than patients.

Because of uncertainty and misunderstanding surrounding the relationship of physicians and examinees in the occupational setting, and the harms that can flow from this situation, a Bill of Rights of Examinees (1996) has been proposed to clarify the relationship and set minimum standards for disclosure (Box 3.1). These or similar provisions have been adopted by several companies as well as in the AMA Code of Ethics. The central elements of this approach are a commitment to disclosure and a willingness to clarify the relationships and processes surrounding medical examinations in occupational settings.

Regulation of Practitioners under Common Law

Law in both the US and Canada may be statutory or common law. Statutory law is written law set down by a legislature or municipality. Regulations are rules developed and enforced

Box 3.1 A Proposed Bill of Rights for Examinees

Each individual subjected to an examination at the direction of his or her employer has a right:

1.   To be told the purpose and scope of the examination.
2.   To be told for whom the physician works.
3.   To provide informed consent for all procedures.
4.   To be told how examination results will be conveyed to management.
5.   To be told about confidentiality protections.
6.   To be told how to obtain access to medical information in the employee's file.
7.   To be referred for medical follow-up if necessary.

Source: Rothstein M (1996) Legal and ethical aspects of medical screening. *Occup Med: State of the Art Rev,*11(1): 31–39.

by competent government agencies in order to implement statutes (see Chapter 4). Common law is case law built on the precedents set by judicial decisions over the years and is constantly evolving. In occupational health, statues and regulations govern what is done for the protection of workers, but common law more often applies to the interaction between health care providers and workers as patients or individuals.

The common law is a body of legal doctrines and principles developed by courts over time in the course of adjudicating cases. Because it originated in England, the common law remains important in countries whose legal systems are based on English law. Common law is fundamental in ordering the conduct of parties in those areas where little or no legislation has been enacted. Few, if any, statutes address the practice of occupational medicine and therefore the common law is the primary basis for defining and regulating the physician–patient relationship. These judge-made rules have developed largely in the course of deciding the following three main types of personal injury cases arising from the practice of occupational medicine.

Negligent Failure to Diagnose or Inform of Diagnosis

Failure to diagnose is the most important category of cases in frequency of litigation and doctrinal significance to occupational health law. Traditionally, the courts have rejected claims by plaintiffs who asserted that an occupational physician's failure to diagnose their condition delayed treatment and adversely affected their health outcome. The courts in rejecting liability generally do so by applying the benefit rule, the treatment rule, or both. The benefit rule provides that if a medical assessment is performed for the benefit of the employer, such as a preplacement or periodic medical examination, then there is no physician–patient relationship. Similarly, the treatment rule provides that if no treatment is contemplated in the medical encounter, then there is no physician–patient relationship. If there is no physician–patient relationship, then there is no legal duty to act with reasonable care. If there is no legal duty, then there can be no legal liability for malpractice.

The traditional legal analysis was applied in *Medical Center of Central Georgia, Inc. v. Landers*, 616 S.E.2d 808 (Ga. Ct. App. 2005). An employee who was exposed to asbestos was given an Occupational Safety and Health Administration (OSHA)-mandated annual chest X-ray.

Although it showed a spot on the employee's lung, the employee was not informed of the result until a year later when he had his next X-ray. He sued the physician and the physician's independent practice group for medical malpractice. The Georgia Court of Appeals held there was no physician–patient relationship, applying both the benefit and treatment rules, and thus no duty or liability. It should be noted that this case involved an independent contractor physician. Legal recovery is even less likely against employer-salaried physicians because workers' compensation law generally bars negligence claims (including medical malpractice) against co-employees.

In the last several years, a growing number of courts have been willing to abandon the traditional benefit and treatment rules and find liability even in the absence of a traditional physician–patient relationship. The first important case to permit liability was *Coffee v. McDonnell-Douglas Corp.*, 503 P.2d 1366 (Cal. 1972). An applicant for the job of airplane test pilot was given a series of preplacement medical tests, including a comprehensive blood test. The results of the blood test indicated a very high blood sedimentation rate, suggestive of a serious inflammatory condition. The examining physician, however, never read the laboratory report and the individual was hired. Seven months later the individual was hospitalized and diagnosed with multiple myeloma. The California Supreme Court held that the company physician's negligence in failing to read the laboratory report was legally actionable because in assessing the applicant the physician and the employer voluntarily assumed a legal duty to act in a reasonable manner.

Another illustrative case is *Green v. Walker*, 910 F.2d 291 (5th Cir. 1990), involving an annual physical examination of a cook on an offshore oil rig conducted by a contract physician. The physician allegedly failed to diagnose the early stages of lung cancer and the man later died. In a lawsuit brought by the man's estate, the United States Court of Appeals for the Fifth Circuit held that even in the absence of a physician–patient relationship, a physician owes a duty to an employee undergoing an employer-mandated medical examination. "When an individual is required as a condition of future or continued employment, to submit to a medical examination, that examination creates a relationship between the examining physician and the examinee, at least to the extent of the tests conducted." Thus, even though the employer had no duty to conduct the examination, when it implemented a mandatory examination policy its agent had a duty to conduct the examination in a reasonable manner, including using ordinary care in reviewing all of the tests that were ordered.

Medical malpractice actions are based on state common law, and the law differs in each state. Although more states have been willing to reconsider the rule barring legal actions because of a lack of a physician–patient relationship, many states still adhere to the traditional rule, thereby complicating the ability to predict the result in any given case.

Negligent Job Placement

Medical examinations are used to determine an individual's suitability for employment in certain positions. Some lawsuits have alleged that harms resulted from negligent assessments. For example, in *Ewing v. St. Louis-Clayton Orthopedic Group, Inc.*, 790 F.2d 682 (8th Cir. 1986), an employee was injured on the job and received workers' compensation benefits. He was later referred to an independent medical examiner for a return-to-work evaluation. The employee alleged that the examination was negligently performed, which led to him prematurely returning to work and sustaining further injury. The United States Court of Appeals for the Eighth Circuit held that, despite the absence of a physician–patient relationship, the examining physician owed a duty of reasonable care to the examinee.

Other lawsuits have been brought by employees who were prevented from working based on an allegedly negligent assessment that concluded the employee was unfit. For example, in *Armstrong v. Morgan*, 545 S.W.2d 45 (Tex. Ct. Civ. App. 1976), an employee, upon being promoted, was required to have a physical examination performed by a company-retained physician. The physician's report indicated that the employee was in very poor health and, as a result, the employee lost his job. According to the Texas Court of Civil Appeals, the facts stated a valid claim for negligence. "If Dr. Morgan negligently performed the examination and as a result gave an inaccurate report of the state of appellant's health, and appellant was injured as a proximate result thereof, actionable negligence would be shown."

In some instances, it has been asserted that a negligent occupational medical assessment caused harm to a third party. In one tragic case, *Wharton Transport Corp. v. Bridges*, 606 S.W.2d 521 (Tenn. 1980), a truck struck the rear of a car parked on the side of the road and occupied by a family, causing the death of one child, severe injuries to three other children, and minor injuries to the father. The truck driver was not hurt. The trucking company paid US$426,000 to settle the lawsuit brought by the occupants of the car and then brought an indemnity action against the independent physician it had retained to determine whether the truck driver was physically fit to drive a truck in interstate commerce, as required by Interstate Commerce Commission regulations. (Department of Transportation regulations began in 1989.) The Tennessee Supreme Court held in favor of the trucking company and against the physician based on evidence of a subsequent examination that showed the driver had a variety of serious impairments, including the following: (1) only 5 percent vision in his left eye and blurred vision in his right eye caused by chorioretinitis; (2) severe osteoarthritis in both legs causing a loss of flexion and range of motion; (3) chronic degenerative disc disease in his neck and lower back that impaired his ability to move his head and neck; and (4) chronic fatigue, depression, and emotional exhaustion.

Negligent Treatment

Several lawsuits have alleged malpractice in providing first aid or continuing health care. Although many of the actions against company-salaried physicians have been barred by workers' compensation laws, some legal actions have been successful. Most common are the cases where there is an alleged failure to diagnose a work-related injury or a claim that treatment aggravated an injury. In one case, the employee asserted that a company physician over-prescribed painkilling drugs for an injury, causing the employee to become addicted.

In *Nolan v. Jefferson Downs, Inc.*, 592 So.2d 831 (La. Ct. App. 1991), a racetrack physician was found liable for the negligent treatment of a jockey's eye injury. The physician, who was under contract to provide medical services at the track, seldom went to the track himself and delegated his duties to a gynecologist, who was a convicted felon. The gynecologist's negligent treatment and failure to refer an injured jockey to an ophthalmologist caused a permanent eye injury. According to the Louisiana Court of Appeals, it was reasonably foreseeable that the physician's unauthorized delegation of responsibility to an unqualified replacement would result in harm to an injured jockey.

Personal injury lawsuits also may be brought by third parties for injuries attributable to the negligent treatment of an employee. In *Homer v. Pabst Brewing Co.*, 806 F.2d 119 (7th Cir. 1986), a night shift supervisor for a brewery reported to the plant medical department with severe cramps, nausea, and diarrhea. The nurse on duty gave him some Kaopectate® and, after a nap in the medical department, he was sent back to work. Still sick at the end of his shift, the employee lost consciousness while driving home and crashed into another car, causing permanent injuries. The United States Court of Appeals for the Seventh Circuit reversed a jury award in favor of the injured party and held that the employer "has not assumed a duty to unidentifiable members of the general public by undertaking to provide occupational temporary health care to its employees."

Statutory Law

There are many federal and more state laws governing employment, most of which have to do with discrimination and benefits. The federal statutes of primary importance in occupational health are addressed in this section.

Americans with Disabilities Act

The Americans with Disabilities Act of 1990 (ADA) is a comprehensive federal law prohibiting discrimination on the basis of physical or mental disabilities. Title I of the ADA, dealing with employment discrimination, covers employers with 15 or more employees. Besides most private sector employers, the ADA also covers state and local government employers and the US Congress. Federal government agencies are not subject to the ADA, but they are covered by comparable provisions in the Rehabilitation Act of 1973.

In prohibiting employment discrimination based on disability, the ADA also regulates the way fitness for duty assessments are conducted. For purposes of legal analysis, the process is divided into three stages, with different legal rules applicable to each stage (see Chapter 23 for guidance on compliance with these rules).

First, section 102(d)(2) of the ADA prohibits all pre-employment medical examinations and inquiries, including questionnaires administered before an offer of employment. This provision was designed so that individuals with disabilities will not be disqualified from employment without being afforded an opportunity to demonstrate they have the necessary abilities to perform the essential functions of the job. The ADA provides that, at this stage, an employer may not "conduct a medical examination or make inquiries of a job applicant as to whether such applicant is an individual with a disability or as to the nature or severity of such disability." The only permissible inquiries are about the ability of the applicant to perform job-related functions. For example, an employer or its designee, including a physician, may ask if the individual is able to climb telephone poles, drive a truck, or manipulate small parts if these are essential job functions. The employer also could ask, more generally, if the individual has a physical or mental impairment that would prevent the individual from performing essential job functions.

The second stage begins after the employer has extended an offer of employment conditioned on successful completion of a medical assessment. Pursuant to section 102(d)(3) of the ADA, an employer may require an "employment entrance examination" ("preplacement", often called "pre-hire" or "post-offer") of unlimited scope so long as (1) all entering employees in the same job category are subject to an examination, regardless of disability; and (2) all medical information is collected and maintained on separate forms and treated as confidential. The only exceptions to the confidentiality rules are that supervisors and managers may be informed about necessary work restrictions and accommodations, safety and first aid personnel may be informed if the disability might require emergency treatment, and government officials investigating compliance with the ADA may be provided with relevant information on request. As part of the post-offer medical assessment process the employer and its physicians are permitted to require as a condition of employment that the individual sign an authorization disclosing all of his or her health records. (As discussed below, genetic information is exempt from disclosure pursuant to the Genetic Information Nondiscrimination Act.) If a conditional offer of employment is withdrawn based on health information, however, the only permissible reason is that the individual is unable to perform essential functions.

The third stage, applicable to current employees, is the subject of section 102(d)(4) of the ADA, which provides that all medical examinations and inquiries of current employees must be "job related and consistent with business necessity." Employers may offer medical examinations of a non-job-related nature, such as comprehensive medical examinations and wellness programs, but employee participation must be voluntary. It is lawful for an employer to offer inducements to employees, such as reductions in health insurance premiums, to participate in health risk assessments or lifestyle modifications, including smoking cessation, but these inducements are closely regulated.

Occupational Safety and Health Act

The Occupational Safety and Health Act of 1970 (OSH Act) does not contain a broad requirement for employee medical examinations, thereby leaving the decision of whether to conduct examinations and their specific elements to employers and their physicians. In one area, however, employee exposure to toxic substances, medical examinations are often required by regulation and their contents specifically detailed. Employee medical examinations are expressly authorized by section 6(b)(7) of the OSH Act. The only statutory exception is section 20(a)(5), which precludes examination, immunization, or treatment of employees who object on religious grounds, except where medical attention is necessary for protecting the health or safety of others (see Chapter 4 for guidance on compliance with the OSH Act and with OSHA standards).

When applicable, OSHA standards dealing with specific toxic substances require physicians to furnish employers with a statement of suitability for each employee subject to employment in the area of potential exposure, conduct periodic (usually annual) examinations, and in some instances conduct examinations on termination of employment. The failure to offer mandatory examinations may lead to the issuance of OSHA citations and proposed penalties.

Section 6(b)(7) provides that medical examinations shall "be made available" to exposed employees. OSHA has interpreted this language to mean that the employer must offer the examination, but the employee may refuse to take it. Nevertheless, OSHA does not prohibit employer sanctions, including discharge, if an employee refuses to participate in medical surveillance, except if the refusal is for religious reasons. In other words, unless it is the subject of a contrary provision in a collective bargaining agreement, an employer may make participation in medical examinations a mandatory condition of employment.

Section 6(b)(7) also provides that medical examinations shall be made available "by the employer or at his cost." OSHA's health standards include language indicating that all costs for medical examinations must be borne by the employer. The employer also may be required to compensate employees for time spent undergoing examinations outside normal working hours and for extra transportation expenses they incur in off-site testing.

Despite several legal challenges, most of the medical surveillance requirements of OSHA standards have been upheld by the courts. For example, in *National Cottonseed Products Association v. Brock*, 825 F.2d 482 (D.C. Cir. 1987), the medical surveillance requirements of the cotton dust standard were challenged on the ground that there was no "significant risk" because only especially sensitive workers were at risk from exposure to cotton dust at the action level. The United States Court of Appeals for the District of Columbia Circuit rejected this argument and held that medical surveillance and monitoring were justified to (1) verify the effectiveness of the standard; (2) develop data to determine whether the standard was sufficiently protective; and (3) ensure that hypersensitive workers are removed from exposure before long-term injury.

Some OSHA health standards attempt to resolve disputes about an employee's fitness for duty after certain exposures by using a "multiple physician review" procedure. Under a few particular standards, if an employee is found unfit by the physician selected by the employer, the employee may obtain a second opinion, and, if the first two physicians disagree, a third physician is chosen by the first two physicians, and the third physician's decision is dispositive. All costs are borne by the employer. In reviewing these provisions the courts have looked to the nature of the hazard and the effects of the procedure, and have reached differing results, striking down the provision in the commercial diving standard but upholding the provision in the lead standard.

Other Laws

A variety of other federal and state laws regulate occupational medical examinations. At the federal level, some laws, such as the Mine Safety and Health Act, provide for medical examinations of employees with hazardous exposures as a way of protecting employee health. Other laws, such as those requiring medical certification of airline flight crews (regulated by the Federal Aviation Administration) and drivers operating motor vehicles in interstate commerce (regulated by the Department of Transportation), are designed primarily to protect the safety of the public (see Chapter 22). At the state level, medical examinations may be required for numerous regulated occupations, including teachers, school bus drivers, police officers, firefighters, and transportation workers. Workers' compensation laws also regulate aspects of medical examinations, including selection of physicians, compensation of physicians, and criteria in assessing work-related disability (see Chapter 2).

Medical Records Access and Disclosure

Despite periodic efforts in Congress since the 1970s, the US still does not have comprehensive federal legislation on health privacy. Instead, there are assorted laws dealing with the privacy and confidentiality of certain kinds of sensitive health information, such as HIV status, substance abuse treatment records, and genetic information. At the state level, a variety of laws also address certain types of sensitive health information, and medical practice and licensing laws add an additional layer of protection for clinical records. Few laws specifically deal with occupational health records. Consequently, to understand health privacy and confidentiality in occupational medicine it is necessary to review several sources of law.

Occupational Safety and Health Act

By regulation, the OSH Act grants employees access to their exposure and medical records to allow them to play a meaningful role in their health management. Unlike other OSHA record-keeping requirements, the access regulation does not require that certain documents be obtained or developed, but only that existing records be maintained and made available to employees and other authorized parties.

Employees have a right of access to their entire medical files regardless of how the information is generated or maintained. Excluded from the definition of "employee medical record" are certain physical specimens, health insurance claims information, and records of voluntary employee assistance programs. A limited discretion is also given to physicians to deny access where there is a specific diagnosis of a terminal illness or psychiatric condition. This exception, known as "the therapeutic privilege," reflects the medical paternalism of 1980, when the regulation took effect, and does not comport with the current view of medical ethics favoring disclosure. In fact, in 2006, the AMA specifically disavowed the therapeutic privilege regarding disclosure of health information to patients.

Other parties besides the affected employees have limited rights of access to individually-identifiable health records. Collective bargaining agents must obtain written consent before gaining access to employee medical records. OSHA has a right of access to employee medical records, but those records in a personally identifiable form are subject to detailed procedures and protections. The National Institute for Occupational Safety and Health (NIOSH) also has a right of access to employee medical records in conducting a health hazard evaluation. Strict confidentiality provisions apply to any records accessed, reviewed, or disclosed.

OSHA's access to medical records regulation provides that, with a few exceptions, employers must preserve medical records for the duration of employment plus 30 years. Employers may keep the records in any form, including electronically. Upon receipt of a request, an employer must provide access in a reasonable time, place, and manner within 15 days. In responding to an initial request an employer may provide a copy without cost, provide copying facilities at no cost, or loan the record for a reasonable time. Administrative costs may be charged for subsequent copying requests.

Genetic Information Nondiscrimination Act

As noted above, after a conditional offer of employment, the ADA permits employers to conduct comprehensive medical examinations and to require access to the individual's complete health records. This general rule has been modified by the Genetic Information Nondiscrimination Act of 2008 (GINA). GINA prohibits discrimination in health insurance and employment on the basis of genetic information. GINA does not pre-empt the numerous state laws that afford equal or greater protection. GINA defines genetic information as information about the genetic tests of an individual applicant or employee, information about the genetic tests of family members, or information about a disease or disorder in family members. GINA applies to employers with 15 or more employees, the same coverage as Title VII of the Civil Rights Act of 1964 and the ADA.

Besides prohibiting employment discrimination based on genetic information, GINA prohibits employers from requesting, requiring, or purchasing genetic information about an employee. Reading the ADA and GINA together, after a conditional offer of employment an employer can require the submission of an individual's complete health records, except for genetic information. Because of the broad definition of genetic information in GINA, including family health histories, and the extensive interspersing of genetic information in health records, it is practically impossible for custodians of health records to comply with GINA's disclosure limitations, regardless of the whether the records are maintained in paper or electronic form. Thus, many custodians respond to requests for disclosure of limited health records by sending the entire record. The development and adoption of electronic health records capable of segmented disclosures represents the best hope of limiting the routine disclosure of genetic information to employers and other third parties pursuant to an authorization.

Another provision of GINA relevant to occupational medicine permits employers to engage in genetic monitoring of employees for the effects of toxic substances in the workplace under the following conditions: (1) written notice is provided to the employees; (2) the employees provide voluntary, written authorization or the monitoring is required by law; (3) the employees are informed of their individual results; (4) the monitoring is in compliance with any applicable regulations; and (5) the employer receives results only in aggregate form. This provision, however, only deals with post-exposure monitoring; it does not permit employers to offer voluntary, pre-exposure genetic testing of employees to detect a genetically-mediated increased risk of adverse health effects.

Health Insurance Portability and Accountability Act Privacy Rule

Many individuals, including physicians and nurses, erroneously assume that the Health Insurance Portability and Accountability Act (HIPAA) Privacy Rule provides comprehensive health privacy regulation. In fact, HIPAA and its Privacy Rule apply only to users of electronic health claims information in the following three classes of covered entities: health providers, health plans, and health clearinghouses (which standardize the format of health data for billing). Employers are not considered covered entities, but employer-sponsored employee benefit plans are. Therefore, employers are required to build a "fire wall" between employee health benefit information (e.g. health claims) and other employment records (e.g. personnel records). Employer health plans also have a responsibility to safeguard the privacy and security of personally identifiable health information through a variety of measures detailed in the HIPAA Privacy Rule and the HIPAA Security Rule.

Occupational physicians often need access to employee health information generated by HIPAA covered entities, such as hospitals, physicians, and physical therapists. The Privacy Rule provides that disclosure of protected health information to health care providers for purposes of treatment does not require any prior consent or authorization by the individual. Occupational physicians, however, generally are not obtaining the information for treatment and therefore the treatment exception to the authorization requirement would not apply. Also, several states have medical privacy laws that apply to all disclosures of health information, regardless of the purpose. Consequently, occupational physicians should obtain employee authorizations for all disclosures of personal health information. The HIPAA Privacy Rule requires authorizations to include the following elements: (1) a description of the information to be disclosed; (2) the name of the person or class of persons authorized to make the disclosure; (3) the name of the person or class of persons authorized to receive the information; (4) the purpose of the requested use or disclosure; (5) an expiration date or event for the use or disclosure; and (6) signature of the individual and date (45 C.F.R. § 164.508(c)).

Common Law

Legislative enactments protecting individual health record privacy and confidentiality, to the extent they exist at all, rarely provide any compensation to the individuals harmed by the unlawful disclosures. The primary remedy for financial compensation lies in bringing a common law legal action for invasion of privacy. Of the four bases of invasion of privacy, public disclosure of private facts is the most appropriate to the factual situation in which health care providers or other custodians of personal health information unlawfully disclose the records or contents. In a lawsuit for invasion of privacy by public disclosure of private facts the plaintiff must prove the following elements: (1) disclosure to the public or a large number of persons; (2) a fact that is private in nature; (3) which would be highly offensive to a reasonable person; and (4) is not a legitimate concern to the public.

Each of the four elements of the tort has been subject to controversy. In cases alleging the wrongful disclosure of employee health information, an important issue is whether the disclosure was made to the public or a large number of persons. Some courts hold that the unauthorized disclosure of employee health information to a limited number of employees is not equivalent to public disclosure. Other courts, however, hold that where a "special relationship" exists between the plaintiff and the individuals to whom the information is disclosed (e.g. supervisors, co-employees), this constitutes sufficient "public" disclosure.

Another important consideration is whether the disclosure is highly offensive to a reasonable person. In some questionable decisions, courts have held that disclosure of exceedingly personal health information was not unreasonable. For example, in *Young v. Jackson*, 572 So. 2d 378 (Miss. 1990), a female laborer at a nuclear power facility became ill at work and was hospitalized, later undergoing a hysterectomy. She was deeply affected psychologically by the surgery and did not even tell her husband. After she returned home, a coworker called and said the company needed to know what type of medical procedure she had; he promised to inform only a company safety official and the Nuclear Regulatory Commission, as required by law. The woman reluctantly disclosed she had a hysterectomy. Subsequently, rumors began circulating at work that she was treated for radiation exposure on the job, and to quell the rumors the company told her coworkers that she had a hysterectomy. The woman was very upset by the disclosure and she sued for invasion of privacy. The Mississippi Supreme Court held that the disclosure was justified and therefore the employee could not recover in her action for invasion of privacy.

Conclusion

The primary ethical and legal issue of occupational medicine for the last century, the legal status of the relationship between the physician and the employee, has not been resolved. The lack of clarity of the relationship still gives rise to ethical dilemmas, questions of trust, and interference with medical practice. Greater disclosures to examinees about the role of the physician and specific medical findings made during a medical assessment may be helpful in mitigating the harms to individuals and their health from occupational medicine encounters. In general, the more the practice of occupational medicine aligns with widely-accepted clinical standards, the greater the likelihood of avoiding misunderstandings and adverse health outcomes.

Recommended Reading and Resources

Lewis KS, Kleper AL (2002) Legal issues confronting the occupational physician. *Occup Med: State of the Art Rev*, 17(4): 625–635.

Postal LP (1989) Suing the doctor: lawsuits by injured workers against occupational physicians. *J Occup Environ Med*, 31: 891–896.

Rothstein MA (2008) GINA, the ADA, and genetic discrimination in employment. *J Law Med Ethics*, 36(4): 837–840.

Rothstein MA (2012) *Occupational Safety and Health Law*. Eagan MN, West Publishing (division of Thomson Reuters).

US Dept. of Health and Human Services, Office for Civil Rights (2011) Summary of the HIPAA Privacy Rule. Available at: www.hhs.gov/ocr/privacy/hipaa/understanding/summary/index.html. Accessed December, 22 2011.

4 Occupational Safety and Health Regulation

Judith Green-McKenzie and Ronda Brewer McCarthy

The regulation of occupational health and safety is historically comprised of two main domains, that of setting evidence-based standards for the protection of workers and that of enforcing those standards, principally through inspection of workplaces and imposing a penalty for lack of compliance. This basic framework, which originated in the UK in 1833 and was refined in legislation over the course of the 19th century in Britain through the Factories Acts, was adopted by individual US states, beginning in the 1870s. A century later, the US passed national legislation for worker protection.

Except for aviation and federal government workers, under the Constitution occupational health remains a provincial responsibility in Canada, with a variety of institutional arrangements. Canadian provinces passed factory inspection laws beginning in the 1880s.

In recent decades, public opinion on the value and effectiveness of regulation has swung widely in North America, reflecting changing political philosophies. Regulatory agencies in occupational health have experimented with a number of systems that de-emphasize "command and control" regulation and have sought to find a more consultative and cooperative relationship between employer and regulatory agency. These have included voluntary worksite responsibility and compliance systems, sometimes audited by third parties, allowing flexibility in achieving performance-based standards (tracking indicators of safety performance), and incentive, reward, or recognition programs for good performance. Such programs have often not met with great success and they are perceived with skepticism by organized labor and large segments of the public.

Within the last few years, however, a new approach has emerged from the European Union that emphasizes a legal requirement to conduct risk assessments (see Chapter 21) and to manage identified risks, combined with new approaches, such as "control banding," to simplify the management of risks and to make compliance more accessible and less expensive to small and medium enterprises. This approach is gaining momentum worldwide, but in North America the standards/inspection/enforcement paradigm remains the norm.

Occupational health care providers are expected by employers to be knowledgeable about occupational health standards and are often called upon as consultants in solving specific problems, in response to a citation for noncompliance, or to establish new programs, especially for surveillance. This requires a working knowledge of the occupational health and safety regulatory system, standards, compliance, and enforcement.

In the US, occupational health and safety regulation is primarily governed by national legislation and enforced either by the national regulatory agency (the Occupational Health and Safety Administration, OSHA) or its delegated state equivalents. In Canada, there is wide institutional variation among provinces, therefore making generalization difficult. This chapter will emphasize the US as a practical matter, and because the basic elements of standards setting and enforcement are similar. However, practitioners in Canada are advised to review applicable provincial or federal legislation and agency organization because they do differ, sometimes considerably, in detail from the American system. A particularly valuable resource for information is the Canadian Centre for Occupational Health and Safety.

The Occupational Safety and Health Act

The bipartisan Williams-Steiger Occupational Safety and Health Act of 1970 (OSH Act) was the most sweeping federal law to govern occupational safety and health in US history. It was the first major piece of legislation passed in the US to govern occupational safety and health across the great breadth of industries. The US Congress declared "its purpose and policy" in passing the OSH Act in 1970 was "to assure so far as possible every working man and woman in the Nation safe and healthful working conditions…" Signed into law on December 29, 1970 by President Richard Nixon, this act led to the establishment of the Occupational Safety and Health Administration (OSHA), the National Institute of Occupational Safety and Health (NIOSH), the Occupational Safety and Health Review Commission, and the National Commission on State Workman's Compensation Laws.

As important as its specific provisions, the OSH Act contains the "General Duty Clause," which places a duty on the employer to provide a safe workplace and was created to cover all possible hazards, not just those that could be foreseen at the time. The General Duty Clause states that each employer "shall furnish to each of his employees employment and a place of employment … free from recognized hazards that are causing or are likely to cause death or serious physical harm to his employees." The General Duty Clause thus places the responsibility for eliminating or minimizing hazardous conditions squarely on the shoulders of the employer.

The OSHA is the agency of the Department of Labor that enforces the regulatory mandates of the OSH Act by setting standards, rules and regulations by which covered employers are expected to conduct business. OSHA was created by Congress one year after the OSH Act of 1970. It is the main federal agency involved with safety and health legislation and governs occupational safety and health regulation in the US. Its purpose is to prevent work-related injuries, illnesses, and occupational fatalities by issuing and enforcing standards for workplace safety and health. OSHA aims to create a better workplace for all workers and to ensure their safety by promulgating and enforcing relevant standards that govern job activities and hazardous substances.

NIOSH, now a part of the Centers for Disease Control, is responsible for conducting research and providing recommendations for the prevention of work-related illnesses and injuries. The Occupational Safety and Health Review Commission is an independent federal agency created for the purpose of addressing contested citations or penalties that result from OSHA inspections of workplaces. The National Commission on State Workmen's Compensation Laws, also created by the OSH Act, was charged with reviewing the state of the workers' compensation system in the US (see Chapter 2).

Standards and Guidelines

Section 6 of the OSH Act gives OSHA the authority to adopt enforceable standards, rules, and regulations governing workplace health. It created NIOSH in large part to advise OSHA in the adoption of regulations and to support standards with research, but did not give NIOSH standards-setting authority, so that NIOSH is part of the standards development process but not part of the enforcement mechanism. The Mine Safety and Health Administration (MSHA) sets standards for the mining sector, under separate authority (the Mine Safety and Health Act). Other federal agencies have limited authority to set occupational health standards in narrowly-defined areas, including the Environmental Protection Agency (EPA, pesticides), the Federal Aviation Administration (flight personnel), and the Nuclear Regulatory Commission (nuclear workers and radiation health).

As a federal agency with rule-making authority, OSHA has been delegated the power to set occupational health standards, with the few exceptions noted. During the first few hectic months of its existence, OSHA adopted guidelines that were available at that time. An example is the adoption of existing standards under the Walsh–Healy Act, a predecessor federal law covering government contractors. This Act mandated that workers on certain government contracts are limited to an 8-hour day, and to a 40-hour week, and that workers must work under safe and healthful conditions. OSHA also adopted new standards governing exposure to chemical and physical agents in the workplace, many within 22 months of the adoption of the OSH Act, as well as adopting recommendations for workplace exposure limits regarding known hazards put forth by organizations such as the American National Standards Institute (ANSI). ANSI standards are arrived at by consensus. OSHA promulgated many of these into standards in 1972, which now carry the force of law.

One of the advantages of rule-making, as opposed to writing standards into legislation (as is done in provincial legislation in Canada), is supposed to be that standards can be changed as needed without legislative action. However, in the specific case of OSHA this has rarely happened and one attempt at rule-making (the ergonomics standard) was even overruled by Congress. Once recommendations for workplace exposure limits are formally adopted as an OSHA standard, any change is difficult and subject to a lengthy rule-making process. As a result, although much new knowledge has been generated about many hazardous substances over the years, most OSHA standards have not changed since the early 1970s. Similarly, few new standards have been promulgated, as the process from conception to rule is arduous. For example, OSHA only issued a historic new rule, the Cranes and Derricks Standard, in April 2010 to replace a 40-year-old rule.

All employees covered by the OSH Act must comply with legally binding OSHA exposure limits. These are referred to as permissible exposure limits (PELs), short-term exposure limits (STELs) and Ceiling limits (Ceil). These standards are regulatory limits on the amount or concentration of a substance in the air. They may also contain a skin designation but do not account for other modes of exposure such as ingestion. These exposure limits also do not take into account absorbed dose or biologically-active dose. Of note, exposures that are in compliance with these OSHA standards are not necessarily "safe," as observance of these limits does not guarantee that no workers will suffer some ill effect at these levels. Similarly, it also does not necessarily mean that all levels out of compliance are "unsafe."

The OSHA PEL is the legal limit for exposure of an employee to a chemical, substance or physical agent. For a chemical substance, the chemical regulation is usually expressed as concentration in parts per million (ppm), or in milligrams per cubic meter (mg/m^3). Units of measure for physical agents such as noise are specific to the agent. OSHA PELs are based on an 8-hour "time-weighted average" (TWA) exposure. The 8-hour TWA means that, for limited periods, a worker may be exposed to concentrations higher than the PEL, so long as the average concentration over eight hours remains lower than the standard. A STEL addresses the average 15–30 minute period concentration of a substance to which a worker may be exposed during a single work shift. A Ceil is the concentration of a substance above which a worker may not be exposed at all, for any period of time.

Existing PELs are published in the Code of Federal Regulations (29 CFR 1910) and 425 PELs have been established, including the most common chemical hazards such as benzene, beryllium, cadmium, formaldehyde, methylene chloride, hydrogen fluoride, mercury, tetrachloroethylene, and trichloroethylene. Many of these standards also mandated surveillance measures, such as blood tests (for example, lead), chest films (asbestos), and audiometry (noise). PELs may be embedded in standards that mandate specific control procedures, such as the asbestos standard and the lead standard which, confusingly, exists in two versions: one for General Industry and one for Construction. These standards often have requirements for the "medical removal" of workers from the workplace in the event of overexposure, for example the 40 µg/dL standard for lead.

Voluntary Standards and Guidelines

The industrial hygiene community does not consider many OSHA permissible exposure limits to be sufficiently protective. Many employers (probably most large companies), have therefore adopted as working standards guidelines that only permit lower exposure and therefore afford a greater degree of protection. The most heavily used, and the most influential internationally, are recommendations of the American Conference of Governmental Industrial Hygienists (ACGIH).

The threshold limit value (TLV®) of a chemical substance, written as an averaged exposure limit over a period of time (usually eight hours), also called a "time-weighted average" (TWA), is a recommendation by the ACGIH. The ACGIH is actually a professional society, not an official agency of the federal government, which since 1938 has been reviewing toxicological data and developing guidelines for exposure based on those data. TLVs® are reviewed every year, updated as needed, and published annually by the ACGIH. Of note, many current OSHA PELs were based on ACGIH recommendations made in 1968. The ACGIH was also the origin of STELs and Ceils adopted by OSHA.

A TLV® stipulates the concentration of a hazardous substance to which a typical worker may be exposed day after day throughout a lifetime without unreasonable adverse risk of disease or injury. A TLV® is *not* intended to be a quantitative estimate of risk, a toxicity threshold, or a diagnostic criterion for a disease or condition. The TLV is an estimate based on the known toxicity of a given chemical substance in humans or animals, and on the reliability and accuracy of the latest sampling and analytical methods. New research may lead to modifications of the TLV®, so they are always provisional, never permanent exposure limits.

Biological Exposure Indices (BEIs®) are also published by the ACGIH and updated yearly. BEIs® are tests on the worker that reflect a worker's exposure to a chemical, and absorption of the chemical, from various sources. For example, blood lead level may reflect not only airborne lead, but also exposure from other routes such as dermal or ingestion. Sensitive methods to determine levels in humans are not available for most substances and this limits the applicability of the BEI approach. Some "biological monitoring" BEIs® provide early warning of response to a chemical or its metabolite, such as monitoring cholinesterase levels. The approach of biological monitoring BEIs® as exposure guidelines is limited in its usefulness due to the wide variability of individual responses.

TLVs® and BEIs® are not standards and are not legally enforceable as exposure limits, unless they are written into a contract. They are guidelines determined by a voluntary body

Table 4.1 OSHA Permissible Exposure Limits and ACGIH and NIOSH Recommended Exposure Levels Compared (Eight-hour TWA for Three Selected Chemicals)

	OSHA PEL	ACGIH TLV®	NIOSH REL
Acrylonitrile	2 ppm	2 ppm	1 ppm
Epichlorhydrin	5 ppm	2 ppm	Carcinogen: lowest feasible exposure
Beryllium	0.002 mg/m3	0.0005 mg/m3	0.0005 mg/m3

of independent knowledgeable individuals who review existing peer-reviewed publications on industrial hygiene, toxicology, occupational medicine, epidemiology, and other relevant disciplines.

Recommended exposure limits (RELs) are guidelines recommended by the NIOSH. OSHA takes RELs into consideration when promulgating new regulatory exposure limits. Unlike the ACGIH, whose TLVs® are published in a small booklet, and whose justifications for setting the guidelines are summarized in only one or two pages for each chemical or physical agent, NIOSH presents documentation in support of RELs in "criteria documents" which are often hundreds of pages in length, take years to produce, and are extensively reviewed. Although RELs are not enforceable standards, they have influence because they are produced by a federal agency and are designed to be used by OSHA in implementing new standards. With reduced budgets, NIOSH has produced fewer criteria documents, and some "current" criteria documents are now well over a decade old. Despite this, however, the thorough documentation behind each recommended standard keeps these documents useful.

Table 4.1 shows a few chemicals, and the differences between OSHA standards and ACGIH and NIOSH recommendations. The table demonstrates that OSHA, ACGIH, and NIOSH may not agree with one another and that the basis for a recommended exposure level may differ. (For example, NIOSH considers epichlorhydrin to be a carcinogen whereas the ACGIH and OSHA do not.)

In Canada, standards resemble TLVs® and are expressed as Occupational Exposure Limits, as they usually are in Europe. They are recommended by provincial occupational health and safety regulatory agencies and incorporated into provincial legislation.

Medical Surveillance

Medical surveillance is the systematic, ongoing assessment of employees who are exposed or who have potential exposure to occupational hazards (see Chapter 20). Workers are monitored for the appearance of early signs of adverse health effects, both to identify early signs of developing occupational disease for secondary prevention in the individual and to assess the effectiveness of exposure prevention strategies for the group. Medical surveillance programs therefore require the analysis of individual and aggregate surveillance data over time, making it critical to use software that allows group-level analysis as well as tracking results for individuals.

Medical surveillance may either be recommended or "mandated" (required by regulation) depending on the type of work being performed, factors such as duration of the task, materials being used, and potential for exposure. Recommended or voluntary surveillance may be undertaken by the employer for various reasons: more stringent protection of the worker, to limit the liability of the employer, when the employer is trying to provide an extra margin of safety under the General Duty Clause, when the actual exposure to a hazard cannot be easily measured, when exposure may be sporadic or unpredictable, where and when occupational exposure standards do not exist, when a hazard is new and poorly characterized, and when negotiated as part of a labor-management agreement.

Many OSHA standards mandate specific medical surveillance practices. An important function of occupational health services is to ensure that workplaces are compliant with federal and state regulations, as detailed in the Code of Federal Regulations, which require surveillance when employees are exposed to specific hazards. Documentation of compliance is essential for the protection of the worker and to address the legal liability of the employer. Examples of hazards for which OSHA has mandated medical surveillance programs include lead (two standards exist, as noted, but they are similar), arsenic, cotton dust, and asbestos. The medical surveillance requirements may include:

- mandatory periodic testing at varying prescribed intervals
- post-hire (baseline) testing
- tests and procedures specific to the potential hazard
- specific methods of performing and interpreting tests and procedures
- long-term records-keeping requirements
- mandated access to records by governmental authorities

Variances

Under the OSH Act it is possible for variances to be granted to a company, exempting them from a particular standard with justification, but they are uncommon. In general, employers should not be encouraged to seek a variance from OSHA standards unless there is documented evidence that it will result in a much higher level of protection, and never to avoid responsibility for worker protection. Cost of compliance is never acceptable grounds for a variance. The request for variance can be submitted at any time, and if it comes after an inspection, it will not affect the citation.

There are several categories of variance:

1   Temporary (limited time) relief, usually when a new standard is phased in but the employer is unable to modify the work environment or obtain the necessary equipment by the date the regulation takes effect. The employer has to submit a viable compliance plan.
2   Interim order, which permits the employer to continue operating under existing conditions while OSHA reviews an application for a variance.
3   Permanent variance, which allows the employer to use methods to achieve health protection for workers that are different from those mandated by a standard; the method must be demonstrated to be at least as effective as standard methods.
4   Experimental variance, which allows an employer to use new and innovative methods of protection, with OSHA's cooperation, for purposes of improving worker protection.
5   National defense variance, which allows "reasonable variations, tolerances, and exemptions from" standards "to avoid serious impairment of the national defense."

Variances from occupational health standards are uncommon. They almost never occur in Canada.

State OSHAs and Occupational Health Regulation at the Local Level

Congress recognized that at the time when the OSH Act was being debated several states had already been operating effective occupational safety and health programs. Many of these states wished to continue their state programs and to have the option of putting more stringent standards in place. The law therefore provided an option for states to run their own "state OSHA" programs. They could apply to OSHA to do so and receive up to 50 percent funding from OSHA for their programs once they received OSHA's preliminary approval. Today, 26 states, Puerto Rico, and the Virgin Islands have OSHA-approved State plans and each has adopted their own standards and enforcement policies. Of these, 21 states (Alaska, Arizona, California, Hawaii, Iowa, Indiana, Kentucky, Maryland, Michigan, Minnesota, North Carolina, New Mexico, Nevada, Oregon, South Carolina, Tennessee, Utah, Virginia, Vermont, Washington, Wyoming), the US Virgin Islands, and Puerto Rico operate comprehensive programs covering private sector and state and local government employees while three states (Connecticut, New Jersey, and New York) have state plans that cover public employees only. For the most part, these States have adopted standards that are identical to federal OSHA. States that do not have state OSHAs, the District of Columbia, Guam, American Samoa, and other Pacific Trust Territories are served by state (or equivalent) offices of federal OSHA.

Participating states must adopt a program comparable to the federal program. State regulations, as permitted under the OSH Act, must be at least as strict as the federal law and may even be stricter in standard setting and policy enforcement. Additionally, states running their own programs are required to cover state and local government employees, although available financial resources pose a limiting factor. OSHA approved the first state plans for South Carolina, Montana, and Oregon in 1972.

Employers (enterprises, regardless of who owns it or how it is organized, with at least one employee) are required to comply with state OSHA standards, with the exception of federal employees covered by federal OSHA directly or indirectly by interagency agreement, miners covered under the Mine Safety Act, agricultural and pesticide workers covered by the EPA's Worker Protection Standard, farmers who employ only immediate members of their own family, self-employed individuals, and, for federal OSHA only, state and local government workers (who are covered by state programs where these exist). Small enterprises that employ less than ten people on the payroll during any 24 hour period are normally exempt from OSHA record-keeping and reporting rules but must otherwise comply with all applicable standards.

OSHA Consultation Branch and Voluntary Compliance

OSHA has both a consultation and a compliance branch, and keeps the two separated insofar as is possible, so that employers will not hesitate to ask for help out of fear of triggering an inspection. The objective, which has only been partially successful, is to assist employers in solving problems before they become compliance problems and to divert issues away from enforcement when solutions are readily available. The service is targeted to small enterprises.

The consultation service is primarily a resource for the employer. The main purpose of the consultation service is to assist management in correcting a health or safety problem by providing information and education to employers and employees. Consultation is confidential but requires consultation with employees and immediate correction of imminent hazards that may be uncovered. In practice, OSHA consultation services may be limited in scope because of limited resources.

As early as 1975, federal OSHA established free onsite consultation programs delivered through state authorities and the consultation branch system is mirrored in state OSHAs.

OSHA has made similar initiatives to encourage voluntary compliance. In 1978, in an effort to encourage voluntary compliance and assist businesses, particularly small businesses, the agency started its New Directions Grants program. This program provides seed money to organizations that then develop and offer safety and health training to employers and employees. OSHA also supports a Voluntary Protection Program (VPP) for recognition of employers with effective cooperative health and safety management programs.

Enforcement and the OSHA Compliance Office

The Compliance Office is in many respects the employee's advocate. The OSHA Training Institute (OTI) was established in January 1972, to train OSHA compliance officers and stakeholders on safety and health topics. State OSHAs operate in a similar manner.

OSHA compliance officers may visit workplaces for programmed (routine) inspections (which have become very uncommon due to a shortage of compliance officers), in response to employee complaints, and in specific situations, such as after fatalities. Inspections are prioritized as follows:

1   Imminent danger—a condition in which there is reasonable certainty that a danger exists, which can be expected to cause death or serious physical harm immediately or before the danger can be eliminated through normal enforcement procedures, as defined in section 13(a) of the OSH Act.
2   Investigation of accidents resulting in a fatality or in the hospitalization of three or more workers. The employer has eight hours to notify OSHA of an accident of this significance.
3   Responses to complaints from workers
4   Programmed inspections

Once a job hazard is recognized by employees, OSHA expects that it should first be brought to the attention of the employer. If no action is taken, any employee may contact the OSHA area office to file a complaint. All complaints are evaluated and priority is assigned by the perceived severity of the hazard. On the basis of the evaluation, OSHA staff decides whether to conduct an inspection. Formal requests for inspection of hazards that are not considered to be serious should be dealt with either by dismissal or by an inspection, which is scheduled within 20 working days. If OSHA decides not to conduct the inspection, the union representative or the employee signing the complaint must be informed, in writing, of the reason the inspection was denied. An informal review may then be requested. There are also programmed inspections conducted at workplaces where there is a high risk of injury, such as construction sites.

An OSHA inspection consists of three parts: the "opening conference," "the walk around," and the "closing conference." During the opening conference the inspector describes the inspection plan to management and to representatives of the employees. The next phase is the walk around and inspection tour. Management and employee representatives are allowed to accompany the OSHA inspector on this tour. The final phase is the closing conference and the results of the inspection are discussed with management. Possible methods of correcting hazards, and possibility of deadlines and fines are also discussed. A representative of the employees can request attendance at this meeting but management has the privilege of vetoing employee representation. If violations are found, an additional follow up inspection may be conducted in an effort to ensure that the company has corrected the violations.

Violations fall into one of three categories: "imminent danger," "serious," and "other than serious." Citations for imminent danger are rare. When they are made, the facility is forced to close down immediately until the danger is corrected. Serious violations are regarded as those which have a substantial probability of causing death or physical harm.

An employer found to be out of compliance with OSHA standards may be issued a citation and given an abatement date, by which time the hazard must be corrected. If the employer does not comply with the citation, the OSHA inspector can apply an injunction to halt further work until the worksite is safe. If abatement dates are missed or ignored by employers, the employer may also be assessed a civil penalty for each day that the violation continues past an abatement date. Extensions beyond the abatement date are common and employees may continue to be exposed to the hazard during this lag period.

Standards are enforced through inspections and citations. If no specific standard exists for a workplace hazard then the employer is expected to adhere to the "General Duty Clause" in the OSH Act, which states "Employers are required to maintain a workplace free from recognized hazards."

Fines are determined by how dangerous the violation is and the seriousness of the violation in OSHA's prioritization, the size of employer's business, the apparent good faith of the employer, and any record of prior violations. If management shows "good faith" in trying to keep the area safe, there may be a reduction in the penalty. There is also a reduction in the penalty for small businesses. Serious violations are subject to the maximum civil penalty. Willful and repeated violations also carry the maximum penalty. The employer can appeal OSHA actions on violations, fines, prescribed clean-up, and deadlines to the OSHA Appeals Board (which is a separate, autonomous body under the OSH Act), and to seek relief from a penalty.

OSHA penalties are not usually large, however. In 2010 the average OSHA penalty was US$1,000. The median initial penalty proposed for all investigations in cases where a worker was killed conducted in financial year 2007 was just US$5,900. However, there are occasional large fines for egregious infractions. In 2011 an OSHA inspection of the second largest refinery in the US, owned by Exxon Louisiana, identified 20 serious violations, with substantial probability of causing death or physical harm, and two "other than serious" violations, resulting in a fine of US$126,000. In 1987, OSHA imposed a fine of US$1.6 million on Chrysler Corporation's Newark, Delaware, plant for multiple violations.

Monetary penalties for OSHA violations are obviously not a deterrent for some companies, as it may be more cost-effective for them to pay the violation fine than to introduce the engineering controls necessary to protect the worker and the environment. By themselves, fines at the current level are not a sufficient incentive to provide a safe working environment. The federal government has therefore developed a program called the Worker Endangerment Initiative (WEI) for companies that serially violate environmental and worker safety laws. The WEI pairs investigators from OSHA, EPA, and prosecutors from the Environmental Crimes Section of the Department of Justice to investigate and prosecute such cases as criminal offenses. For example, in 2001 a Motiva Enterprises facility explosion killed one worker and injured eight others. The explosion resulted in 99,000 gallons (375,000 liters) of sulfuric acid draining into the Delaware River. The OSHA penalty for the violation was US$175,000. In 2005, the company pleaded guilty to a Clean Water Act violation and was fined US$10 million dollars. In 2007, British Petroleum agreed to pay a record fine of

US$50 million under the Clean Air Act for the 2005 explosion at a Texas refinery that killed 15 workers and injured more than 170 others.

National Institute for Occupational Safety and Health

NIOSH is not an enforcement agency, although employers often confuse it with OSHA. NIOSH is part of the Centers for Disease Control and Prevention, in the US Department of Health and Human Services. NIOSH was established in 1971 by the OSH Act of 1970 with the charge to provide research, information, education, and training in the field of occupational safety and health. It is the primary federal agency conducting research on the safety and health of the workplace. One of NIOSH's responsibilities is to review chemical, toxicology, and process-control data to arrive at "criteria for a recommended standard" of exposure and control. These criteria have been published as "criteria documents" by NIOSH.

NIOSH draws from several public health disciplines such as industrial hygiene, epidemiology, nursing, engineering, medicine, statistics, psychology, the social sciences, and communication in order to conduct its programs. As directed by the OSH Act, NIOSH works to maintain adequate numbers of occupational safety and health professionals and researchers by establishing, strengthening, and expanding graduate and undergraduate educational programs and special training grants.

Although NIOSH does not have a direct role in enforcement, in carrying out its research, NIOSH can request and subsequently obtain confidential medical and exposure records. This is necessary as NIOSH often relies on access to both medical records and human subjects in private industry in order to carry out its work. NIOSH does have rules concerning confidentiality and records management, which must be followed (42 CFR Parts 85 and 85a). In general, when NIOSH requires access to private records, it is for purpose of studying the effects of exposure on human beings, in order to make appropriate recommendations.

Recommended Reading and Resources

Note: OSHA, NIOSH, and state OSHAs and the Canadian Centre for Occupational Health and Safety have voluminous and comprehensive documentation on the internet and in hard copy covering every topic likely to be of interest to health care providers and occupational health services.

American Council of Governmental Industrial Hygienists TLV/BEI Resources. Available at: http://www.acgih.org/tlv/. Accessed November 15, 2011.
Canadian Center for Occupational Health and Safety. Available at: http://www.ccohs.ca/. Accessed December 25, 2010.
Centers for Disease Control, National Institute for Occupational Safety and Health website. Available at: http://www.cdc.gov/NIOSH/. Accessed November 15, 2011.
Centers for Disease Control. Workplace Safety and Health Topics. Available at: http://www.cdc.gov/niosh/topics/hazards.html. Accessed December 25, 2011.
European Agency for Safety and Health at work. Available at: http://osha.europa.eu/en/front-page. Accessed November 15, 2011.
Guidotti TL (2010) *The Praeger Handbook of Occupational and Environmental Medicine*. Santa Barbara CA, Praeger ABC-Clio. See especially Chapters 14 and 24.
Hartnett J (2009) *OSHA in the Real World: Maintain Workplace Safety While Keeping Your Competitive Edge*. Aberdeen WA, Silver Lake Publishing. There are many "OSHA compliance guides" for employers but they are usually irrelevant to health care providers, except as they may be employers themselves. This one may be particularly useful for recalcitrant or skeptical managers.

Moss DA (2002) *When All Else Fails: Government as the Ultimate Risk Manager.* Cambridge MA, Harvard University Press. An academic treatise on the basis for regulation.

Occupational Safety and Health Act of 1970. Public Law 91-596 84 STAT. 1590, 91st Congress, S.2193, December 29, 1970, as amended through January 1, 2004. Available at: http://www.osha.gov/pls/oshaweb/owadisp.show_document?p_table=OSHACT&p_id=3355. Accessed August 29, 2011.

United States Department of Labor, Occupational Safety and Health Administration. Timeline of OSHA's 40 year History. Available at: http://www.osha.gov/osha40/timeline.html. Accessed October 15, 2011.

United States Department of Labor, Occupational Safety and Health Administration. OSHA at 30. Three Decades of Progress in Occupational Safety and Health. Available at: http://www.osha.gov/as/opa/osha-at-30.html. Accessed November 7, 2011.

United States Environmental Protection Agency Worker Protection Standards for Agricultural Pesticides. Available at: http://www.epa.gov/agriculture/twor.html. Accessed November 15, 2011.

5 Ethics

Tee L. Guidotti and M. Suzanne Arnold

Codes of ethics guide professionals in their behavior and define what is appropriate in practice. All health professions have codes of ethics. Those for the occupational health professions characterize their relationship with the employer, the workers they protect, and society as a whole. These codes of ethics are fundamental to good practice and place an obligation on the occupational health professional to practice in a manner that is respectful of others, appropriate to their role and training, protective of workers' rights, and helpful to progress in the field.

Codes of ethics are not laws but they have application in law in that they define standards of acceptable practice. Breaches of ethics may result in discipline by professional organizations or may result in legal action against the professional. Codes may also help to resolve conflicts when they arise and protect the occupational health professional from pressure to compromise on workers' rights or interests. This inappropriate pressure may come from any side—employers, unions, or government agencies.

The basic ethics of occupational health must apply to all occupational health professions, in order to coordinate their ethical obligations and to prevent those who do not have the best interest of the worker in mind from exploiting differences. For example, if there were a difference between nurses, physicians, and administrative staff in the ethics of protection of medical records, supervisors or others who sought information to which they were not entitled would simply go to the profession or occupation with the weakest code and demand to see the record.

The occupational health service staff includes at a minimum physicians, nurses, and clerical support staff working under the direction of the licensed physician or nurse. It is important to recall that all these staff members in the organization, not just the licensed health care professionals, enjoy a position of trust. They are all expected to act ethically. Some, including the licensed health care professionals, have the capacity to balance the rights and obligations of the employees with those of the company as a whole without compromising ethical codes. Others, who lack their training, do not. It is critical, therefore, that office and field staff be trained in the ethics of occupational health, subject to an unambiguous policy, provided with explicit guidelines, monitored, and that ethics be part of their performance review. Likewise, when licensed health professionals are not in charge, managers must be educated in the ethics of occupational health practice, if they are not already.

The ethics of occupational health practice are universal in coverage but not absolute. They are constrained by local laws. They should be observed equally in rich or poor countries and for workers at all levels of skill and income. However, codes are not laws, and when local laws exist contradicting them, the occupational health professional must naturally obey the law.

Similarly, ethical principles sometimes are in conflict. This happens most often when the rights of an individual conflict with the rights of the group. For example, if an individual worker has a condition or illness that presents a serious risk to coworkers or to the public (such as untreated or resistant tuberculosis in a workplace with other employees or a seizure disorder in someone who is operating a train), then under certain very specific circumstances, their right to privacy is not absolute. When the potential harm is grave (for example, potentially causing serious injury or death) and almost certain to occur, the worker may be removed from work or denied a job or reported to competent authority. However, the interests of the worker can only be compromised legitimately when the potential harm is grave.

Common Ground

Codes of ethics for the occupational health professions have been promulgated by professional organizations such as the American College of Occupational and Environmental Medicine, the Occupational and Environmental Medical Association of Canada, the American Association of Occupational Health Nurses, and by organizations, safety professionals, epidemiologists, and many others. Consistency among these various codes is essential. If every organization's and each profession's code were different, there would be confusion and room for unscrupulous employers or powerful interests in labor or government to play one profession off against another to get what they want. Fortunately, these specific codes of ethics derive from a common set of ideas about fairness, justice, responsibility, and professionalism which are recognized by all occupational health professions.

The closest thing to a model or universal code is the Code of Ethics for Occupational Health Professionals of the International Commission on Occupational Health (ICOH, http://www.icohweb.org/core_docs/code_ethics_eng.pdf). This document, which is revised and updated periodically, is a foundational document against which the other professions harmonize their professional codes. Unfortunately, this code is rather long and in its current version is not clearly written but it is undergoing revision. Some provisions reflect Covenants of the International Labour Organization which most of the world uses for guidance, but because the US has not ratified some of the more important covenants, a few provisions, on such matters as mandatory joint worker–management safety committees (which are mandatory in Canada), are not always applied in the US (see Chapter 6). Some of the most fundamental provisions of the ICOH Code follow.

An ethical framework for occupational health rests on certain principles, some of which are obvious and others implicit in the discussion. The primary principle is that the health of workers must be protected and that this protection is the responsibility of the employer. This means that the employer may not require the worker to work in an unsafe environment. This principle is embodied in the right of refusal and in the "general duty clause" of the US Occupational Safety and Health Act, which requires the employer to provide safe and healthful working conditions (see Chapter 4).

When serious occupational hazards are identified, there is a tendency to wait for the ideal solution, or for a convenient time (such as a building renovation) rather than to correct the problem immediately. The ICOH Code states that the rapid application of simple preventive measures that are technically sound and easily implemented is preferable to delay, which prolongs the unacceptable risk.

Occupational health professionals have an obligation to avoid conflicts of interest. There is, however, an inherent conflict of interest when an occupational health professional, providing services to the worker, is employed or works under contract to the worker's employer. The struggle for the occupational health practitioner is to be a true professional, remaining independent, honest, and objective in his or her opinion.

Occupational health professionals and employers have an obligation to avoid discrimination, intended or otherwise, whether or not management policy or actions are discriminatory.

Working Conditions

It is the responsibility of the employer to provide a safe and healthy workplace. If there is a problem, the workplace should be changed to correct it rather than screening workers to find those who can tolerate existing conditions. Occupational health professionals should share information about issues in the workplace accurately, honestly, and completely, with employer and worker alike. However, they should not disclose company secrets or proprietary information unless the safety of a worker or the community is threatened.

Workers have a right to be informed of the hazards and risks that they may be exposed to in the workplace. They can learn of the hazards and risks by individual instruction or by the hazards and risks being posted in the workplace and on any materials being used. (This principle is the basis of the OSHA Hazard Communication standard.)

Biological monitoring involves obtaining exposure-related information through testing workers rather than, or along with, environmental monitoring. This is not considered to be medical practice. As a general rule, levels of substances that can only be present due to an occupational or environmental exposure and which are not normally found in the body (for example, blood lead) can be disclosed when the purpose is environmental monitoring, not diagnosis. However, the level of a substance (e.g. blood glucose) that is normally present in the body remains confidential. If a worker is a participant in a biological monitoring program he or she must be informed of the results of any tests. Abnormal results from such a program should always lead to a thorough review of the worker's health, the working conditions, and the way in which a job is being done. It is not ethically defensible to conduct a monitoring program that has no purpose but compliance with rules, and for which no follow-up action is taken, because the purpose is false.

The results of a biological monitoring program should not adversely affect an employee's employment relationship. If a level is high enough that the employee needs to be removed from the job, it represents a failure of protection. Ethics and good business practice require that the employee's income be maintained and that he or she not be penalized.

Disability and Accommodation

Occupational health professionals should assist workers who have health problems or an impairment to do the job and keep their employment to the extent possible, given their impairment. In the US, this is covered by the Americans with Disabilities Act (see Chapter 23) and in Canada by the Charter of Rights. The worker has an absolute right to know the nature, name, and probable cause of any disorder that is found, and of the hazards and risks to which he or she has been exposed—occupational health professionals have an absolute duty to inform the worker of these findings.

Professionalism

The ICOH Code is very explicit that the occupational health professional has an obligation to know what hazards (and their related risks) are in the workplace and to understand the process and working conditions. Ignorance is not an excuse.

Occupational health professionals should speak up and not let control of potentially serious hazards and risks be deferred due to lack of commitment by management. Sometimes, this will place the occupational health professional in an uncomfortable situation, but that is part of his or her role. However, the importance of the hazard and its related risks must be taken into consideration when management is deliberately ignoring the problem or becomes hostile, jeopardizing the effectiveness of the occupational health professional in other matters. A risk of minor injury does not rise to this standard but an exceptional and substantial risk clearly does, for example an order to a worker to sandblast with silica sand in the absence of reliable respiratory protection.

Decisions, advice to management on hazard and risk control, the technical rationale for programs, screening tests, fitness to work determinations, communications with workers, and other important occupational health information should be documented in writing. This protects the occupational health professional in the case of a legal problem, OSHA inspection, or review by senior management.

The ICOH Code, in particular, is explicit that occupational health professionals have an obligation to maintain professional competence and autonomy. The practitioner is expected, as an ethical obligation, to be adequately trained and to keep his or her education and training up to date. (This provision falls most heavily on two groups of practitioners: safety officers who are thrust into their jobs without adequate training, and physicians and nurses who treat occupational injuries and illness without learning about the occupational health care system.) By making adequate preparation an ethical requirement, the ICOH Code is serving notice to these practitioners that they must know their limitations, and to their employers that they must provide opportunities for training. Otherwise, workers may not be protected and the practitioner will not only be ineffective but cannot truly function with the independence and autonomy that occupational health professionals must have.

Closely related to this is a provision in the ICOH Code that the employer has an ethical obligation to provide the occupational health professional with adequate resources to do his or her job. Although not spelled out, there is an implied duty on the part of the occupational health professional not to become the "fall guy," completely ineffectual, and used as cover for abuse or for perpetuating poor practices. Here again, a balance must be struck, because a decision must sometimes be made whether it is better to provide inadequate protection or none at all, and this will vary with individual circumstances.

Medical and Nursing Practice

Ethical principles for medical practice and nursing practice in occupational health services are often different than those for medical and general nursing practice. The reasons can best be appreciated by studying the history of occupational health in practice and certain differences that exist in law which also apply in ethics pertaining to the physician– or practitioner–patient or –worker relationship (see Chapter 3).

There has been a long history of inappropriate testing for preplacement evaluation, screening, and periodic health surveillance. For example, some employers in the days before the Americans with Disabilities Act required low back X-rays as a pre-employment screen for workers who might be at risk for low back pain, a test that is not only useless but that subjects the worker to unacceptable radiation. Others have allowed the use of screening tests that have not been validated for the purpose, leading to lost job opportunities for no good reason and de facto discrimination. Thus, a substantial part of the ICOH Code is taken up with provisions that may seem strange in light of current evidence-based medical practice. Even so, these provisions are directly relevant to proposals that have periodically come from employers to introduce genetic testing (in the US, before the Genetic Information Nondiscrimination Act of 2008), or to require screening for G-6-PD deficiency, or sickle trait (which remains controversial in high-altitude work).

Tests to screen for health effects (periodic health surveillance, fitness for duty, preplacement evaluation, return to work, and other testing, often collectively called "medical monitoring") should be evidence-based and should perform with good predictive value in the working population being tested. The results of examinations carried out within the framework of health surveillance must be disclosed and the significance of the findings must be explained to the worker concerned. The ICOH Code states that participation in medical monitoring should be voluntary and based on informed consent, such that a worker can opt out unless the testing is required by law. In the US and Canada, however, workers cannot opt out of testing when it is a contractual requirement for employment or in compliance with an OSHA standard (except for religious reasons).

Fitness to work evaluations for a given job must be based on the specific job demands and workplace conditions, and the health standards required of the worker should be relevant to the specific job requirements (often called "bona fide occupational requirements" or BFORs). The occupational health professional who is working on behalf of an employer or insurance carrier has an obligation to report such information as is directly pertinent to the employee's work capacity or accommodations that are needed, but no more. The employer is entitled to a determination of "fit," "unfit," and "fit with accommodation" (with the accommodation specified) but not to the diagnosis or medical history of the employee. (These principles also underlie the Americans with Disabilities Act.)

Confidentiality of Information

The occupational health professional should always treat the individual worker's exposure records and medical record as confidential, just like any other medical record, securing it and limiting access to qualified health professionals. Aggregated and anonymous information, however, can be shared on a statistical basis, as long as it is not possible to identify an individual worker. Paper records should be kept locked and secure. Electronic records should be protected with access controls and audit trails, so that alterations can be traced.

Health care providers have a responsibility to protect the confidentiality of medical records, subject to law. The individual worker may give consent for this information to be available to anyone, but in the absence of written informed consent the health care provider is only permitted to share it with those who are legally entitled to receive it, such as OSHA or workers' compensation carriers. This does not include managers outside the occupational health service of an enterprise. Employers have an obligation to respect the confidentiality of personal medical information of their employees. Unless informed consent is given by the worker, confidential medical information must stay within the occupational health service and cannot be shared, for example with human resources, or with management, or with coworkers. Legal requirements override this principle, of course, when required by statute, workers' compensation, or discovery during litigation.

Although the injured worker's consent is generally required to release confidential medical information, he or she cannot prevent the treating physician from reporting information as required by law, for example to the government or in a workers' compensation claim. The worker is entitled to be informed of what information will be conveyed to third parties.

The informed consent process is best handled, in order to prevent ambiguity and misunderstanding, by using a specific form (see Exhibit 5.1) that is dated and signed by the worker (and witness) and should specify the segment of information that the worker is consenting to release, the individual who may release the information, to whom the information is to be released, and the specific reason for the release. In addition, the consent should have a stated period of validity (dates).

"Attorney–client privilege" allows lawyers to refuse to reveal information given to them in confidence by a client. Physicians and nurses do not legally enjoy the same privilege as lawyers, but they have traditionally practiced their profession as if there were a legally recognized physician– or practitioner–patient privilege. In day-to-day practice, it is assumed by both the patient and the health care professional that information passed in the course of a medical interaction will remain confidential, but in legal proceedings and insurance reviews confidential, compromising, and even embarrassing medical information is not protected, although it may be ruled irrelevant. This has led some observers to declare that it should simply not be collected. However, the consequences of an incomplete or censored medical evaluation may easily be omitted from the record of relevant or important information that happens to be inconvenient.

How occupational health information is handled is central to the ethical behavior of the occupational health professional. To avoid conflict and mistrust, it is essential that a written policy and written procedures be available to everyone in the organization, from the chief executive officer to the newest of recruits, and that the clerical and administrative staff be trained. The policies and procedures must safeguard the rights of employees, recognize the rights and obligations of the occupational health professional, and specify the information that can be shared (basically, functional capacity) to allow employers to make responsible decisions and achieve productive results. These policies and procedures must be in place whether the occupational health services form part of the organization or are being contracted from outside. The critical questions that must be addressed in the policy and procedure documents are: who are the members of the occupational health staff, what is the content of the occupational health record (i.e. occupational health information), who has ownership, where and for how long is it stored, who has access, and what may be disclosed to whom.

Confidentiality of medical records is a major issue in occupational medicine, as it is in medicine in general (see Chapter 3). Ownership is the simplest part of the issue. The general rule in most countries is that the physical medical record itself is the property of whoever owns the file or the platform in which it is recorded and causes the record to be made, but that the information it contains belongs to the person who created it and is at all times available to the worker or patient and available for correction or supplementation. In practice, this means that the employer or, if community-based, the occupational health service actually owns the physical or electronic record.

Access to this record, however, is strictly limited to the occupational health professionals and their support staff. Not even the employee has full and unrestricted access to the physical medical record; a worker cannot demand to take it home with him or to destroy her file. The employee has a complete right to any laboratory and biological monitoring results that pertain to him or her, medical diagnosis, and fitness for duty judgments. Clinical notes, preliminary opinions, and consultants' reports that are not ultimately relevant to the employee's working relationship and personal health, however, should be revealed only at the discretion of the occupational health professional in charge of the record, after review to ensure that information on third parties is not mentioned, or on subpoena by a court of law. In the situation in which a private physician provides consultative occupational health services to an employer, the record often remains in the possession of the private physician. Arrangements should be made so that these records will not be destroyed, and for confidential storage by the employer upon demand, because under OSHA regulations such records should be maintained for at least 30 years after the employee has left the company.

Employers must establish strict procedures for the maintenance, storage, and disclosure of health information. If this is done well, employer–employee trust will be established and the occupational health professionals can function in a highly professional and ethical way. Such procedures serve and protect the legitimate rights of all three parties.

The Practitioner–Patient Relationship

Unlike other branches of medicine, where a straightforward two-party relationship exists between doctor and patient, in occupational medicine third parties are always involved. This reality requires strong ethical codes to manage potential conflict and also to define the difference between what is and what is not a physician–patient relationship, which is the model for medical and other professional ethics, and similar relationships between workers and other practitioners. Where there is a relationship of trust between the practitioner and the worker, usually in the context of medical treatment, the relationship is said to be "fiduciary," most importantly the physician–patient relationship. Where the relationship is not one of assumed trust, the relationship is "not fiduciary." Some relationships in occupational medicine and nursing are fiduciary and others are not. The distinction is critical.

Fiduciary relationships

The physician–patient relationship is based on the assumption that the physician (or other health care giver) is providing care for an individual (the patient), usually by mutual consent (except in an emergency where the patient or a responsible guardian cannot express his or her wishes), and that there is trust between the treating physician and the patient, making it a "fiduciary" relationship. There is an expectation that the physician will act professionally, in the patient's personal interest, and will guard medical information from disclosure to others without consent of the patient but will share findings completely and truthfully with the patient.

The physician–patient relationship is never quite so simple in practice. Medical ethics governs fiduciary relationships reasonably well but there are still problem areas. For example, when a physician treats several members of the same family, the family members' interests may not be aligned. For example, there may be evidence of spousal abuse, a parent may make the wrong decision for a child, or one member may have secrets (such as a communicable disease or an embarrassing condition such as a sexually transmitted disease) that they do not wish to disclose to other family members.

The fiduciary relationship is not absolute but it must never be broken unless required by law or to prevent serious consequences. In a typical medical practice, the physician must sometimes (although rarely) break confidentiality against the patient's or family's wishes when reporting confidential information to third parties (such as public health authorities), warning others of specific expressed intent to kill or maim (vague or lesser threats are not sufficient), and when reporting family secrets to the authorities (such as evidence of child abuse). This is never done lightly, of course, and always causes great anguish.

Many physicians, on the other hand, see themselves as unconstrained advocates for their patient's stated (although not always real) interests. In occupational medicine, the most common manifestations of this are exaggeration or even untruthful statements on workers' compensation claims and disability applications, and in certification of time off work (the "note from the doctor") in excess of what is actually required. These actions are taken on the assumption that they do not matter, that they benefit the patient, and that the primary care physician is obliged to trust the patient. In fact, these casual abuses are wrong and cost a great deal in unnecessary time off work, show a lack of trust in the primary care provider, and account for delayed rehabilitation and reintegration of the worker into productive work life. Sometimes the assumptions that primary care physicians make that justify these abuses are just a rationalization of a wish to maintain a good ongoing relationship with the worker or family. These practices have been going on a very long time and are the main reason that occupational physicians (and occupational health nurses), in general, often have little confidence in the trustworthiness of family physicians on such matters.

In occupational medicine and nursing practice, many clinical encounters have this fiduciary element and are typical physician–patient relationships, such as providing acute care for injured workers. Even in fiduciary relationships, the physician, especially, is not always obliged to act in the perceived, narrow interest of the patient. When acting as the treating physician or attending nurse, the occupational health practitioner cannot always put the interests of the patient or injured worker first, when to do so would be at the expense of truthfulness, against the law, or where there is a risk of grave harm to others. This is not unique to occupational medicine. Many countries and states have laws requiring physicians to notify the department of motor vehicles if the patient has a seizure disorder or failing vision; the physician cannot refuse and the patient cannot legally prevent it.

Relationships that are not Fiduciary

Many medical and nursing encounters in occupational health practice do not involve an expectation of treatment and are not fiduciary in nature. These include the many functions of occupational health professionals that do not have the characteristics of a physician–patient relationship, such as fitness for duty evaluations, independent medical examinations, and periodic health surveillance. Similar non-fiduciary relationships exist for insurance evaluations, induction examinations in military service, and screening programs for public health for which treatment is not offered. No physician–patient relationship exists, in the ethical sense. In such encounters, the physician is not accountable to the worker, except in the most general terms of professional responsibility (as noted below and discussed extensively in Chapter 3). The worker in this case is not truly a patient, either, because there is no expectation of treatment. In these situations, the occupational health professional is accountable to the sponsor of the service, such as the employer, insurance carrier, or government agency. There is nothing unethical with this arrangement, which stands at some remove outside of the usual code of medical ethics, but such circumstances are covered by the ethical codes of occupational health.

Licensed health professionals, physicians and nurses in particular, have to be clear at all times on whether a "physician/nurse/healthcare provider– patient relationship" exists with the worker. When the worker is being assessed and treated by the physician for an occupational injury, for example, a physician–patient relationship exists. When that same physician is conducting an evaluation for the employer for fitness to work, or for an insurance company for impairment assessment, a physician–patient relationship does not exist, because the service is being performed in the interest of a third party. A medical evaluation that is conducted solely for the purpose of a third party—such as a fitness for duty evaluation, disability evaluation, an independent medical evaluation, or periodic health surveillance—and does not constitute a provider–patient relationship. The provisions in codes of ethics with respect to honesty, integrity, and the disclosure of health risks that may be discovered still apply but not absolute confidentiality, as medical information discovered by the physician may be disclosed to third parties in such situations. This situation is so common that it is worth printing a notification on forms, and confirming it for legal purposes by obtaining the worker's signature on it, to document that he or she was informed that a provider–patient relationship did not exist.

Where there is no provider–patient relationship, the occupational health professional still has an obligation to meet professional and legal standards: inform the worker that no practitioner–patient relationship exists, obtain consent for the examination, tell the worker about significant findings, recommend medical follow-up when something abnormal is found, and manage any medical emergencies that arise during the course of an evaluation, although there is no obligation to treat the patient otherwise.

Protecting workers' rights and health is fundamental, but there are times when a competing right or public health interest forces a balance to be made. This applies most often to physicians and nurses who detect a serious health problem that the worker would rather conceal or refuses to acknowledge. The ethical principle is that neither the confidentiality of medical information nor the duty to warn of possible risk is absolute. The standard for disclosure of information without the protection of law or consent is very high: serious injury or risk to life, which is likely (not just possible) to occur without disclosure. Disclosure may also be allowed when it would be in the worker's own interest (for example, if the worker became seriously ill at work and cannot give consent), or when disclosure is necessary to prevent highly likely and unacceptably severe risk against the public interest (for example, if a worker had an active and highly communicable disease such as tuberculosis). Likewise, impairment of workers in safety-sensitive jobs (such as an untreated seizure disorder in a bus driver or continuing alcohol abuse in a tanker captain), may require disclosure for protection of the community, despite the worker's refusal. Judgment is required. The risk of a minor illness (such as influenza) or the unlikely possibility of a minor injury (for example, the risk that a worker would drop a wrench on someone's foot) is not severe enough to warrant breaking confidentiality.

These situations require the occupational health professional to balance individual and collective interests. In such situations, occupational health professionals should try to persuade the worker to disclose the information voluntarily. In case of conflict, it is always best to make the balance clear to each party and to document the situation in writing. Legal advice may be required.

Applying Ethical Codes

Ethical codes are intended to be guidance. They cannot anticipate all possible situations or problems. At the same time, when there is a gap or a conflict, that does not mean that anything goes and that the parties with power can do what they want. The provisions of codes of ethics should always be interpreted conservatively, with an emphasis and weight in decision-making on protecting the rights and health of the worker whenever there is doubt or conflict. The occupational health professional who finds him- or herself in a difficult situation should seek objective help wherever it can be found: from legal counsel, the competent authority (a government agency), colleagues, or organizations, while at the same time keeping the matter confidential to the extent possible. Complete and extensive documentation is essential to resolving these difficult issues. Sometimes they cannot be resolved and the occupational health professional has to make difficult choices. This is part of being a mature, adult professional in a responsible position on which workers' lives and health depend.

Increasingly, the practice of medicine, generally, is being constrained by powerful forces, such as managed care (including utilization review), insurance-driven preauthorization and utilization reviews, Medicare guidelines, defensive medicine (and its flip side, intimidation and capitulation to patients because of fear of malpractice actions), and directive state legislation and common law (most obviously law affecting abortion but also involving determination of death). Individually, these factors may be positive or negative but in the aggregate they constrain the practice of medicine in ways that affect the interests of patients in ways that were unthinkable a few decades ago. Physicians in primary care, especially, are much more likely to practice in situations in which the physician–patient relationship is heavily influenced and sometimes effectively pre-empted by third parties. This has caused great anguish in the medical profession. On the other hand, the fundamental issues inherent in occupational medicine are more or less settled and have not changed for decades. The ethical situation of general medicine is therefore converging with that of occupational medicine, rather than vice versa.

Recommended Reading and Resources

American Board of Industrial Hygiene. Code of Ethics. Available at: http://www.abih.org/downloads/ABIHCodeofEthics.pdf. Accessed May 16, 2011.

American College of Occupational and Environmental Medicine. The ACOEM Code of Ethics. Available at: http://www.acoem.org/codeofconduct.aspx. Accessed December 22, 2011.

American College of Occupational and Environmental Medicine. The Seven Ethical Principles of Occupational Medicine. Available at: http://www.acoem.org/uploadedFiles/About_ACOEM/Code%20of%20Ethics%20-%20Condensed%20Version.pdf. Accessed December 22, 2011.

American Occupational Health Nurses Association. Code of Ethics. Available at: https://www.aaohn.org/for-your-practice-items/code-of-ethics.html. Accessed May 16, 2011.

American Occupational Health Nurses Association. Standards of Practice. Available at: https://www.aaohn.org/for-your-practice-items/standards-of-occupational-and-environmental-health-nursing.html. Accessed May 16, 2011.

Board of Canadian Registered Safety Professionals. Code of Ethics. Available at: http://www.bcrsp.ca/ethics.html. Accessed May 16, 2011.

Board of Certified Safety Professionals. Code of Ethics. Available at: http://www.bcsp.org/pdf/ASPCSP/code_of_ethics_July2010.pdf. Accessed May 16, 2011.

Brandt-Rauf SI, Brandt-Rauf E, Gershon R, Brandt-Rauf PW (2011) The differing perspectives of workers and occupational medicine physicians on the ethical, legal, and social issues of genetic testing in the workplace. *New Solut*, 21(1): 89–102.

Guidotti TL (2005) Ethics and skeptics: what lies behind ethical codes in occupational health. *J Occup Environ Med*, 47(4): 168–175.

International Commission on Occupational Health. Code of Ethics. Available at: http://www.icohweb.org/site_new/ico_core_documents.asp#. Accessed May 16, 2011.

London L (2005) Dual loyalties and the ethical and human rights obligations of occupational health professionals. *J Occup Environ Med*, 47(4): 322–332.

Occupational and Environmental Medical Association of Canada. Code of Occupational and Environmental Medical Ethics. Available at: http://www.oemac.org/?page=72. Accessed December 22, 2011.

Rosenstock L, Hagopian A (1987) Ethical dilemmas in providing health care to workers. *Ann Int Med*, 107(4): 575–578.

Toulmin S (1986) Divided loyalties and ambiguous relationships. *Soc Sci Med*, 23(8): 783–787.

Westerholm P, Nilstun T, Øvretveit J (2004) *Practical Ethics in Occupational Health*. Milton Keynes UK, Radcliffe Publishing.

Exhibit 5.1. Model Authorization for Release of Medical Information

---

Authorization for Release of Medical Information

I, _____, hereby authorize _____

to release the following medical information about me:

_____
_____
_____

to the following person(s)/organization(s);

_____
_____

I give my permission for this medical information to be used for the following purposes:

_____
_____
_____
_____

I do not give my permission for any other use or re-disclosure of this information and this authorization is not effective beyond the following date: _____.

_____
Signature of person authorizing release

_____ _____
Signature of Witness   Date of Signature

---

6 Corporate and In-House Occupational Health Services

Joel Bender and Paul Joos-Vandewalle

Managing occupational health, and resolving conflicting demands at various levels within any large organization, is becoming more challenging and complex as global companies expand and extend their manufacturing, distribution, and service capabilities both locally and abroad.

The most critical factors for a successful occupational health program in any company are a caring philosophy and a public commitment from senior leadership that will resonate throughout the organization. Everything else is process and without this commitment it is all hollow and likely to collapse. Strong leadership, integrity, and social conscience can be articulated in a clear and unambiguous vision statement such as this: "The company leadership is committed to providing all employees with safe and healthy working conditions and recognizes the value of promoting the health and well-being of employees, their dependants and retirees. The company acknowledges its responsibility for the environment and to the communities in which its facilities are located; it is also committed to producing products that are safe and reliable when properly used."

There are five universal core components of a company health and safety policy. Whether a company explicitly addresses all five in their policies or not, and whether they separate or combine them as responsibilities in the organization chart, the employer must always manage these five dimensions of health in their workforce and operation:

- *Health.* To guarantee a safe and sound workplace by prevention of occupational health risks.
- *Safety.* To prevent injury, accidents and loss of property, through the provision of a safe workplace.
- *Environment.* To prevent health risks beyond the "fenceline," or boundaries of company facilities, including product safety and preventing and mitigating environmental hazards.
- *Sustainability.* The effective use of materials and energy, reducing waste and prevention of pollution in order to minimize the impact on the environment, originating from production.
- *Wellness.* To enhance the health and well-being of employees through education and providing opportunities to enhance their personal and family health.

The terminology of corporate health and safety must be understood for clear communication and in order to appreciate the usual lines of conflict and cooperation in large organizations. "OH&S" (ampersand optional) is universal shorthand for "occupational health and safety" and refers to health protection (both occupational medical services and industrial hygiene, which are generally in staff positions serving the entire organization) and to safety (safety officers are usually closer to production and line responsibility). In some organizations, health and safety are under different managers and are separated in the organization chart, frequently leading to conflict, but when they are united in one unit or department it is usually called OH&S or "health and safety" and is managed by a more senior manager. "HSE" (no ampersand) is universal shorthand for "health, safety, and environment," and refers to professionals and company units or departments that manage all three. (Note that HSE may also stand for the Health and Safety Executive, the UK occupational health regulatory agency.) This model is replacing narrow "OH&S" departments across industry with departments that have been given broader responsibility, which sometimes includes security when emergency management is a major concern for the company (see Chapter 31). "Environment" always refers to environmental health protection and compliance with environmental standards, but may include sustainability. Sustainability, from the business perspective, assumes that there is always a link between the health of the environment and human health, however indirect, and that this is reflected in the public perception that health and sustainability go together. It is also generally more efficient for companies to have environmental issues all under one management unit. Some companies have appointed "sustainability officers" to manage and track their performance on issues such as recycling, fair trade, pollution reduction in excess of environmental regulations, and carbon emissions. "Wellness" is oriented to prevention and healthy living and covers health promotion, issues of health and productivity, achieving work/life balance, and management of health expense other than work-related injuries and illness (which can be viewed as the management of disability and chronic disease). As a management function, responsibility for wellness is often combined with "Health" in an occupational health service but may be contracted out (see Chapter 30).

Exhibit 6.1 (at the end of this chapter) is a model corporate policy for HSE. A foundational policy becomes the authority within the company for subsidiary policies and a template for policies that address specific hazards, risks, and functions, as outlined in other chapters.

Portfolio of Responsibilities

OH&S management systems are designed to manage risks and protect workers throughout the global business, applying consistent company standards and complying with national or local regulations (see Chapter 7). This can be challenging for a large organization with operating units around the world. In emerging economies and developing countries, local regulations are usually weaker than those in the home country or the countries where the company operates and are often poorly enforced. Not infrequently, company standards play a role in improving the standard of occupational health protection in emerging economies.

The objectives for any medical department, regardless of size, are to optimize the health and well-being of employees, direct resources, and provide solutions to achieve the company's health, safety and environmental goals:

- Compliance with governmental regulations, corporate mandates, and organized labor agreements, both globally and locally, and the documentation to prove this and preferably to provide assurance that the company is not only compliant but proactive.
- Comprehensive, professional, medical, and ancillary clinical services that meet and anticipate the needs of the company.
- Enhancement of work/life practices that allow people and the company to achieve full potential.

Table 6.1 Typical Business Portfolio for Occupational Health Services

Compliance	Clinical Services	Work/Life Enhancement	Operations Management
• Hearing conservation • Blood borne pathogens • Metal working fluid • Drug screening • Mobile equipment operation	• Personal • Urgent care • Primary care • Surveillance examinations • Flu immunizations • Travel medicine	• Disability management • Disease management • Health maintenance • Employee assistance • Behavioral health benefits • Wellness programs • Health care benefit consulting	• Hazmat • Plant/staff/safety • Consultation • Communications • Staffing management • Resource/finance management • Joint health and safety • Supplies and equipment • Occupational health and safety • Labor relations • Health research • Medical file management • Training and education • Information systems • Global platforms

- Management of occupational health service operations in a manner that is consistent with core values and business priorities and exceeds customer expectations of quality and value.

Through experience, companies have identified certain key functions or services to be necessary to meet these objectives. Table 6.1 shows a typical business portfolio of occupational health services provided to employees, some of which also protect their families and communities. Some of these functions are best done in-house and some are better done by outsourcing to contractors or purchasing services individually from vendors. In order to achieve greater effectiveness as well as efficiency, however, these functions must be managed in a coordinated way as part of a total system, not simply provided piecemeal by contractors to meet the lowest regulatory requirements.

With an increasingly mobile workforce and global company reach, maintaining a comprehensive occupational health system for all employees is difficult but essential. Apart from the impact on human performance, having a comprehensive system and plan also protects the company against liability issues and helps to reduce escalating costs. Therefore, it is prudent to have a sound organizational structure to manage occupational health issues on a consistent basis.

Organizational Structure

The organization and reporting arrangements for OH&S depend upon the size and structure of the company, and, to a certain extent, the industry and the geographic location and distribution of the company. The positioning of OH&S in the organization is critical.

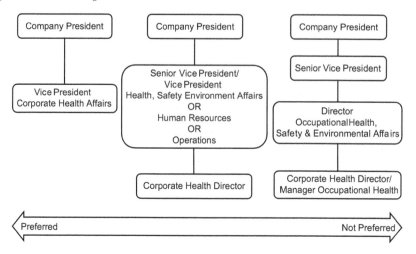

Figure 6.1 Placement of occupational health and safety in the structure of a large organization

Figure 6.1 shows three common structures for the placement of OH&S, and therefore internal occupational health services, in a large organization.

The Corporate Director

The leadership position for an occupational health department within an organization has traditionally been, and is currently most often held, by an occupational health physician (MD or DO). The most frequent title for this leadership position has been "Corporate Medical Director" (CMD). This implies that specifically medical expertise is required for the position and that is not always the case. More recently, two other scenarios have developed that have changed this nomenclature in some organizations. In the first instance, some corporate physicians may have an expanded role that could include industrial hygiene, safety, and, in some situations, environment. In these cases titles such as "Corporate Director (or Vice President) Occupational Health and Safety," or "Corporate Director (or Vice President) Health, Safety, and Environment," are appropriate. Some physicians also prefer the title of "Corporate Director – Occupational Health" as this wording is felt to have broader implications than a purely medical one – implications that suggest a broader preventive approach to health. In the second instance, as the leadership of occupational health is evolving and is not necessarily limited to physicians, some multinational organizations have appointed other occupational health professionals to head their corporate departments. These leaders are often from other occupational health disciplines, such as occupational health nursing, industrial hygiene, toxicology, and safety—so titles such as those noted above are, again, appropriate. Corporate Medical Director continues to be reserved for the lead physician in the organization.

For the purpose of this chapter, the leadership position will be referred to as the "Chief Health Officer" (CHO) of the organization. No matter what the title, the person responsible for the organization's occupational health should be an individual with proven competencies in occupational health and with advanced knowledge and training in corporate administration, including policy development and successful program implementation. If the person also has responsibility for other disciplines, knowledge in these areas is also essential.

The corporate OH&S should be led by a senior manager reporting as high up in the organization as is practical. A physician with a strong administrative and professional background should ideally occupy the management position, providing leadership as well as technical expertise, but this requires a management and leadership skill set well beyond mastery of clinical medicine. Some CHOs are also vice presidents of the company, but most are not. Rarely do they report directly to the President or Chief Executive Officer of the company, as in the model on the left in Figure 6.1. CHOs more frequently report, as in the middle model, to a vice president or senior vice president of health, safety, and environmental affairs; to the vice president or senior vice president of human resources; or very occasionally to an executive or senior vice president of operations.

The position of CHO is one of great responsibility. The corporate Vice President or CHO is responsible for developing, supporting, coordinating and auditing the Health, Safety and Environment programs, reporting to management council at least biannually. This individual is also responsible for coordinating, reviewing, and approving external communications on issues that relate to the health, safety, and environmental concerns. Exhibit 6.2 (found at the end of this chapter) outlines the responsibilities of the position and can also be used as a draft position description for recruitment to this position.

Most companies (other than banks) reserve the title of Vice President for very senior level positions. Layered underneath and reporting to Vice Presidents are directors, and beneath that managers. In the example on the right in Figure 6.1, the CHO might have the title of Manager, Occupational Health, reporting to the Director of Occupational Health and Environmental Affairs.

The Corporate Medical Director, if not reporting to a vice president of OH&S, should at least report to someone at the policy-making level and have sufficient authority by virtue of the position to be able to influence or set policy and to establish standards of practice. At whatever level he or she is placed, the CHO becomes a resource for management on a wide range of health-related issues, including insurance options, product safety, and liaison with government agencies. The CHO drives the business philosophy for health and safety within the company by providing guidance for policies used to establish organizational goals. It is the responsibility of senior management to support efforts of the medical director to maintain a healthy and sustainable workforce by providing adequate resources. This support will foster successful implementation of policies and lead to a sustainable health, safety, and environmental culture within the enterprise.

The CHO, aside from developing policies and procedures for the standard occupational health services, may manage a professional team that deals with a number of complex occupational health and related issues including the prevention of work-related disorders. The ability to do this goes beyond medical training and experience and requires the CHO to have mastery of basic business skills (management, financials, budgeting, strategic planning, even marketing) as well as personal leadership qualities and effective communication skills that can span and shift instantly among interaction with technical experts, highly assertive and often skeptical senior officers, workers on the shop floor, and the general public (usually under stressful conditions). The CHO must learn to apply OH&S solutions to a global context through innovative thinking, best-in-class practice, accurate information, and insightful technical analysis. Within the company, this requires the CHO to win trust and credibility in order to influence consensus among diverse groups. The road to success is often one of constructively challenging conventional wisdom through education, but doing so in a manner that is not confrontational. Ultimately, the CHO must be able to translate the vision and mission of the corporate medical department into actionable plans and measurable objectives that have clear milestones.

Many companies, particularly in highly technical fields, use a matrix form of organization, in which employees report to a manager for the department or division in which they are permanently assigned and a project manager for the duration of the project they are working on. CHOs experience this when they are based at a corporate headquarters but their work ranges widely across divisions of the company. Living within a world of matrix management can present challenges for the medical leader because incentives and priorities are not always aligned. The medical director must learn how to navigate issues successfully when support is needed from organized labor, human resources, finance, administration, compensation, and benefits. Health care delivery systems, risk management, product stewardship, and issues of health and productivity bring another level of complexity to the job and the CHO adds value to the company by optimizing outcomes and managing these issues in an integrated fashion. Mastering managerial skills, promoting teamwork, and strengthening business acumen will contribute immensely to the success of a CHO.

Regional and Group Medical Directors

Whether or not the CHO is also the CMD (that is, the Chief Health Officer is the Corporate Medical Director, which is usually the case), it is advisable to have a CMD as lead medical director or at least a group medical director positioned over at least all licensed health providers, to provide professional leadership for occupational health programs (Figure 6.2). This position is particularly important in companies with a number of manufacturing units distributed over a large geographical area, or where occupational health nurses and contract physicians provide most of the occupational health services at the local, operational level. A group medical director can also provide more direct supervision to part-time occupational health physicians, who usually are not able to give the local staff direction on programming or broader issues of management, especially in complex manufacturing environments.

At the next level down, senior and regional medical directors who report directly to the CMD (and for this level of complexity a corporate medical director with stronger authority is preferable to a senior "group medical director" who serves in a coordinating role) are

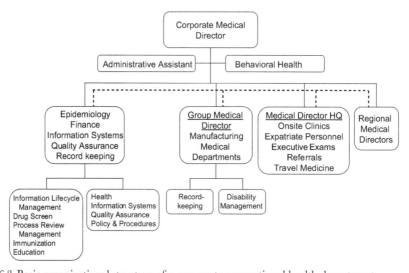

Figure 6.2 Basic organizational structure of a corporate occupational health department

Box 6.1 Roles and Responsibilities of Group and Regional Medical Directors

Reporting to the corporate medical director, the group/regional medical director will:

- Develop and manage a medical business plan and budget in conjunction with units.
- Act as liaison with corporate health services, plant medical departments, and plant/regional leadership.
- Assess medical team capabilities and make staffing recommendations.
- Define, collect, analyze, and report regional/plant medical and hygiene metrics.
- Ensure regulatory compliance and ensure adherence to occupational exposure guidelines (shared responsibility with industrial/occupational hygiene).
- Evaluate quality assurance data, analyze customer feedback surveys, and coordinate corrective actions as necessary.
- Act as liaison between company and appropriate government and community agencies.
- Ensure that periodic health surveillance is up to date and compliant, and monitor patterns of positive findings and anomalies.
- Lead or coordinate local outbreak investigations and participate in health hazard evaluations.
- Collect and analyze ergonomics related injury and illness data, recommending corrective action; coordinate common corporate, regional, and local ergonomics processes; and provide ergonomics training and support.
- Identify existing and emerging plant/regional medical and hygiene issues and develop appropriate action plans: SARS, AIDS, avian influenza, etc.
- Lead contact for any local, regional, or country expatriate and family health-related issues.
- Monitor emergency management preparedness on the part of units.

generally needed to lead medical services in larger geographical regions, especially when their responsibilities include industrial hygiene, and ergonomic activities. (In companies without a CHO, they usually do not and these occupational health functions are placed in another department, often creating problems of coordination.) The purpose of these positions is to provide strategic leadership in delivering common occupational health processes and procedures and to deliver adequate and eventually world-class industrial hygiene, ergonomic, and occupational safety standards throughout the company. Additional roles and responsibilities are shown in Box 6.1.

It is imperative that senior and regional medical directors develop a solid working relationship with their regional or country medical teams. This means overcoming unique, local challenges regarding language, culture, educational level, and economic support, often by forging personal relationships and trust (and doing so quickly, before the next turnover in personnel).This helps to ensure compliance with company standards at a national level in locations far from the corporate office, where there is often a tendency to relax or follow the lead of less vigilant companies in the country. The smaller and less complex the enterprise at the local level, the smaller the corporate health and safety group required in country or onsite. However, irrespective of size, strong professional leadership is still needed to support OH&S functions, and to ensure that audits and reporting are accurate and complete. Staff who are employed locally, particularly in different cultures, may have different attitudes and priorities, may not appreciate why audits and reporting are important, or may have limited experience. Communication is often a problem across cultures.

Consultant Medical Directors

Companies that have neither a senior manager nor a company medical director responsible for OH&S sometimes use external part-time medical consultants for medical functions. More often, companies will use part-time consultants as regional medical directors. Many consultants can do an adequate job but to add value to the company the objective should be to find a consultant who understands how their task fits into the big picture and is committed to quality, consistency, and accurate reporting. Consultants must be carefully selected for their ability to provide the necessary services at every level within the organization. On the other hand, their limitations and inevitable lack of familiarity with the corporate structure and priorities must be appreciated. Engaging a consultant for medical functions should therefore be the beginning of a long-term relationship in which information will be shared and communication is easy.

In-House Occupational Health Services

Occupational health services provided within the company to employees will differ across regions and within each country and sometimes from location to location. Whether particular services are provided onsite or offsite for all employees will depend on the size of the workforce, the nature of the work, the location of the site within the community, and the availability of suitable nearby medical facilities, although the explosion of internet applications is making it much easier to provide some services, such as wellness and training, online. Which services are provided will also depend on government or local legislative requirements and corporate sustainability policies. If onsite clinical medical services are to be provided, it is imperative that the medical department be included in the initial planning or the planning of any appreciable changes to determine the requirements for design, staffing, equipment, and supplies. Working in other countries within joint ventures complicates the delivery of occupational health services, and the roles and responsibilities for medical care need to be clearly delineated.

Occupational health services should include some form of personal health care management whenever possible in order to contain costs and to assist with health- and wellness-related productivity and performance issues. Many onsite clinics, domestic and international, with large work populations are often used for primary care to avoid absence from work and for better control related to the cost of medical care. Even if these services are provided onsite the employee may still visit a personal physician out of the company network. However, the onsite medical staff should at least able to interact with offsite providers to monitor employee health, well-being and absence. Onsite urgent care centers and clinics run by contractors are an increasingly popular model for employers (see Chapter 1).

Return-to-work, disability evaluations, and medical certification of absence following injury or illness, may not be available at all in some emerging markets, making it difficult to determine the actual cost of health care and productivity issues. In large multinational corporations with a significant mix of expatriate and national employees, particularly those that have grown by acquisition, work-related injury rates, workers' compensation claims, and absence records for personal injury or illness are often not centralized. Usually, only the former is monitored closely, in order to adhere to government regulations. This deficiency may make it difficult to track the company's productivity and performance.

Small Enterprises

Small business enterprises employ up to 60 percent of the workforce in developing or newly industrialized countries. These establishments, which include restaurants, motels, retail shops, automobile repair shops, and machine shops and cross all sectors of the economy, may have 1 to 50 employees, by definition. Although often characterized by limited capital investment, smaller annual revenue, or fewer numbers of employees, they are critically important to national economies. The US Small Business Administration has reported that all small enterprises in the US, taken together, employ just as many workers as all large companies (60 million). These businesses drive employment, adapt quickly to changing market conditions, produce goods or services nearer to the customer, and provide jobs for those who are often under- or unemployed. As well, many important innovative companies have started small and grown quickly to become major employers, establishing (in the case of microelectronics and information technology) entire new industries.

There are special challenges to providing occupational health services to small businesses. Many are marginal enterprises that cannot afford increased operating expenses, even though the future savings might be substantial. Smaller businesses may be exempt by legislation from occupational health regulation and workers' compensation. Formal links with governmental agencies, trade associations, and local chambers of commerce may be non-existent, especially if it is a family business.

It is much easier for small enterprises to access good medical care than adequate occupational health services. Unfortunately, in many instances small enterprises are unaware or may be reluctant to seek help.

There have been a number of pilot and demonstration programs around the world to reach out to small enterprises. Excellent occupational health services can in fact be supplied to small enterprises and to small units of large organizations or small, independent employee groups of any size. However, for this to take place the owner or president of the small business must take an interest in occupational health services, which is difficult when they are often struggling to survive financially and to stay in business. This requires education and insight into their problems. They must also have access to affordable services.

Services to small enterprises are a substantial opportunity for an occupational health service that is flexible and willing to educate and market to small businesses. It is a tremendous asset for any employer to have a knowledgeable physician available to care for injured employees, conduct pre-placement examinations, provide health evaluations, and provide advice on controlling workplace hazards. Community-based occupational health services can provide a wide range of medical services to smaller businesses. Guidance on how to reach small enterprises and adapt services to their needs can be obtained from many sources: the American College of Occupational and Environmental Medicine, the Canadian Centre for Occupational Health and Safety, the National Institute for Occupational Safety and Health, and the Occupational Safety and Health Administration. Services to small enterprises has been a major priority for international agencies and very useful publications are available online from two United Nations organizations, the International Labour Organization and the World Health Organization, many of them organized around the long-running campaign for "Basic Occupational Health Services for All." Table 6.2 provides a few of the

Table 6.2 Key Occupational Health Services Offered by Physicians and Other Health Care Providers Consulting for Small Businesses

Needs Assessment	Control Strategies	Clinical Services	Record-Keeping
Identify health and safety hazards common to the workplace	Communicate results of assessments to owners, management, and workers	Conduct pre-placement, screening, and periodic exams	Understand and comply with record-keeping requirements
Conduct workplace inspections through walkthroughs	Identify control strategies needed and available	Promote ergonomic solutions	Enforce policy on confidentiality of medical records
Rank risks in terms of urgency and prioritize ("risk assessment", see Chapter 21)	Assign relative priorities based on feasibility and urgency	Provide for delivery of diagnostic, therapeutic, and rehabilitative services	Complete or provide medical assessment for workplace injuries and diseases
Conduct repeat assessments with changes in production, equipment, and materials	Provide oversight of remediation including installation	Provide first aid, blood borne pathogen, and emergency response training	Maintain exposure and surveillance records
Advise management on needs and priorities	Provide education, training, and awareness for owners and employees	Manage medical aspects of occupational and non-occupational absence issues	Monitor and report effectiveness of hazard control measures
Advise management on need for specialized expertise for problem-solving (e.g. industrial hygiene)	Monitor effectiveness (through surveillance and health experience)	Promote health and well-being for high-performance workforce	Prepare and maintain workers' compensation reports and claim records

key occupational health services that should be provided and thoroughly understood from the point of view of owner–managers by physicians offering consultations to small businesses.

Employee Participation

Worker participation in OH&S decisions varies widely across industrial sectors and countries, by provisions under contracts with organized labor, and by local custom. The form of participation can range from just suggestion boxes to joint (labor and management) health and safety committees all the way to "works councils" (a partial workplace shared-governance model popular in western Europe) at the local or enterprise levels. Regardless of legal obligation, successful companies generally encourage direct participation of workers to prevent injuries and illness, improve quality, enhance productivity, and to enrich workplace culture. CHOs or local full-time medical staff (but usually not consultants) are often deeply involved in these participatory practices as they pertain to OH&S, ergonomics, wellness, and health care delivery.

The relationship of labor and management in works councils is often spelled out by legislation and further clarified by collective bargaining. All Canadian provinces and territories, and the federal government require employers to have joint worksite health and safety committees, although rules regarding their operation vary. In Germany, the interests of employees have been institutionalized in the works council (*Betriebsrat*), which has certain rights to information, consultation, and co-determination. In fact, there is a legal obligation for collective "co-determination" (*Mitbestimmung*) in areas of injury prevention, health protection, work rules, hazards, and training. Some observers credit the works council model for contributing to Germany's recent economic resiliency, competitiveness, and flexibility in response to changing demand by reducing friction between labor and management, and managing the conditions of work with less conflict.

Joint groups or semi-autonomous workgroups have also been used to determine best practices for workforce health and safety, ergonomic enhancements, productivity improvements, or even reductions in workplace exposures. These are usually one-off task forces that are convened to address a particular problem or to map out a new direction for the company. The medical director is usually a key member of these groups as they work through issues such as new technology, the organization of work, training, and general work conditions.

Even in the absence of organized labor, successful companies seek to engage workers in health and safety processes. This may be accomplished through health and safety committees in which management might select representatives or through existing Total Quality Management teams (as described below) where management and employee representatives rotate through assignments such as OH&S.

Acceptance of worker participation in OH&S on the part of managers in North America has been facilitated by the popular management concept called "Total Quality Management" (TQM). TQM is a structured process of continuous quality improvement that has led to job enrichment and more autonomy for workers, in which all employees participate in quality improvements. Health and safety processes have been included into TQM quite effectively. The advantage of this is that production management is often intimately familiar with the TQM process, so worker participation is not viewed as threatening or unusual.

The medical director and every physician involved in the in-house occupational health service must understand and accept the various forms and extent of employee involvement in order to implement successful prevention strategies. The following principles of joint cooperation are essential to improving health and safety performance:

- Workers on the shop floor are in the best position to identify potential hazards and to contribute to preventing occupational incidents involving loss, injury, or health risk.
- Employees have the right to be involved in decisions that impact their health and well-being.
- Employees have greater motivation to promote safe practices and healthy behaviors if they are involved and educated.
- Equal partnership, with a well defined process for engagement, results in cooperation between labor and management, and drives improvement in working conditions.
- Experiences and ideas from workers for health and safety improvements should be highly valued by management.

Occupational Health and Safety Policies

An OH&S policy should reflect the company's business philosophy, articulate its commitment to employee well-being, recognize relevant laws, define roles, and assign responsibility. The template shown in Exhibit 6.1 is a good starting point for developing an OH&S policy.

The key strategic principles of an OH&S policy include:

- Protecting the health and safety of employees by optimizing working conditions, establishing programs, and providing services designed to provide safe technology and avoid hazards (primary prevention).
- Protecting the health and safety of persons living or working areas near company operations by establishing programs that minimize the impact of the operations on the environment.
- Acknowledging the local government's responsibility, authority, and competence in the development and control of working conditions, wherever the company has operations.
- Recognizing employees' own interest in OH&S, through the cooperation and collaboration of employers and workers.
- Continuous follow-up and development of OH&S.

OH&S, HSE, and the entire panoply of health-related issues faced by a company cannot be managed by a corporate medical department acting alone and is not the exclusive responsibility of the OH&S staff. It is a "line" responsibility, part of the operational reporting and accountability of managers up and down the organizational chart, from the corporate leadership through division directors to shop foremen. The implementation of these principles requires appropriate support, legal provisions, administrative enforcement, and OH&S management systems within the organization. The corporate leadership, including the chief executive officer, is responsible for the policies that allow the OH&S system to be effective, for the culture of the organization, and for providing the tools and systems that allow senior managers to solve problems. Senior management is responsible for the directing of resources and implementation of programs to achieve company health, safety, and environmental goals. Ultimately, it is the senior manager at each location who is responsible for managing these issues.

The OH&S team should have a clearly documented staffing plan that identifies required services, inventories resources (including a staffing headcount), delineates responsibilities and reporting, assigns staff based on services provided, and articulates a rationale for determining whether assigned staff are full-time or contract. The staff members of the occupational health program are employees of the organization, too, and their careers are bound up with the occupational health service. They need opportunities for training and peer interaction, normally through attendance at conferences, and support for professional commitments, such as licensing and continuing education. Ideally, the plan should include a clear progression or succession plan for advancement of these employees, with a suitable mentoring program in place.

Recommended Reading and Resources

There are very few current titles on the topic of corporate occupational health services management, which is one reason for the production of the present book. There are many titles in occupational medicine generally, occupational health and safety generally, the management of specific occupational health problems, and the management of OH&S departments. Some of these have chapters on corporate medical departments but they are mostly out of date because of widespread changes in corporate organization and management.

Moser R Jr. (2008) *Effective Management of Health and Safety Programs*. Beverly Farms MA, OEM Press.
Smith I (2007) *Occupational Health: A Practical Guide for Managers*. London, Taylor and Francis.

Exhibit 6.1 Example Occupational Health and Safety Policy

<COMPANY NAME>
Occupational Health and Safety Policy

<COMPANY NAME> has a responsibility to protect the health and safety of each individual at all times. **<COMPANY NAME>** health and safety policies and practices affect an individual's physical and psychological health and safety.

The Occupational Health and Safety Policy relates to all individuals who enter the company premises or uses the company's equipment.

Federal, state and local governments have their own Occupational Health and Safety (OH & S) legislation and regulations, which govern the standards of health and safety in the workplace; **<COMPANY NAME>** must comply, as a minimum, with all the relevant governmental OHS legislation.

<COMPANY NAME> should review policies regularly in collaboration with all stakeholders, seeking recommendations from recognised authorities. The review date of this policy should be clearly documented on the policy.

Policy Number   **<NUMBER>**

Policy statement

- **<COMPANY NAME>** has a duty of care to provide all persons[1] with a safe and healthy environment.
- This Occupational Health and Safety (OHS) Policy adheres to the **<TITLE OF LOCAL GOVERNMENT LEGISLATION[2]>**
- **<LOCAL COMPANY NAME>** also complies with the **<CORPORATE REGULATIONS OR STANDARDS>** that reflect additional health and safety requirements.

The **<LOCAL COMPANY NAME>** is also committed to:
- – providing a duty of care that protects all employees from injury, illness or abuse;
- – developing and administering OHS risk management systems;
- – auditing OHS procedures and practices;
- – consulting with all stakeholders when reviewing OHS policies;
- – maintaining and storing OHS documentation and records in accordance with **<OHS LEGASLATIVE REQUIREMENTS>;**
- – providing stakeholders with OHS professional development and training;
- – developing policies as OHS legislation changes;

---

1   For the purpose of this policy, "persons" include <management, employees, ancillary staff (part-time staff, kitchen staff, cleaners, maintenance personnel), volunteers, visitors, local community>.

2   There are legislative Acts and regulations for each country/state and local government that address the issue of OHS. The local company is advised to seek information that is relevant to their area of jurisdiction.

- developing a program for employees returning to the workplace. This includes rehabilitation programs due to workplace injuries/illness, extended personal leave (illness, stress or bereavement); and
- ensuring that all OHS policies are transparent and available for all personnel to access.

- The OHS Policy applies to all hazardous chemicals, events, situations, tasks, buildings, equipment, methods, materials, substances, products and vehicles used for transporting employees.
- It is understood that there is a shared legal responsibility and accountability between, and a commitment by, all persons to implement the OHS Policy, procedures and practices.
- The company also complies with **<OHS INTERNATIONAL STANDARDS, CODES OF PRACTICE, COUNTRY STANDARDS>** and best practice recommendations from recognised authorities.
- The procedures relating to the OHS Policy are clearly labelled and displayed on company premises for all stakeholders to read. *(OHS policies, procedures and practices should be easy to read and interpret. The local company must consider translating all information in to applicable local languages to meet the language needs of all their employees.)*

Rationale

The rationale represents a statement of reasons that detail why the policy and/or procedures have been developed and are important to the service.

Please refer to:
- Duty of care

<The company can outline its duty of care position statement>

- Public liability insurance

<The company may decide to provide details regarding public liability insurance. For example, name of insurer; policy number; policy expiry date; insured amount; and insurer contact details. This may also be a requirement in licensing regulations>.

Responsibilities of different stakeholders

- Stakeholders are legally bound to comply with OHS responsibilities.[3]
  The company's stakeholders
- **<This section can include information regarding the induction procedures for each stakeholder listed below>:**
  Employer, owner/s (in joint ventures)
  Employees

---

3   The company should contact their local OH management agency to clarify their OHS obligations and seek further information and advice as required.

Visitors[4]
External contractor[5]
Special consideration[6]
* There are legislative requirements specific to the health and safety of pregnant women, such as risk to injury (manual handling); risk of infection (rubella); or illness

The Occupational Health and Safety Committee

The company can document their OHS legislative requirements regarding OHS representatives and committees.

<COMPANY NAME> has established an Occupational Health and Safety Committee. The names of the committee members are:

```
.............................................................................
.............................................................................
.............................................................................
.............................................................................
```

The roles and responsibilities of the committee are:

* to facilitate co-operation between the employer and employees with a view to ensuring the health and safety of the employees
* to provide employees with information including standards, rules and procedures relating to health and safety which are to be carried out or complied with at the workplace
* to deal with any other relevant matter as agreed
* to assist the OHS representative and the President to ensure the OHS responsibilities of management and staff are met on a regular basis
* to assist in the communication to staff of OHS practices and awareness
* minutes of meetings will be kept and made available to all staff
* to provide advice to the President on the induction of new staff on Occupational Health and Safety matters.

The health and safety committee meets monthly. The activities and issues with which the Occupational Health and Safety Committee deal are reported regularly at senior leadership meetings.

---

4   For the purpose of this policy, a "visitor" is defined as an individual who has been invited to the company for non-employment purposes.
5   For the purpose of this policy, an "external contractor" is defined as an individual who has been invited to the company to perform a specific function.
6   For the purpose of this policy, "special consideration" includes pregnant women or persons with additional needs.

Strategies and practices

These are examples. The company is encouraged to develop and adapt the following strategies and practices as required by individual circumstances and best practices.

OHS legislation focuses on the workplace addressing health and safety risks before they become a hazard, resulting in the development of procedures and practices that aim to eliminate or minimize risks from occurring or controlling them as they arise. Therefore, the company needs to develop risk management strategies; this is a comprehensive process that identifies, assesses, controls, minimizes, or eliminates risks that can potentially cause injury or illness to persons or damage to the environment.

Risk management strategies

An effective risk management strategy is a step by step procedure which:

- aids decision making;
- controls the cost of resources;
- increases the knowledge of risks and hazards;
- encourages the collaboration process; and
- prepares the company for external audits and reviews.

Identifying risks

Risks are identified by considering:

- What is the risk?

A risk can be a situation, event, task, material, service, method, or substance.

- What is the nature of the risk?

Risks can be environmental, physical, psychological, chemical, biological or financial. A risk can also affect company reputation or can be related to critical events, such as a natural disaster or pandemic.

- What is the history of the risk being a near miss?

The company may have recorded near misses or only actual incidents, which detail how many times the identifiable risk almost occurred and what were the outcomes.

Assessing risks

Risks are assessed by considering the:

- Probability of the risk occurring in normal conditions.
- Probability of the risk occurring in abnormal conditions.
- History of incidents and emergencies relating to the risk.
- Past, current and planned strategies to control the risk.

Controlling risks

Once risks have been identified and assessed, they are either eliminated, controlled, or minimized. The step-by-step hierarchy to controlling risks is as follows:

- Eliminate the risk.
- Find a substitute to the risk.
- Engineer control mechanisms to diminish the likelihood of the risk.

There may be no way of eliminating or substituting a risk and the company will need to develop control mechanisms to minimize the risk from occurring.

- Administer controls to minimise or eliminate the risk.
- Implement the use of Personal Protective Equipment (PPE).

Each step in the hierarchy may not be relevant to every risk. If a risk cannot be eliminated, address step two and find a substitute. If the risk cannot be substituted, move to step three, and so on. If the risk can be eliminated in the first instance, then there may be no need to find a substitute. For example, the risk is a toxic substance for employees. The control method is to remove substance, therefore eliminating the risk and preventing employees from coming in contact with the substance. If the process cannot do without the particular substance in the manufacturing process, find a suitable less/non-toxic substitute. If not possible to substitute try to establish control mechanisms to reduce exposure, etc.

Evaluating risk management strategies

The effectiveness of risk management strategies and OHS procedures and practices are evaluated by:

- reviewing and dating strategies every **<TIMEFRAME>;**

This includes changes to legislation or recommended practices.

- consulting with stakeholders; and
- maintaining records which document the history of:
    - building and equipment safety checks;
    - Material Safety Data Sheets (MSDS);
    - incident reports; and
    - emergency response plans and evacuation drills.

Documenting OHS procedures and practices

- The maintenance of OHS records complies with OHS legislation and regulations.

Effective documentation improves the communication between all stakeholders and ensures consistency of accurate information. Examples of OHS documentation include incident reports, safety checklists and evacuation procedure floor plans.

Maintaining safe environments

The number of risks that can potentially cause harm, injury, illness and damage is extensive, especially when there are unique circumstances. The list below identifies some examples of key areas of potential risk.

Emergency Response
Please refer to the Emergency Response Policy.

First aid
Please refer to the First Aid Policy.

Food safety
Please refer to the Food Safety Policy.

Hazardous Materials
Please refer to the HAZMAT Policy.

Hygiene and Infection control
Please refer to the Hygiene and Infection Control Policy.

Maintenance of buildings and equipment
Please refer to the Maintenance of Buildings and Equipment Policy.

Policy created date   *<DATE>*

Policy review date   *<DATE>*

Signatures   *<SIGNATURES>*

Exhibit 6.2 Responsibilities of the Chief Health Officer

The **[chief health officer <*INSERT APPROPRIATE TITLE*>]** provides global medical and strategic leadership in the development and ongoing support of the organization's business plan with respect to health issues. The incumbent manages or controls the departmental budget and headcount with the objectives of continuous improvement, creating value, and cost reduction. The medical director establishes and administers corporate medical and occupational health policies in collaboration with other departments or staff playing a key role in integrating the various health-related activities into a Total Health Management (THM) team. Here, the emphasis should be on quality improvement, efficiency of services provided, productivity improvement, absence management, and meeting specific health outcomes. The medical director plays a key leadership role in developing a culture where the occupational health employees can identify and articulate key business plan objectives and strive to achieve these objectives as members of a broader corporate team. The director must also foster understanding and support for the THM team, which includes a proactive effort aimed at improving health through risk identification, risk reduction, and illness prevention. He or she is also expected to provide leadership in the areas of human resources management and diversity.

In addition to business plan development and management at a corporate level, there are three operational areas of focus for the CHO:

1. Medical Department Oversight **[through a corporate medical director <insert appropriate title> if the CHO is not a physician]**
    1.1. Directs and supports the company strategy to integrate medical and other health related activities at the plant level and supports local medical personnel to achieve the business plan objectives.
    1.2. Ensures that an appropriate level of medical care is provided and oversees record-keeping practices and quality assurance activities to identify and address improvement opportunities in the distribution of medical care.
    1.3. Establishes process controls to ensure proper plant level medical department and health program administration of government programs, corporate mandates, labor agreements and special projects.
    1.4. Provides for the development of appropriate training for medical personnel.

2. Supervision of Group and Regional Medical Directors
    2.1. Directs the activities of the group and regional medical personnel and provides support for initiatives so that there is consistency with the business plan. **[through a corporate medical director <insert appropriate title> if the CHO is not a physician]**
    2.2. Conducts audits, evaluates OH&S results and provides candid, constructive feedback.
    2.3. Fosters effective communications between the corporate staff, group or regional management, and manufacturing facilities.

2.4. Drives common processes and systems within and across the groups and regions to maintain the required standards.

3. Corporate and Community Services

3.1. Directs activities related to epidemiology, finance and information systems to improve health and well-being of employees and in some instances dependents.

3.2. Provides health leadership for corporate occupational health and safety policies, recognizes patterns suggesting health or safety issues, and develops sufficiency plans to correct them.

3.3. Directs activities related to wellness and behavioral health programs for employees and interacts effectively with industrial hygiene, health and safety, ergonomics, disability management, labor relations, benefits staff and other functions as appropriate.

3.4. Provides health leadership in joint management-labor activities and establishes a positive relationship with organized labor representatives.

3.5. Actively engages community institutions, such as medical societies, hospital staff, health care coalitions, educational institutions, and others to establish and maintain rapport with external medical leadership and opinion leaders.

3.6. Acts as a spokesperson on behalf of the company to promote key messages within the company and community that extend beyond health, safety, environment and improving the health care delivery system for employees, retirees, and families.Coordinates specifically medical functions required in the organization (such as standing orders, physician reports). **[Through a corporate medical director <insert appropriate title> if the CHO is not a physician.]**

7 Global Occupational Health

Joel Bender and Paul Joos-Vandewalle

Globalization is the umbrella term that economists and thought leaders use for a bundle of economic changes that have transformed the world economy. These changes, and some of their implications for occupational health, include:

- Free trade, which allows individual countries to specialize in commodities or productive activity that best suits their resources and the skills of their people, whose productivity depends on health.
- Competition, which favors the most productive workforce, and therefore good health and low health care costs.
- Export-oriented national economies, which earn countries greater income but may also make them dependent on the stability of certain commodities and markets; companies are now more dependent on export than before, even in the US, and that means more travel and transportation.
- Rapidly emerging markets that attract investment and require a company to have a local presence, but that also have different occupational health standards.
- Free flow of capital, so that investment options are not limited to local markets and companies regularly set up manufacturing operations as well as sales offices around the world, challenging employers to be consistent in their occupational health services.
- Globalized management, so that managers in occupational health now oversee large decentralized networks of health care providers from ever-smaller corporate medical departments.
- Travel as a routine business practice, such that for many executives and professionals it is no longer useful to think of "going on a trip" because for all practical purposes they are in continuous travel, with their home office just one more stop.

As economic growth escalates in emerging markets, many multinational and national companies are focusing their efforts on manufacturing in these countries, not just making sales and shipping finished goods. With this extra demand for permanent local facilities in developing countries, occupational health and wellness must now be managed on a global scale, and increasingly in areas that are outside major cities and company enclaves or camps.

In addition, managing access by employees and their dependents to acceptable general medical and emergency dental care is essential for both long-serving expatriate workers and visitors to operations in less developed, poor, conflict-prone, challenging, and remote sites. Failure to manage global health issues effectively may result in serious and avoidable consequences for the injured or ill employee or family member and also directly affects the employer through its effect on morale, the threat to key personnel, and expense, since the cost of even a single emergency evacuation from a remote part of the world can exceed the budget for management of an entire global health department. However, all developing countries have a general health care infrastructure of greater or lesser capacity, but not many have a well developed occupational health infrastructure.

Incidents are being reported of unsatisfactory occupational health care, environmental conditions, product safety, and process safety issues. Some of these incidents have taken place in large multinational companies or even smaller enterprises that have had good health, safety, and environmental track records. The challenge faced by these companies is global reach with ever-expanding product lines, and complex manufacturing processes with supply chains that stretch across many countries that have vastly differing standards.

For companies with manufacturing and service facilities in both emerging and developed countries, there are unique challenges related to labor laws, cultural nuances, health care, language, product stewardship, workplace health and safety, and environmental regulations. Corporations need to provide sound global medical services within the framework of existing country laws and regulations, corporate stewardship, global sustainability initiatives, and corporate governance. They also need to balance standards within their home country and what is practical "in country" outside of North America, in places where there may be a shortage of occupational health and safety (OH&S) personnel and no history of good work practices.

A structured process, such as that described below, is helpful in guiding implementation of global occupational health initiatives in order to protect both individual employee and company interests. This requires a full understanding of global and local medical service requirements, and a deep understanding of the company's goals, operations, and the nature of the workforce in each country.

Local conditions do require flexibility and responsiveness, however. Everything cannot be rigidly standardized. For example, the presence of onsite nurseries (crèches) or childcare centers depends on the makeup of the workforce. In many emerging markets in certain industries, especially those requiring assembly, the majority of employees are female from dual income families, where there is little or no other support for childcare. Such support for families is of particular importance in China, with the one child policy and lack of family support due to migration of workers from rural areas.

Leadership Commitment

The health and well-being of every employee within the work environment, wherever situated, is the responsibility of the global leadership team, who are held accountable for events in the workplace environment. A culture of good "health, safety and environment" (HSE) practices should prevail throughout the organization, from the executive suite to manufacturing divisions to sales and service. The leadership team should be held accountable for poor HSE performance with specific requirements included in job descriptions, and incentive programs that are consistent with maintaining or improving health and well-being. In the face of increasing competition and the demand for ever more productivity, continuous improvement for health as well as business processes must now become the normal course of business.

There must be a commitment from leadership down to the employees, to establish a successful HSE culture within the company and this should be reflected in a written corporate policy that is enforced for the purposes of evaluation and advancement within the company (see Chapter 6 for a model policy). Specific goals should be established within each region and individual country to demonstrate that there is a genuine commitment within the organization. This is also demonstrated when the entire senior leadership team is involved in the process and accepts responsibility for the results.

HSE is global in terms of individuals, departments, companies, and regions with the framework for success being similar across the board. Emerging countries should be afforded the same attention irrespective of the labor force, and not just bound by locally acceptable values. As these countries continue to expand production capacity and market share, transparency and adherence to HSE global regulations will be an increasingly important business imperative. Metrics, in the form of performance indicators, must be developed for each organization to show management that HSE practices improve health, safety, environmental conditions, productivity, and human performance.

In emerging markets, health professionals with local knowledge are essential but usually in short supply. Consultants and senior staff from the home office will be required over the short term to mentor national staff and to ensure implementation of adequate standards, and close supervision may initially be required. However, eventually suitable talent at a regional and local level must be identified and delegated responsibility to sustain progress and adapt new approaches as business develops. This may be a protracted and incremental process, as team members gradually acquire the knowledge and expertise needed to operate independently from headquarters while maintaining both corporate and local standards.

Management Structure

A designated "Global Medical Team" (the name is not important) consisting of the key managers and providers from occupational health, human resources, safety, and managers in charge of major "off-shore" (outside the home country) contract providers can be established as a convenient and effective way to provide necessary stewardship throughout the organization. Adequate resources and suitably qualified staff should be deployed to implement the occupational health program globally, requiring carefully attention in the budget to travel, communications, and training expenses.

In many organizations the medical department reports to human resources and HSE reports to manufacturing. The "health" in the latter title sometimes refers to occupational health or industrial hygiene. A single independent department for both medical, and health and safety provides a more streamlined approach with appropriately defined roles and responsibilities, and control at both administrative and operational levels. It also facilitates communication, as hygiene can talk to the medical department about surveillance and problems they spot in various departments and the medical department can talk easily to hygiene and safety about hazards they learn about through encounters with injured workers or interviews during medical services.

Some companies precisely document reporting structures and delineate roles and responsibilities in a well-ordered organization chart (universally called an "org chart" in business). This affords less opportunity for incongruous reporting and poor process implementation. It may also create a more cohesive team, leaving less margin for error within the HSE organization where absolutely unambiguous reporting and authority is required, as in military medical departments. However, it also runs the risk of becoming inflexible and impeding communication among operating units and between departments with closely-related responsibilities, such as occupational medicine, safety, industrial/occupational hygiene, and security.

Larger organizations often prefer to operate within a matrix organization. However, employees often dislike matrix organizations intensely because the lines of authority are often unclear. This is particularly true in occupational health, which is a staff (cross-cutting corporate service) responsibility serving many line (production) divisions. There is often less control and a greater margin for error and confusion about responsibilities in matrix organizations, which can negatively impact the entire company. Such deficiencies may only become evident after a major incident that requires legislative reporting or regulatory oversight. Therefore, it is critically important to have very clear communications and recognized divisions of responsibility within the organization.

Relationships among related departments are the key to long-term success in recognizing when old problems are out of control, monitoring quality of the overall OH&S/HSE effort and anticipating new problems. There should be a defined and structured relationship between the global corporate medical services department and the decentralized teams at regional and country level. The corporate entity should be primarily responsible for maintaining company standards and the regional offices should demonstrate accountability in having the team implement these standards locally. Ideally, a Regional Medical Director responsible for a particular continent or group of countries should report to the Global Medical Director at a functional level, emphasizing problem-solving and coordination. At an administrative level the Regional Medical Director should be part of a leadership council that reports directly to the Regional President or Chief Executive Officer (CE)O, similar to the Global Medical Team for the corporation as a whole.

Team Structure

There are great advantages to the company to have an integrated team comprised of experienced medical, health, safety, and environment professionals focused on improving the health and well-being. In some cases where HSE reports through the manufacturing or production divisions independent of the medical team, there can be strong pressure to under-report lost-time incidents and lost work days in order to attain safety performance goals (see Chapter 17). An independent team provides the authority and expertise to monitor data-gathering and compliance for accurate reporting; it protects the integrated occupational health department and allows it to operate without prejudice and undue influence. This is in the best interest of the employees and allows the company more accurately to identify gaps in health and safety, and to take corrective actions. Such interventions ultimately improve productivity and performance in the workplace. Having a suitably qualified medical leader accountable administratively to a very senior executive at a regional level and functionally to the Global Medical Director will enhance confidence and trust.

It is important to understand cultural nuances and develop an appreciation of local regulations for HSE processes, in addition to corporate policies and procedures. Sometimes local habits and cultural attitudes are serious impediments to the delivery of quality occupational health services. For example, in countries that view expatriate workers as servants, contract workers are particularly at risk because neither the contracting company nor the contractor puts a priority on their well-being. On the other hand, some cultural attitudes can support quality of care, if skillfully manipulated. Countries with a Confucian tradition of family-oriented ethics may be amenable to an appeal to the local manager's responsibilities for workers because they would be shamed and lose face if an incident happened.

Occupational Health Management System

Business plans should be developed by medical service leadership within each global region starting with each manufacturing unit in a given region. A business plan should be developed for the country or region that includes objectives, designates a champion for each objective, and has well-defined targets. Broad corporate objectives in areas such as safety, human resources, quality, responsiveness, and cost will have to be integrated into the business plan for medical services in each global region. Key performance indicators are then derived that reliably reflect progress toward those objectives (see Chapter 17).

Business plans need to show incremental improvements over time, as every medical unit will be starting at a different level of quality and commitment. Attaining corporate and regional objectives under these circumstances will require auditing and mentoring within the organization. Convergence to the highest standard among the countries in which the employer operates is the ultimate goal but it takes time to reach that goal.

Occupational health management systems should apply to both employees and contractors. These management systems and performance standards should be part of the bidding and selection process for contractors/vendors. Vendors should ensure that these requirements are specifically met. Health and safety of all workers, including contract workers, visitors, and those of joint ventures are imperative. Medical examinations as part of pre-placement, during periodic check-ups and for post-sickness/injuries constitute a critical aspect of the occupational health management system.

Medical surveillance should be consistent from one manufacturing unit to the other whatever the national or local standards may be, even though the facility may be legally responsible only for local government regulations. Standard setting may be extremely decentralized in some countries, with marked differences in standards. More often, less developed countries will have strong regulations in their legislation but weak enforcement. Minimum standards that reflect global best practice (such as the current standards in North America or Europe, and that are applied in the home country) should be adopted for all operations, irrespective of local requirements. This is a necessity in order to protect workers in countries where occupational health standards are relatively new, inadequate, or non-existent. Medical surveillance, being a backstop to hazard control (see Chapter 20), is particularly important in situations where management cannot be sure that global standards are being followed.

Medical services must ensure that control measures being implemented are consistent with the workplace risk assessment. This is usually the responsibility of HSE, loss prevention, or some department other than occupational health. However, the occupational health service has much to offer in workplace risk assessment and management. An integrated, comprehensive department can best manage all the functions required to identify hazards, evaluate them, assess their implications for health, control them, and monitor the effectiveness of controls (see Chapter 21).

Disaster planning, pandemic preparedness plans, and business continuity plans in the event of supplier disruption, office closures, or absence of a critical mass of workers are essential in modern business, wherever operations are located (see Chapter 31). Emergency response procedures (ERPs) and first aid training are often particularly important in emerging markets and developing countries because public services are often lacking or inadequate. For example, even in rich developing countries, such as in the Middle East, ambulance services are generally not public; they are usually provided by individual hospitals, do not provide in-transit emergency medical treatment, and often leave much to be desired in service. Provisions should be made for expatriate or foreign employees who may not necessarily be covered under local government emergency crisis plans, especially provisions for evacuation to safe havens. Evacuation is exorbitantly expensive and should only be used as a last resort but costs can be controlled by having contract arrangements for emergency medical care and stabilization, evacuation, and repatriation in place for expatriate and traveling employees, especially those in remote or unsafe locations. Clear policies and procedures should be maintained with concise roles and responsibilities within the company on how to deal with extended families and local national staff. At the same time, nationals without special arrangements should have no expectation that care will be provided outside their own country, unless this is a contract benefit. This will avoid any unrealistic expectations from the workforce in cases of catastrophe.

Indicators and Monitoring Performance

The central problem of global health management is to ensure that the regional occupational health services are consistent in following the guidelines and standards established by the corporate medical department. There is a natural tendency in a decentralized system to fall back on local custom and standards and "the way we've always done it" and to resist or even demonize occupational health professionals and managers from corporate headquarters as out of touch, irrelevant, and interfering. The result can be a catastrophic disconnect between the way things should be done and the reality on the ground.

Monitoring adherence to corporate guidelines and standards is generally done by reporting (typically more often than quarterly, because things can go wrong too quickly) and by audit. Reporting is necessary but should never be approached with an attitude of confirming that things are going well; data should always be viewed skeptically with a view to finding "numbers that don't look right," as these anomalies are often the first indicators of problems or deviations from required procedures. The audit procedure, as will be discussed, should be conducted onsite and should always be intrusive. The aim is not to reassure management. It is to ensure that important things that can harm employees, interfere with operations, and damage the reputation of the company are not left unaddressed and that local or regional operations have not adopted irregular practices that are unsound.

The most common indicators in use for occupational health management are lost-time injury rates, lost work days, and absence. These are flawed lagging indicators and should be supplemented by leading indicators, such as number of educational sessions provided, number of workers trained in CPR, and periodic health surveillance services provided (see Chapter 17).

In most countries, both developed (including the US) and in emerging markets, employees sometimes return to work prematurely after serious injuries in order to prevent lost-time incidents or lost work days from being counted against the company or the operating division. This is an ongoing problem. The occupational health service must not allow itself to be coerced or persuaded into going along with inappropriate return-to-work certification.

This is in contrast to other countries in which employees with minor injuries are automatically classified as lost-time incidents and may be absent for many days, weeks, or even months, approved by their personal physicians. Sometimes employees are hospitalized for minor injuries or required to have unnecessarily frequent medical follow-ups in order for doctors/medical institutions to generate additional revenue. Many companies merely accept these practices as inevitable and do not monitor the number of days off; only the specific number of lost-time incidents is recorded. Others are proactive and see this as an opportunity for education, training, and consultation with local physicians regarding best practices globally.

Absence should be monitored for both occupational and non-occupational injury and disease. However, absence is not the whole story. Pushing absence too low, by creating penalties or incentives for coming into work, often has unintended consequences, such as encouraging workers with contagious illness (such as colds and the flu) to come to work when they should not and risk infecting others. Likewise, workers who come to work while impaired temporarily with episodic illnesses like asthma or severe allergies, migraine, irritable bowel syndrome, and diabetes often work poorly and have low productivity despite being at their posts. There is therefore a reciprocal relationship between absence and presenteeism when absence is pushed too low. More often, however, unexplained absence is excessive (relative to community illness and context) and uncontrolled, and a certification system for absence (for example, requiring medical clearance by the occupational health service if the worker is off more than three days) is required. Just the existence and consistent use of an absence monitoring system is usually enough to reduce absence rates substantially, without onerous enforcement (see Chapter 24).

Auditing

Data generated by the regional or local occupational health service are important for day-to-day management and monitoring. However, data are too easily manipulated, or biased, or distorted in the reporting to rely upon for due diligence and to ensure full compliance with corporate policy. At some point, onsite inspection is necessary.

The audit team must ensure that corporate policies for health and well-being are available, implemented, and aligned with country laws and regulations but also conforming with minimum acceptable company standards. Examples include areas such as smoking, drug and alcohol policies, HIV/AIDs in the workplace, and child labor.

Such inspections, conducted as an audit, should be approached as detective work, not as a "show and tell." Medical and safety teams should be allowed access to any part of a manufacturing facility for auditing purposes at any time. This can be an issue in all operations but is most common in emerging markets due to lack of transparency and attempts to conceal non-compliance with medical and safety standards. Audit teams should never allow themselves to be persuaded by management to be "guided" or to make arranged visits, because they will inevitably be taken through compliant areas and not trouble spots by local personnel who wish to make a good impression. The teams should strike out on their own and visit facilities and departments unexpectedly.

Environmental control particularly with regards to toxic waste that may affect employees and local communities is a growing area of concern. Environmental stewardship and sustainability initiatives play an important role in this area. In many developing countries, vector control for mosquitoes to prevent diseases such as dengue and malaria should also be a priority for environmental control because it has a direct public health impact on the workforce and surrounding populations.

In developing countries, the public health infrastructure is usually inadequate to guarantee protection for the health of expatriate workers and corporate travelers. It is therefore necessary for the Global Medical Team to take on some functions of a public health board. This includes inspecting or reviewing living accommodations, surveillance of nutrition/cafeteria standards and food preparation staff (onsite as well as offsite kitchens), water quality, and exposure to toxic hazards, such as pesticides, that are commonly used in the community as well as in a plant. Sport and recreation facilities, and accessibility for employees should be based on the appraisals done in conjunction with employee feedback. Simple measures such as walking paths or "taking the stairs" programs can be implemented at very low cost.

Employees in emerging countries are often migrant laborers who are accommodated onsite in dormitories. These facilities should be open to audit staff, who should have access to all areas related to employee health and welfare. Work camps for expatriate workers are often neglected and may present poor sanitation, fire hazards, and infectious disease risk from poor vector control (mosquitoes that carry malaria and dengue are common problems), and from local prostitution (a major concern in countries where HIV/AIDS prevalence is high). These work camps are often under the management of contractors or subcontractors but their problems reflect back on the company.

There are often producer collectives or cooperatives in emerging markets where products are sourced from many different manufacturers, particularly in the textile, apparel, and electronics sectors. Some of these collectives may only manufacture one part of or one particular item for a company. The collectives are usually small and can be family run businesses or be very small informal enterprises. Tracking medical or product safety issues under these circumstances can be extremely difficult. However, increasingly corporations are held accountable by shareholders, the public, legal action, and politicians for ethical and responsible practice all along the value chain for their products, including the behavior of their suppliers and contractors. Every effort should be made to audit their operations and procedures as well.

Vendor Selection

Large employers often contract with organizations that can provide either direct services (such as evacuation) or fine-grained screening services to identify local health care providers. One such vendor, and the standard of comparison because of its size, coverage, and market dominance, is International SOS™, which provides health care, medical assistance, and security services worldwide. There are also regional networks that cover a part of the world or a large country such as China, and that because of their local connections also specialize in sorting out financial arrangements and payment disputes. Most of these services are oriented toward general and emergency health care but a few (including International SOS™) are developing occupational health services as a business line.

It is desirable for vendors providing occupational health services to be able to provide reliable support across the region being serviced. If different vendors are required serving different regions or countries, one should ensure that the baseline reporting information required by the company at a global level will be comparable and accurate, so that services to the particular population or region can be accurately evaluated. Particularly in developing countries and emerging markets, where much of this is novel, one must ensure that vendors are carefully vetted for their true capabilities, rather than their stated capabilities, before embarking on any formal contracts. It is helpful to interview a variety of vendors to ensure that they are capable of providing the services under the contract.

Employee assistance programs (EAPs), in particular, are almost non-existent in most developing countries and many emerging markets. Selecting an appropriate vendor can be very difficult. Tolerance of substance abuse, especially alcohol, varies greatly from country to country. In some countries, alcohol abuse may not be perceived to be a problem requiring attention, especially binge drinking on weekends. In many countries, drug possession or use is a capital or prison offence and so employees are understandably reluctant to accept referral to EAPs for this reason.

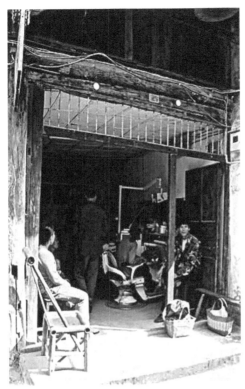

Figure 7.1 A dental clinic in a third-tier city in China. Access to safe, clean, professional dental services is a serious issue in the developing world

Dental services are a particular problem in developing countries. In many developing societies, dentistry has not been considered a profession like medicine and is practiced on the street or in shops by itinerant or traditional practitioners using crude and unsterilized implements (see Figure 7.1).

Local Vendors and In-Country Care

Occupational health care differs between countries. The corporate and regional medical directors of a global company should be aware of these differences, as should providers who offer travel medicine services to expatriate workers. For example, in emerging markets the onsite medical facility at a plant is usually regulated by government and in addition to primary care may include extensive rehabilitation facilities. In many of these countries, an onsite facility is often not capable of dealing with work-related injuries, other than minor injuries for employees who can return to work immediately. Most cases are referred offsite to nearby medical facilities. In such situations, it makes little sense to invest in sophisticated equipment but some means of tracking injured employees through the local health care system and monitoring quality of care may be essential.

Trained occupational health physicians are usually in short supply but in some countries they are virtually absent and care must be provided by other means. In South Korea, in many large locations, only minor incidents and emergency care cases are attended to onsite, and then by nurses or paramedics with a limited scope of work. However, extensive rehabilitation

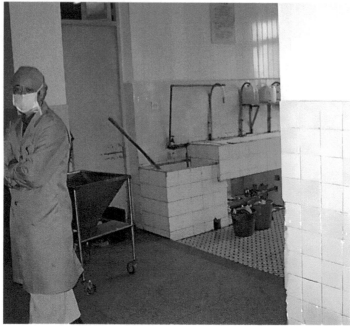

Figure 7.2 A hospital scrub room in a second-tier city in China. China's health care system is developing very rapidly in the major cities but remains problematical in the regions

is often available onsite at the same locations, treating both work and non-work-related injuries with little control by company-hired physicians. These circumstances may result in conflicts with regards to whether an injury is counted as work- or non-work related (with the question of who pays) or recordable as lost-time (with the question of whether reporting is accurate).

On the other hand, in China there is often an onsite physician, but this person may only be qualified in traditional Chinese medicine and may have little or no western medical training, let alone occupational health training. In such cases, all work-related injuries would be referred offsite and the onsite facility should be used only for basic primary and chronic care. The local health care facilities may or may not achieve an international standard of hygiene (see Figure 7.2). Many hospitals in large cities have clinics or wards specifically for foreigners. The global health division of the employer should monitor these conditions carefully at the corporate level, because they change rapidly, especially in China.

Industrial parks are particularly popular in light manufacturing, the electronics industry, the chemical industry, and other industries in which companies want to be near each other as vendors and suppliers. Such parks often provide onsite facilities for a number of different companies. (See Chapter 1 for a discussion of this model.) The challenge is that where the level of medical care is not comparable to that in developed countries, the company has little control over the standard of health care provided by the local facility. There may be deficiencies in basic hygiene practices, blood borne pathogen protection (see Figure 7.3), infection control (see Figure 7.4), use of personal protective equipment, and emergency care management of critically injured or ill personnel. In these instances, some companies prefer to retain an onsite occupational health professional to provide direct medical assistance in cases where the local facility is inadequate or unreliable, to monitor clinical or rehabilitation services, and to facilitate and direct offsite referrals.

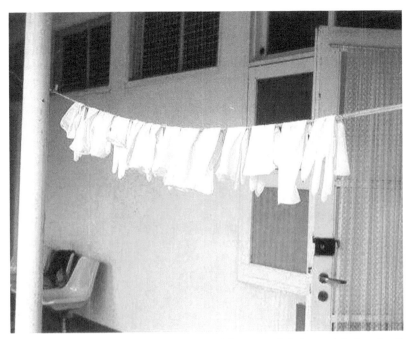

Figure 7.3 Latex gloves hanging out to dry on a washline at a clinic in rural Indonesia after being washed for reuse. Compliance with blood borne pathogen precautions cannot be taken for granted, especially outside urban areas, in developing countries

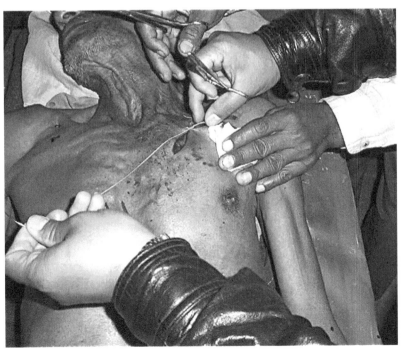

Figure 7.4 A superficial wound is sutured by medical staff who are not wearing gloves, at this clinic in rural India. Infection control precautions are often not observed in developing countries

Recommended Reading and Resources

Guidotti TL (2010) *The Praeger Handbook of Occupational and Environmental Medicine*. Santa Barbara CA, Praeger ABC-Clio. See Chapter 26 on "Global Occupational and Environmental Health."

Guidotti TL, ed. (2011) *Global Occupational Health*. New York, Oxford University Press. This book approaches global occupational health from the point of view of economic development.

Hendrick DJ, Burge PS, Beckett WS, Churg A, eds (2000) *Occupational Disorders of the Lung*. London, W.B. Saunders. See Chapters 35, 36, and 37 on "Legislative Controls and Compensation" in regions of the world.

Herzstein JA, Bunn WB, Fleming LE (1998) *International Occupational and Environmental Medicine*. St. Louis MO, Mosby.

8　Strategic Planning

Tee L. Guidotti, M. Suzanne Arnold, and Marion Stecklow

Provision of specialized occupational health services, including preplacement, surveillance, and preventive services, to a high degree of reliability, differentiates a health care provider that delivers an occupational health service from an occupational health care provider. To do it well requires a knowledge of occupational health practice, efficiency, and attention to detail in workers' compensation and other important dimensions of occupational health care. This demands preparation and planning.

The delivery of occupational health services is hyper-local, in the sense that these services draw their patients and subjects from the immediate area. The most important components to successful strategic planning for any business is knowing your customer, being in the right location, having sufficient and appropriate staffing, providing ample funding and most importantly, knowing the strengths and limitations of the organization and of the vital individual members of the company.

Strategic planning for corporate-level and employer-sponsored on-site occupational health services is addressed in Chapter 6. This chapter pertains to community-based services.

This chapter should be considered complementary to other chapters in the book.

Strategic Planning

A few basic principles underlie the strategic planning of occupational health services at the community level and make it different from the strategic planning of personal health services.

Location

- Locate the facility where the workers work, not where their families live.
- Distance from work sites should ideally be 20 minutes or less by car or public transportation. Employers will not send their employees farther than is necessary to get adequate care.
- The site should be easily accessible and preferably visible from the road.
- Look for space near a local hospital, medical center, or multi-physician practice without its own occupational health service, if a free-standing occupational health center (see Chapter 19). In many cases, after the occupational health provider develops a relationship with the hospital emergency department, the emergency room (ER) physician will refer the patient to the center for follow-up.

- Locate the facility near other specialists and specialty services (particularly physical therapy), unless provided in-house. It will make referral and specialty care more convenient for injured workers and will create referral opportunities from the specialists.

Facilities

- A light, clean, and well furnished space with a welcoming reception area shows respect for the injured worker.
- Plan free-standing clinic facilities for injuries, not for illness.
- The facility design, whether taking over an existing space or designing a new space, should be laid out for the primary type of service expected to be provided. If injury treatment is generally expected to produce the highest patient volume, then the facility must be designed to promote an efficient treatment process. If injury care is not the main focus of the clinic, think through traffic flow and make this compatible with testing procedures.
- Substance abuse testing must be performed in complete privacy and restrooms must meet Department of Transportation (DOT) standards (see Chapter 22). If commercial driver medical evaluations are expected to be a significant part of service mix, design the facility with this in mind.
- If the volume of DOT evaluations is expected to be as high as or higher than injury treatment (many companies also require substance abuse testing at the initial treatment of an injury), then the facility and staffing should be designed to support two or more tracks for multiple examination and testing simultaneously, without staff or workers getting in each other's way.
- Consider providing dedicated space for physical therapy, either with own staff or through a contract provider.
- Plan for referral of difficult, complicated, and disease cases. Occupational disease cases usually require referral to specialists anyway and take a long time to sort out; they should be identified but not necessarily diagnosed or managed in acute care facilities. Consider referral to occupational medicine training and teaching programs, where these exist.
- Adapt to local needs and prepare the facility to give good service to local employers and their workers. (This often means having staff who are fluently bilingual in Spanish or another language of the local workers.)

"Customer Service"

- The employee is the recipient of service, whether a "patient" or a "subject" of a screening test; the employer is the client. The expectations and satisfaction of both are critical to the business side of the occupational health service.
- Hire bilingual staff fluent in the language of the local workers. (In Canada, bilingual in English and French throughout the country.)
- Some employers are very particular about the appearance of the facilities where they send their employees.
- Constantly seek to reduce waiting time for employees, for reporting, and for paperwork. Time off the job and uncertainty over scheduling workers cost the employer money that the smaller business, in particular, can ill afford to lose.
- Cultivate clear lines of communication with employers. If employers are not satisfied, they will simply send injured workers elsewhere and feel that they owe the health facility no explanation.

- Cultivate an attitude on the part of the staff of respect and interest in the workers using the facilities.
- Avoid combining the provision of occupational health services with general health care services—contrary to usual expectations, it rarely works.
- Where politics and economics require the combination of services, keep them completely independent in name, entrance/reception/waiting area, forms, etc.
- Prepare sales and account services representatives well (see Chapter 15), taking great care that they understand the services being offered and do not promise what is unrealistic.

Plan the Business

- Plan volume on the basis of injury rates (refer to Chapter 10), not on the basis of the most visible or valuable industry in the region.
- Labor-intensive, low-technology industries, particularly those employing large numbers of untrained or partly-trained workers with a high turnover, produce more acute injuries and can support high-volume occupational health services.
- Look at the number of employers who are hiring, have warehouses and commercial drivers to calculate volume of preplacement physicals, DOT physicals, and required substance abuse testing.
- It is dangerous to rely on a single contract with a large employer. Loss of the contract will put the occupational health service out of business overnight.
- Dependence on small employers is also not desirable because the cost and effort to maintain these customers is high.
- One or more large customers with a mix of injury treatment, physicals, and substance abuse testing along with several medium to small size customers is ideal.

Starting Up

Most occupational health services start by buying out an existing practice, investing in a franchise, setting up within a hospital or medical group with whatever resources they are given, or starting from scratch. Each option is explored below. Choosing an option depends, of course, on available finances, obtainable staffing, the marketplace, and, in the case of hospitals and medical groups, already-planned master strategies imposed from above.

Option 1: Purchase a Franchise or an Existing Practice

A franchise provides the right to practice in a certain territory under a given brand and with standardized systems. The market leader in franchises at the moment appears to be Doctor's Express®, a network of urgent care centers that includes basic occupational health services. A franchise from this company costs approximately US$600,000 in 2012, according to the website, and no medical background is required to invest. The parent company will then supply business training, equipment (with volume discounts negotiated with vendors), advice, and marketing support. Other franchise operations seem to be moving into the field of network- or employer-based services. Interim HealthCare®, which previously focused on home health care and assisted living for seniors, also offers what it describes as "occupational health services and vendor management to hospitals, prisons, schools, corporations and other health care facilities." This trend is too new to evaluate and presents obvious risks and benefits.

Any existing practice has its own strengths and weaknesses that determine the best path for development, and every situation is different. In evaluating a practice for purchase, it is important to project the trend in business it is likely to experience, given its location and position in the community and the prospects of local employers.

Option 2: Build with a Local Hospital or Medical Group

An occupational health provider may start up as an entirely new occupational health service embedded within or (as a wholly-owned subsidiary) using assets initially provided by a hospital or medical group. Proponents (the champions of this project) should be fully aware of the challenges this option presents:

- Lack of understanding about the market. (In many cases this is compounded by false impressions based on data for general health care.)
- Lack of enthusiasm and support because the financial incentive is limited, in their view, compared to high-revenue specialist care. (The opposite can also be true, that the hospital or group management has unrealistic expectations for spin-off revenue from occupational health care.)
- Lack of understanding about occupational health as a specialty. (In many cases this is compounded by misinformation and outdated impressions.)

The single most important task for the proponent of a new occupational health service embedded in a network is to educate the management on just what is required and to achieve clarity on the goals and objectives of the new service.

Occupational health services may be started in a community by a hospital or medical group for any number of reasons. The occupational health proponent and the management of the hospital or group must be clear on why the organization is doing this in the first place:

- To develop an additional source of revenue (the usual reason).
- To attract patients for general or specialty care (usually with disappointing results).
- To generate revenue through spin-off diagnostic or specialty treatment services (which rarely happens to any appreciable extent, except for physical therapy).
- To meet a need for service in the community (sometimes at an employer's invitation).
- To develop relationships with employers (which requires balance with worker interests).
- To establish a base for education and training (for example, at a medical school).
- To satisfy personal interests (by providers motivated by interest in the field).

The management of the hospital or group must be fully educated and in agreement that while occupational health services may not generate many millions of dollars in referrals and advanced medical treatment to the hospital or medical group (although it may happen with physical therapy), they can be very profitable if managed by their own internal business logic. The community outreach is positive and referrals to specialists and departments over time can become significant. However, occupational health services should be developed for their own value.

A hospital or medical group-based occupational health service will work best if the following steps are taken:

- Identify or recruit a knowledgeable occupational health professional to manage the start-up.
- Define personal and practice objectives.
- Review the profile and needs of local industry.
- Develop a fee and billing system that is separate from the hospital or group.
- Become knowledgeable regarding local occupational health problems, hazards, and risks.
- Become thoroughly familiar with the ethical framework of occupational health.
- Plan the proposed service carefully.
- Recruit or reassign facilities and resources.
- Create a strong, positive working relationship with the hospital/group physicians and administration.

Ideally, these steps should be taken in the order given. However, the usual sequence is precisely the reverse. In other words, a hospital, group, or health maintenance organization (HMO) typically first is brought the idea of opening an occupational health service by a consultant or internal champion, usually without sufficient discussion on the part of busy, distracted managers. It then decides to open an occupational health clinic using whatever resources are at hand, next conducts a market survey to determine how to sell the service, and only then puts an individual in charge who may or may not have a clear idea of the objectives of the service and of the occupational health field as a whole, and is unlikely to have the total confidence of management. Even worse, the hospital or group may skimp on investment or compromise on the quality of assets or staff assigned to the new venture "until it proves itself," which is a formula for disappointing results. All too often, occupational health facilities are started up in underutilized space (usually for a reason), with spare equipment, and staff who are not working out well elsewhere. If the organization is not prepared to invest properly in the service, providing the same support due any other department or organizational activity, it should ask whether it should enter the field at all.

The actual start-up of a hospital- or medical group-based service is similar to Option 3.

Option 3: Starting from Scratch

This is often the best option if the financial support is available. A complete start-up requires close attention to preparing and maintaining a strict budget and careful planning. A systematic, promising start-up can be achieved in phases.

Phase 1: Planning

- Establish financing and budgets.
- Implement a market survey.
- Develop a banking relationship—open account.
- Design and prepare marketing tools.
- Develop a customer base and service mix.
- Develop a strategic plan, as described above.

Phase 2: Implementation

- Hire qualified and experienced occupational health professionals, sales/marketing, and support staff (see Chapter 10).
- Design and furnish the facility.
- Design and post signage.
- Establish clinic hours.
- Establish a relationship with a local medical supplier.
- Develop a good working relationship and referral processes with local specialists and industrial hygiene services provider, if necessary.
- Set up appointments to visit local employers, perhaps a site visit with employers, involving the occupational physician and/or a selected industrial hygienist. (After a firm opening date has been set.)
- Purchase equipment, supplies and materials—both for clinical and office requirements.
- Purchase software and information technology (IT) systems.
- Design procedure and communication protocols specific to each type of service. (For example, one procedure for injured workers, another for preplacement evaluations, another for DOT commercial driver evaluations, and so forth.)
- Establish accounting systems.
- Purchase and integrate communication systems.
- Develop a modern, attractive, informative website.
- Create forms, filing systems, and internal/external communication processes. (Do as much online as possible.)
- Review processes, procedures, occupational health services goals, and customer service policies with staff.
- Plan and prepare an open house for the community and customers.
- Open for business!

Phase 3: Establish Market Presence

- Enhance sales and marketing capabilities.
- Grow customer base.
- Establish relationships with employer workers' compensation providers.
- Develop in-depth knowledge of how each workers' compensation insurer and adjuster operates.
- Develop strong relationships with customers to maintain long-term business.
- Provide continuing education for staff.
- Review policies and procedures annually and update as necessary.
- Review equipment, supplies, medications, software—stay on top of the "latest and greatest."
- Maintain superior cleanliness and appearance in all areas of the facility.
- Promote site visits, at least annually.
- Provide consistent, quality services to customers.

These three phases also assist and apply to the successful development and operation of a hospital based or medical group occupational health service, if the issues discussed in Option 2 are addressed.

Strategic Planning for Growth

A sound strategic planning strategy requires knowledge of the range and levels of services that can be provided, and the potential users of these services. Figure 8.1 is a diagram known as a "strategic planning cube" that allows a three-dimensional representation of the possible combinations of levels of service, range of services, and users or "consumers" of these services. Each subdivision of the cube represents a particular level of a particular service provided to a given category of user. Bringing these three dimensions into one illustration helps one to visualize the possibilities and to identify opportunities for growth.

The range of services, presented in the horizontal dimension, is the easiest to conceptualize. "Primary occupational health care" includes acute injury care, rehabilitation, and workers' compensation services. "Industrial hygiene" services are provided on site in the workplace, usually with a laboratory elsewhere as a base of operations, but these specialized services are not provided by physicians or occupational health nurses. Specialty medical care is rendered on a referral basis for specific problems. Surveillance and fitness for duty refers to periodic health surveilance, screening services oriented toward secondary prevention, and fitness for duty evaluations. "Specialty occupational health care" includes specialty care provided by occupational physicians (and/or occupational health nurses), usually emphasizing toxicology, administrative functions, and the design of programs rather than basic medical care.

Community-based occupational health services, such as hospitals, multispecialty groups, and occupational health centers, usually emphasize basic acute medical care and a basic level of employer-requested screening and preventive services.

Relatively few facilities provide industrial hygiene services in the same group together with medical care. Industrial hygiene services are usually provided by consultants hired for

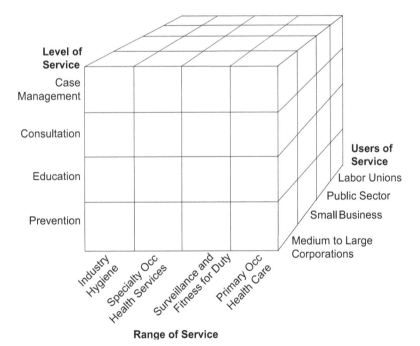

Figure 8.1 A "strategic planning cube" for occupational health, depicting types and levels of medical services, and potential clients (Adapted from *The Praeger Handbook of Occupational and Environmental Medicine* © Tee L. Guidotti. Reproduced with permission of ABC-Clio, LLC, all rights reserved.)

the purpose by the employer, if they are not available in-house. This split between health and hygiene services may not be logical from the standpoint of resolving the problem but it reflects the different professional roles of the physician or occupational health nurse and the hygienist. In rare cases in which industrial hygiene services have been offered by clinics in the past, they have often been undervalued or subordinated to the health services, despite their critical role in controlling hazards. Consulting hygienists, understandably, usually prefer to work alone but may form partnerships with an occupational health service. Industrial hygiene services are usually provided on the case management or consultation level but in recent years there has been a strong emphasis on "risk assessment" to identify hazards early for the purposes of prevention and to ensure compliance with government regulations (see Chapter 21). Notwithstanding the independent roles of the industrial hygienist and of the occupational health professionals (physician and nurses) there is also an interdependent role wherein these complementary professionals work together and communicate on an ongoing basis regarding the health risks of hazards identified in the workplace, the control of the hazards and their related risks, and the means of protecting the health of the workers.

The level of services, on the vertical axis, represents a continuum from direct case management to prevention. Diagnosis, treatment, rehabilitation, and follow-up are familiar as the medical model but problem solving requires more emphasis on hazards and risks than on the outcome. Consultation is a less direct intervention requiring particular insight and expertise, not only into the problem but also into the needs, motivations, and resources of those asking for the assistance. Education includes not only formal training sessions but opportunities to increase the awareness and sophistication of clients so that the services used are more highly valued. Fundamentally, prevention is the foundation of sound occupational health practices.

Each level of service can be matched with each service type in Figure 8.1. The health services may deal, for example, with treatment of individual cases or preventive services to groups of workers. These are the most common types of occupational health services but opportunities to provide consultative and preventive or educational services are often overlooked. While expensive physician time may not be well utilized on a cost-effective basis in providing many educational programs, site-specific health promotion program development and delivery is a specialization of occupational health nurses.

The users of the services, shown along the base of the cube in Figure 8.1, may include larger businesses, small businesses, public agencies, and, potentially, labor unions. Individual workers do not constitute a market for occupational health services in the same way that they and their families are a market for personal health care. The "consumers" of health care are those who use the system, the workers, and those who make the choices, who are called "clients" throughout this book and are mostly employers. In the occupational health care system, it is usually the employer who makes the initial choice (in some states directing the worker to a provider for injury care) and who purchases (directly or through workers' compensation) health services on behalf of the worker. Even when an individual worker changes physicians or seeks care for an occupational health problem from his or her own doctor the system constrains the choice by allowing only a limited number of charges and refusing to pay for unauthorized referrals. In strategic planning for occupational health services, therefore, the essential target is usually the employer. As a practical matter, the workers' needs must always be met but the employer's needs must also be reasonably satisfied or the relationship between provider and client may be brief.

Most occupational health care services are limited to a narrow corner of the cube, the upper right-hand corner. While no occupational health service is ever likely to develop fully all potential strategic planning possibilities, an appreciation of what can be done may lead the facility into a profitable and worthwhile new direction. At every step, however, the providers should be prepare themselves to deliver the service at a high standard of quality before committing themselves to providing it.

Labor unions, in the back tier of "users of service" in the service cube, may have their own insurance plans (in the trades) and sometimes have their own medical consultants or services. They are potential sources of referrals, often for disputed or difficult cases and for medicolegal services. Members tend to rely on their unions for advice on medical referrals for occupational problems. Unions sometimes contract for educational and preventive services for their members but usually prefer to work with academic or non-profit organizations whenever possible. They are excellent sources of referral for medicolegal or workers' compensation appeals services, if the occupational health provider is oriented toward supporting the worker as plaintiff or claimant.

Recommended Reading and Resources

Guidotti TL (2010) *The Praeger Handbook of Occupational and Environmental Medicine. Santa Barbara CA,* Praeger ABC-Clio.

Moser R Jr. (2008) Effective Management of Health and Safety Programs: A Practical Guide. Beverley Farms MA, OEM Press, 3rd ed.

Newkirk WL, Jones LD (1989) OHSs: A Guide to Program Planning and Management. Chicago IL, American Hospital Publishing.

Rest K, Ed (1986) How to begin an occupational health program—administrative and ethical issues (entire issue). Semin Occup Med, 1(1): 1–96.

Smith I. (2007) Occupational Health: A Practical Guide for Managers. London, Taylor and Francis.

9   Hospitals and Medical Groups

Judith Green-McKenzie and David J. D'Souza

Hospitals play several critically important roles in the delivery of occupational health services but not because of the inpatient services that define them as institutions. Few occupational injuries require hospitalization and so occupational health care is almost exclusively an ambulatory care field. This chapter addresses hospitals and large medical groups, which have many similar characteristics and are often affiliated in networks. Where "hospital" is used, it should be understood to apply equally to large medical group practices, unless qualified as a specific reference to hospitals as institutions. Increasingly, hospitals and large medical groups are affiliated into networks, usually with multiple sites.

The most important role played by hospitals and large multispecialty groups is as a sponsor of services for local employers. Hospitals are probably the single largest subsector of providers of occupational health services in the US today, directly and through their health care networks. They are often the dominant provider in their area. (Chapter 1 discusses the various modes of delivery of occupational health services.)

A second important role is as a center for teaching and education of occupational medicine and nursing. This role is mostly confined to teaching hospitals and academic medical centers.

Hospitals and large medical groups are also employers. Most have well-developed occupational health services for their own employees, as a result of stringent requirements for accreditation and longstanding attention from the Occupational Safety and Health Administration (OSHA). As major employers, often the largest in their areas, hospitals have responsibilities to their own employees and to patient safety, which is closely related.

Each of these roles will be discussed in turn.

Hospital-Based Occupational Health Services

Hospitals and multispecialty group practices, which are similar in many respects and often affiliated, are the framework and umbrella for many occupational health services serving employers in the community. They may be organized as hospital or group departments, as a wholly-owned satellite occupational medicine center, or as an outpatient clinic, separate or combined with an urgent care center. Administratively, the occupational health service may be set up as a division within the departments of internal medicine, family medicine, emergency medicine, or as part of urgent care. Each hospital and medical group seems to have its own organizational twist, reflecting the institutional history of the occupational health service.

Those hospital units that are run semi-autonomously and in satellites operate similarly to "occupational medicine centers" (see Chapters 12 and 19, which discuss efficient procedures). Reflecting its roots in acute medical and surgical care, hospital-based services generally operate from 8:00 to 5:00 or 6:00 providing care for injured workers and employer-sponsored screening and surveillance for employees. Occupational health services divert low-intensity injuries from the emergency room and provide acute care at much lower cost when they are open. After hours, the emergency room is available for coverage and most hospitals with this type of arrangement refer the follow-up of injured workers seen in the emergency room to the occupational health service the following day or as appropriate.

The range of services provided by hospital-based and group-based providers is similar to that of other occupational health providers (see Chapter 16), and includes the diagnosis and treatment of injured workers and the provision of screening (surveillance and fitness for duty) and preventive services (including immunization) for employees of local employers. Many of them conduct drug screening and even offer employee assistance programs through their health care network.

Most hospitals and large medical groups use electronic medical record (EMR) systems. In general, hospitals and group practices use the same system for all their services, outpatient and inpatient, as the EMR system is designed to keep information safe, protected, and readily accessible within the system. One should note, however, that few commercial EMR systems for large health care systems provide the features optimal for occupational health services. As such, occupational medicine providers must frequently improvise. Depending on the system, this task is variably challenging. Some of the difficulties include inability of the "one-size-fits-all" EMR to generate needed forms and reports to produce return-to-work or fitness-for-duty reports in the proper format, and lack of important diagnosis codes used in occupational medicine. However, many suitable occupational health software packages do exist and are available on the market (see Chapters 13 and 19) that allow surveillance data to be tracked and case management to be monitored, and that use appropriate terminology. Ideally, hospital-based occupational health services use one of these systems rather than an unsatisfactory institutional EMR system. The hope is that in time software that incorporates the needs of occupational health services will be developed and incorporated into the EMR systems used by large institutions.

The great advantage of hospitals and large medical groups is that referral for specialty care and for physical therapy services is relatively easy to arrange and to document within the system. Follow-up can be arranged quickly and many times the EMR systems can link the injured worker to his or her personal medical record if he or she is also a patient in the same network. Specifically occupational surveillance programs (see Chapter 20) and impairment assessment evaluations (see Chapter 26), although necessarily maintained in a separate record, can easily be related to the worker's personal history if there is a question.

Well-managed dedicated occupational health services based at hospitals have clearly thrived in the marketplace on the basis of their own revenues, especially when their overhead expense has been separated from total hospital or group overhead expense. Indeed, hospital-based occupational health services have led to the establishment of relationships with local employers, who in turn may encourage their employees to go the hospital for non-work-related injuries and illnesses, providing downstream revenue to the hospital system.

In some regions, such as Ohio, hospital-based and free-standing occupational health services have organized into associations. For the most part, however, hospital-based occupational health services are fiercely competitive within their own areas and do not hesitate to use the power of their networks to establish dominance in the market.

Teaching Hospitals and Academic Medical Centers

Academic medical centers, linking hospitals, medical schools, faculty-based medical groups, and often schools of public health, are critical to occupational health care beyond their numbers and their capacity for patient care and services. They are the intellectual centers of the field, supporting training programs for occupational medicine and nursing, producing the best research, providing expert consultation on difficult cases, and disseminating knowledge about occupational injuries and illness to other medical specialties through interaction with teachers and trainees in other fields. Many also provide occupational health services to the hospital and local employers. Others are not staffed or equipped for primary care occupational health care (see Chapters 1, 8, and 16), leaving their local emergency room and primary care or outpatient services to play that role and emphasizing consultation and evaluation of difficult cases, which then become available for teaching and research, Rotations through an occupational health clinic are common for residents in family medicine, internal medicine, and emergency medicine. They are also an important component of training for medical toxicology programs.

An example of an academic occupational medicine clinic that provides not only secondary and tertiary care but also operates a more comprehensive occupational health service is St. Paul-Ramsey Medical Center, an affiliate of the University of Minnesota. This institution has provided primary injury care for many years, which has the advantage of giving trainees a representative experience with occupational health care rather than referred cases, which are often esoteric. Likewise, Beth Israel-Deaconess, in the Boston area, provides basic injury care as well as consultation, and sophisticated services such as ergonomics evaluation. The occupational medicine clinic at the University of Pennsylvania also provides injury and illness care as well as consultation services for environmental exposures.

Research at the population level becomes possible when academic medical centers capture the primary care level of occupational health care or become referral centers for a particular problem. An example is the occupational health service of Johns Hopkins Medical, which has produced a long and impressive list of studies documenting improved outcomes and reduced costs for the employers it serves in the area around Baltimore.

Their Association of Occupational and Environmental Clinics (AOEC, www.aoec. org) consists of a group of approximately 65 member clinics in the US and Canada, and a general membership of several hundred professionals. Although for the most part relatively small operations, member clinics play a disproportionate role as centers for the evaluation of difficult cases, sponsors of educational programs, and advocates for injured workers. Many of them are associated with federally-funded Education and Research Centers (ERCs) supported by the National Institute for Occupational Safety and Health (NIOSH) and so have access to industrial hygiene and other services. AOEC also administers the network of Pediatric Environmental Health Centers, funded by the US Agency for Toxic Substances and Disease Registry (ATSDR), and offers individual memberships, and provides support for the OEM List, the indispensable online virtual community of practitioners in occupational health.

The states of New York and California support a regionalized network of such clinics, based at university medical centers serving major centers. The model was adapted by the Canadian province of Alberta in the 1990s but did not last longer.

Occupational medicine and nursing training programs are highly vulnerable to budget cutbacks, changes in development priorities, partisan political favor, and administrative reorganization. As such, the position of occupational medicine and nursing within academic medical centers and teaching hospitals has been tenuous over the years. John H. Knowles, the legendary chief executive officer of the Massachusetts General Hospital during its period of rapid growth, once called the modern teaching hospital the most complex single institution ever devised. Since he wrote that in 1966, academic medical centers have become much more complicated, expensive, and networked, to the detriment of small programs with limited revenue potential. Occupational medicine and nursing training programs rely on these academic institutions for academic, administrative, and in-kind support but constitute only a tiny part of their operations and generate only modest revenues from consultative clinical activities. Extramural funding from NIOSH is limited and primarily flows to the ERCs. Their unusual characteristics, small size, restricted funding, modest revenue-generating capacity, and low visibility in the community contribute to their dependence on the parent institution.

Most postgraduate training programs in American medicine are supported through funds to hospitals providing Medicare services, through the Center for Medicare and Medicaid Services (CMS, the second M is omitted). The rationale for this is to support the supply of health providers, as clinical trainees (residents and fellows) are directly involved in providing clinical service, and as such are part of the health care labor pool on which Medicare depends to provide care to its beneficiaries. The exceptions are the three preventive medicine specialties, under the American Board of Preventive Medicine (see Chapter 14): general preventive medicine, occupational medicine, and aerospace medicine. (Aerospace medicine training is mostly supported by military programs and will not be further discussed.) The rationale for the exclusion is that preventive medicine specialists are not directly involved with inpatient care and so are not providers of hospital-based clinical services.

Instead, general preventive medicine training is mostly supported by a separate, unique, and highly uncertain Congressional allocation that could disappear in any year, because it requires Congressional action for renewal every year, separate from budget approval. The same rationale is applied to occupational medicine trainees, because CMS does not differentiate among the three preventive medicine specialties, notwithstanding that they have been demonstrably distinct since 1952. The result is that occupational medicine training is limited to scarce NIOSH funding and a few ad hoc arrangements leaving the current residency training programs perennially unable to meet the demand to train an adequate number of occupational medicine specialists. The only legitimate way to access Medicare-based hospital funding has been to involve trainees in the occupational health services for hospital networks, since this puts them into a function that clearly supports clinical care by supporting the needs of providers. However, this is a patch, not a solution to the funding problem. It constrains the experience of the trainee and is insufficient to support an entire training program.

More fundamentally, one could argue that both preventive medicine and occupational medicine among medical specialties (and public health nursing and occupational health nursing among nursing specialties) should have a much larger role in the health care system and merit assured funding. One demonstrated reason is that they reduce the demand for acute care services, and may also reduce the burden of chronic disease. More specifically, in the case of occupational medicine, health care expenditures are rationalized by preventing the shift of costs from work-related chronic illness and disability to Medicare after retirement. Thus far, these arguments have not been persuasive.

Occupational Health Services for Health Care Workers

Hospitals, specifically, are major employers in their communities. They and large medical groups have the same duty to protect their employees as any other employer and are covered by workers' compensation. Occupational health services for hospital employees are ubiquitous because of accreditation requirements. Health care workers in large medical groups may be served by in-house occupational health services or may be served informally by a single health care professional designated to coordinate compliance with accreditation requirements.

Appropriate occupational health for hospital and health care employees has a direct bearing on medical safety in hospitals, in several different ways. Hospital and health care workers are much more likely to comply with patient safety measures when they believe their own safety (and that of their families) is protected. Compliance/adherence to best practices is expected of licensed health care workers. For example, many hospitals launch large "flu campaigns" in an effort to immunize health care workers each year. The success is variable, with some larger institutions boasting greater that 90 percent compliance. The Centers for Disease Control estimates that during the 2010–2011 influenza season, coverage for influenza vaccination among health care workers was only 63.5 percent. Coverage was 98.1 percent among health care workers who had an employer requirement for vaccination. Realizing the importance of hand washing in preventing nosocomial infections among hospitalized workers, hospitals in recent years have also launched "hand washing" campaigns, in some cases involving the patients, who are encouraged to report providers not observed to wash their hands. With the advent of alcohol-based antiseptics, there are fewer barriers to hand hygiene, as these dispensers are now commonly found throughout hospitals. However, the challenge of achieving high levels of compliance among hospital personnel remains. Although inroads have been made on the problem, these measures may have variable success depending on management commitment to safety, as well as other factors.

Occupational health and safety is part of a much larger culture of safety that needs to be seamless and uniform to be effective. Occupational health is therefore a role model, a training ground demonstrating good work practices for hazard control, with a mission beyond infectious hazards to include chemical hazards, sensitizers (latex), physical hazards (lasers), and work organization.

Reporting arrangements within the hospital organization, which is always complicated, varies by institution. Some hospitals place the occupational health service within the human resources (HR) department, with direct reporting to a vice president responsible for HR. Others attach it to a clinical service, such as internal medicine. Some have dual reporting structures, with management supervision for personnel issues (see Chapter 24, on absence) and clinical supervision for delivery of care. One innovative structure (the University of Massachusetts Medical Center, in Worcester MA) has divided occupational health services into the "employee health service" (which attends to fitness-for-duty and preplacement evaluation, compliance issues, and surveillance) and the "occupational health service" (which deals with workers' compensation, fitness for return to work, and long-term disability), each reporting to a different manager, one responsible for human resources and the other loss prevention. Many hospitals marry the two missions, reporting to one medical director. Increasingly, occupational health services offered to employees includes wellness initiatives. The name "employee health service" is giving way to names such as "occupational health services" and "wellness and prevention center" and "employee health and wellness."

Hospital occupational health services are similar, in principle, to other employer-sponsored, on-site occupational health services (see Chapters 1 and 6). In practice, however, they are complicated by the dual clinical and management hierarchies inherent in hospital systems. Since health is the business of the employer when it comes to hospitals, hospital employee occupational health programs cross the boundary between the two, sometimes uncomfortably when there is an inconvenient recommendation to management. This is not too different from other settings such as industry, however, where return to work decisions regarding employees can leave management equally unhappy. The occupational health service is also readily bypassed in hospitals because employees often get provisional care or opinions from their colleagues in informal "corridor consultations," which are usually inadequate for the purpose and does not get documented in the record.

About 20 years ago, OSHA recognized that hospitals were not experiencing the same drop in injury rates as other sectors and that the magnitude of major hazards, such as blood borne pathogen exposure, created a risk equal to or in excess of many industrial sectors that were considered to be at high risk. The result was a regulatory emphasis program focused on the health care sector.

Historically, the health care field has been a relatively high risk sector but the emphasis has been on protecting patients, not health care workers. Modern hospitals demonstrate a high rate of musculoskeletal injuries and for those injured a high rate of permanent impairment leading to disability, largely from claims for back pain, often due to lifting injuries while manipulating patients or equipment. Realizing that nursing staff and transport suffer a disproportionate incidence of lifting injures and with the obesity epidemic upon us, NIOSH conducted a comprehensive lab and field study, first based in nursing homes but then in hospitals, which showed that lifting equipment can reduce these injuries. Effective, safe and cost-effective alternatives to manual patient handling are available for use in the hospital setting.

In addition to the typical hazards of a large and technically complex operation, health care institutions have unique hazards: exposure to chemical hazards; latex allergy; exposure to physical hazards (such as lasers and ionizing radiation); mechanical and ergonomic issues such as due to lifting patients; slips, trips, and falls; and intense psychosocial issues such as due to shift work among nurses, and burnout in intensive care and oncology services. Blood borne pathogen exposures and other infectious hazards are also well known to health care professionals.

Compliance

One of the primary responsibilities of hospital-based clinics that serve the employee is to ensure compliance with regulations from competent authorities (e.g. federal or state OSHA, see Chapter 4), compliance with accreditation requirements, and adherence to various guidelines.

The primary accreditation body for hospitals and large health care facilities is the Joint Commission (JC), formerly the Joint Commission on Accreditation of Healthcare Organizations (JCAHO). The Joint Commission does not specify in detail what occupational health services should be provided to hospital employees but requires that they be provided. The JC reviews the employee health service during scheduled site visits over the course of the three-year accreditation cycle. The JC exerts considerable power because its accreditation (or equivalent accreditation) is necessary for a hospital to qualify for payment under the Medicare program. However, its authority also comes from the assurance of basic standards of quality that accreditation represents, which is demanded by health maintenance organizations and private insurers as well. Hospitals find themselves on the defensive in legal actions and pay higher insurance rates if they are not accredited.

The JC's interest in occupational health primarily stems from the risk to patients but also includes the responsibilities of the hospital as an employer. Accreditation representatives are likely to ask about immunizations of health care providers on site visits, for example. The Joint

Commission International is the accreditation body for hospitals and health care institutions outside North America and is increasing its influence as standards improve worldwide and as "medical tourism" becomes more popular and contract services (see Chapter 7) become more competitive.

The JC is dominant in the field of health care accreditation but there are other agencies that perform similar functions. It is not the only accreditation agency for health care facilities recognized by CMS. Accreditation organizations, mostly non-profit, have proliferated in response to the expansion of health care and quality assurance initiatives, as well as to measures within CMS to introduce competition and alternatives, and to privatize review for eligibility for Medicare and Medicaid. Other agencies include:

- Accreditation Association for Ambulatory Health Care (AAAHC), which accredits outpatient services, federally-qualified community health centers (supported or recognized by the Health Resources and Services Administration and located in underserved areas), managed care organizations, ambulatory surgery centers, and occupational health centers, both on-site and community based.
- Accreditation Commission for Health Care, Inc. (ACHC), which accredits home health providers, hospices, and medical device and prosthetics suppliers; specifically requires surveillance and preventive services for staff.
- Commission on Accreditation of Rehabilitation Facilities (CARF), which focuses on human services, behavioral health, addiction services, and rehabilitation; does not have a specific requirement for occupational health services.
- Community Health Accreditation Program (CHAP), which accredits federally-qualified and other community health centers, home health providers, and hospices; specifically addresses safety of employees.
- DNV Healthcare, a for-profit US subsidiary of Det Norske Veritas, a well-known and highly reputable international standards organization with a long history in occupational health; specifically addresses occupational health issues.
- Healthcare Facilities Accreditation Program (HFAP), which focuses on hospitals, laboratories, and suppliers of durable equipment in health care; specifically recognizes occupational health services.
- URAC (acronym only, with no name spelled out; previously the "Utilization Review Accreditation Commission"), which focuses on staff training and responsibility, including health information protection, and covers any health care enterprise, including managed care organizations, health benefits programs, pharmacies, optometrists, and occupational health services.
- "Exemplary Provider Program" of The Compliance Team, a for-profit organization that accredits small health enterprises such as single-office providers and also suppliers of durable medical equipment and supplies.
- Healthcare Quality Association on Accreditation (HQAA), which focuses on small providers, such as physician offices, home health care services, pharmacies, and suppliers of durable medical equipment and supplies.

Hospitals are required to be in compliance with federal (CMS) requirements set forth in the guidelines for Medicare-qualified providers, called Conditions of Participation (CoP), in order to receive Medicare or Medicaid payments. The hospital or medical group is also responsible to the city or state department of health (DOH), particularly for reporting communicable diseases, and for adhering to state public health laws. State DOHs also conduct their own inspections to ensure compliance. An example is the requirement of many states that health care providers be immune to certain infectious diseases, namely measles, mumps, and rubella, in order to prevent transmission of infection to patients. Proof of immunity may be by titer or by documentation of vaccination. Some states require that health care providers be screened regularly for TB, although some states in which the incidence of TB is very low have waived this requirement. State DOHs may conduct their own surveys to review compliance with CMS guidelines, on behalf of the state, which administers Medicaid.

OSHA standards apply to hospitals, which are responsible for the management of regulated hazards, prevention of work-related injuries and illness, mandated surveillance programs for recognized workplace hazards, and records retention. There are several OSHA standards designed specifically to protect health care workers. Prominent ones are the OSHA Bloodborne Pathogen Standard and the Ethylene Oxide Standard. Other standards have particular relevance and application in health care settings. The Respiratory Protection Standard has played a key role in occupational health protection against airborne TB infection and was important during both the 2002 SARS epidemic and the 2009 H1N1 influenza pandemic. OSHA standards relevant to health care workers and their essential requirements are listed in Table 9.1.

Services

There are many resources available regarding the clinical management of occupational health services for hospital and health care employees. The American College of Occupational and Environmental Medicine *Guidance for Occupational Health Services in Medical Centers* is a key source.

One advantage of having employees centrally monitored in an employee health service is that trends can be identified, especially with occupational health software. For instance, if more than one health care worker from a hospital floor reports with a febrile respiratory illness or the same type of injury, it is easier to detect whether a cluster exists, to identify a possible cause, and to institute preventive measures, such as contact precautions to avoid further spread or ergonomic interventions. This "syndromic surveillance" has also been found effective in emergency rooms to detect new or spreading illnesses in the community.

The hospital employee health service can also provide data collection for the evaluation of safety interventions. For example, back injury, one of the most common occupational injuries, nursing staff being no exception, has been addressed with the use of patient lifts and slings. In the event of an injury, whether or not the lift was employed and employed correctly can be assessed. Outcomes data thus generated have shown that the lifts, if used correctly, can reduce the risk of low back injuries.

Allergy to natural rubber latex (NRL) in the hospital setting, which increased in incidence with the advent of "Standard Precautions," related principally to the increased use of NRL gloves. Employee health service data identified the rise in latex allergy and justified both changes in glove manufacturing and the availability of substitutes where latex was not required, limiting the epidemic (which even so lasted 20 years). Another ingredient in latex gloves, thiuram (an accelerant), can also cause allergy, although it is much less common, and can be found in non-latex gloves as well as nitrile and vulcanized products. Without data from monitoring in occupational health services, the role of thiuram as an independent sensitizer would not be as obvious.

Some hospital-based occupational medicine clinics now offer primary care services for employees, much like on-site medical clinics in industry (see Chapter 1). This is a return

Table 9.1 OSHA Standards that Apply to Health Care Workers

Standard	Coverage and Exposure	Other Provisions
Blood Borne Pathogen Standard 29 CFR 1910.1030	All workers with potential exposure to potentially infectious blood and body fluids, the main infectious organisms being HIV, hepatitis B virus and hepatitis C virus.	Safe needle devices must be available. Needlesticks and splashes must be recorded in OSHA log and type of needle device used must be recorded.
Final rule in 1991, updated 1999 and 2001	Workers must be offered the hepatitis B vaccine free of charge.	
Ethylene Oxide (EtO) 29 CFR 1910.1047	All workers potentially exposed to EtO above the action level or who wear respirators in performing their duties: Action Level: 0.5 ppm (= ½ PEL) PEL: 1 ppm (8-hour TWA) STEL: 5 ppm	Preplacement and periodic surveillance.
Formaldehyde 29 CFR 1910.1048	All workers exposed to formaldehyde at or above the action level and any employee who experiences signs and symptoms of overexposure: Action level: 0.375 ppm (= ½ PEL) PEL: 0.75 ppm (8-hour TWA) STEL: 2 ppm	Preplacement and periodic surveillance.
Inorganic Mercury 29 CFR 1910.1047	Workers potentially exposed, such as those who make dental amalgams, at or above the action level: Action level: 0.05 mg/m^3 (= ½PEL) PEL: 0.10 mg/m^3 8-hour TWA No STEL or Ceil applies	Preplacement and periodic surveillance.
Noise 29 CFR 1910.95	Workers exposed to noise levels above the PEL.* Action level: 85 dBA (most employers use 80 dBA) PEL: 90 dB 8-hour TWA	A standard threshold shift must be reported on the OSHA 300 log and the employee must be offered retraining and follow-up testing among other things.

| Respiratory Protection 29 CFR 1910.134 Standard | Health care workers who provide care to patients with tuberculosis are required to be fit tested for N-95 respirators. | Employers must establish and implement a written respiratory protection program with workplace specific procedures and must always select NIOSH certified respirators. |
| General duty clause (GDC) Section 5(a)(1) of the OSH Act (see Chapter 4) | All workers

Covers hazards and risks not covered by specific standards. | "Each employer shall furnish to each of his [sic] employees employment and a place of employment which are free from recognized hazards that are causing or are likely to cause death or serious physical harm to his employees." |

Notes:
* The action level is not 45 (½ PEL) because the decibel scale is fundamentally logarithmic.
Key: dBA, decibel; PEL, permissible exposure limit; ppm, parts per million; STEL, short-term exposure limit; TLV, threshold limit value.

to decades past, when primary care services were common. The objective is more timely care, less time away from work, and reduced absence. Wellness programs (see Chapter 30) are present in virtually all hospitals but vary among institutions and can be quite diverse. Smoking cessation programs helped a generation of hospital workers to quit when bans on smoking inside hospitals began in the 1980s. Current programs are similar to those in general industry and may feature a health risk assessment (HRA) questionnaire.

EMR systems (see Chapters 13 and 19) are becoming ubiquitous in hospitals. Some vendors offer well-tailored systems that the employee health staff can use efficiently and with limited training, immediately, both for tracking individual employees, and to identify patterns in the workplace, by exposure or occupational groups. However, in a hospital-based employee health service, occupational health services are a part of a larger whole. The employee health service may have to adapt to the EMR system purchased by the institution, requiring it to keep a parallel data system, such as data on Excel, for tracking purposes. Some EMR systems are readily adaptable, allowing the provider to customize notes and orders to reduce the typing necessary as well as the repetition. However, this requires time and effort and for large institutions any modification to the software can be very expensive. In general, hospitals and large medical groups tend to be resistant to requests for dedicated occupational health software, partly because they wish to avoid the expense of purchasing another system, partly because they want to avoid "bolt on" software that interfaces with their system and might compromise it in some way, and partly because they do not want to undermine confidence in the system. Most hospital and medical group EMR software, however, may not be well suited to occupational medicine services.

Immunization

The Advisory Committee on Immunization Practices (ACIP), through the Centers for Disease Control and Prevention (CDC) and the Hospital Infection Control Practices Advisory Committee (HICPAC), a federal advisory body, provide authoritative infection control guidelines to health care facilities regarding immunizations for health care workers. While this is not a legal mandate, health care institutions usually comply and insurers use the guidelines to determine which immunizations they will reimburse. There are three levels of recommendations: (1) those for which active immunization is strongly recommended because of special risks for the health care provider; (2) those for which immunoprophylaxis is or may be indicated in certain circumstances; and (3) those for which protection of all adults is recommended. The goal is maintenance of immunity as a barrier to transmission. The rationale is that health care workers who have contact with patients may be exposed to infection from patients and as such are at risk for exposure to vaccine-preventable diseases. On the other hand, health care providers with patient contact may transmit vaccine-preventable diseases to patients (see Table 9.2).

Hospital-based employee health services are usually charged with providing employees with the required immunizations. Strategies range from administering all immunizations and screening efforts on location in the employee health clinic, to having central control but employing the help of nursing supervisors or nurses traveling from floor to floor providing vaccine to employees. Nurse managers may perform "push pods" on their immediate staff, in which every employee on the floor is approached and must consent or decline the vaccine, with documentation. A push pod team may consist of pharmacists, who in many states can administer vaccine, along with nurses, infection control personnel, nursing education and occupational medicine (OM) staff.

Table 9.2 Vaccines Recommended for Health Care Workers

Pathogen	Periodicity of Immunization
Hepatitis B	3 doses at day 1, in one month and in five-month series, with specified spacing. The titer must be documented one month after the third vaccine. The series may be repeated twice if there is no serological evidence of immunity
Influenza	Annually
Measles, mumps, rubella (MMR)	2 doses 4 weeks apart for health care workers born after 1957 without serological evidence of immunity
Varicella	2 doses 4 weeks apart for health care workers without serological evidence of immunity
Tetanus, Diphtheria, (acellular pertussis)	One-time dose of Tdap as soon as feasible to all health care workers who did not receive it previously, then give Td boosters every 5-10 years
Meningococcal	1 dose to microbiologists routinely exposed to isolates of N. meningitides
Vaccinia	1 dose to laboratory workers who directly handle cultures with vaccinia, recombinant vaccinia viruses or orthopox viruses that infect humans

Surveillance

Periodic health surveillance (see Chapter 20) for hospital employees in North America has been largely reduced to annual testing for the presence of latent TB. TB surveillance is probably the most common surveillance activity in the hospital setting. Surveillance programs may also be created for employees exposed to chemotherapeutic agents, lasers, and other potential hazards for which specific OSHA standards may not exist, under the General Duty Clause (see Chapter 4).

Preplacement fitness-for-duty examinations include color vision screening performed on all employees who do point-of-care testing, where test interpretation is color based. The provisions of the Americans with Disabilities Act (ADA, see Chapter 23) apply. The same preplacement evaluation protocols should be applied to clearance procedures for non-employees, including vendors in the operating room (OR), visiting students and observers, non-staff (voluntary) attending physicians, and volunteers.

Hospital Policy

Like other employers (see Chapter 6) occupational health services in a hospital should be governed by an explicit and overarching general policy which confirms the hospital's commitment to a safe workplace and to continuous improvement in controlling hazards and reducing risk. The hospital policy manual should also include specific policies, preferably one each for easy revision and updating, on all required services, including compliance with OSHA standards, mandatory public health measures, and CDC guidelines, cross-referenced where appropriate to the hospital's infection control policy. Other important policies include substance abuse, monitoring re-entry programs after employees have returned to work following treatment for substance abuse, return to work and absence management (see Chapter 24), employees with communicable diseases, and hand washing.

Having an explicit and clear written policy reduces or eliminates ambiguity and offers transparency and legal protection. Policies should anticipate and address specific problem issues, preferably before they happen in order to support sound management when they arise. This may involve, for example, counseling of a worker who is pregnant regarding exposure to reproductive hazards, such as chemotherapy, ethylene oxide, or lab exposure to cytomegalovirus.

In recent years, there has been increased realization that health care workers occupy safety-sensitive positions no less than truck drivers and train engineers, and that providers with physical or mental impairments may pose a risk to patients. Therefore, it is becoming more common for hospital administration to refer physicians/providers for fitness-for-duty evaluation (see Chapter 22) even before a patient-related occurrence or complaint. It is advisable that policies do not punish staff who are injured or ill or who report a substance abuse problem voluntarily, but they must provide a high level of protection to the patient, and to health care workers who work alongside them and cover their duties.

Two hospitals in Hawaii, on different sides of the same island and rivals for referral cases, once entered into an innovative arrangement. Since they were easily accessible to one another by a connecting highway but their local communities were widely separated, the two hospitals took one another's employees into their employee assistance programs, but never into their own. This allowed them to maintain a higher level of confidentiality and trust in the process.

Employee Health Services as a Starting Point

Many occupational health professionals have their first exposure to the professional field by participating in a hospital-based occupational (or employee) health service. (Chapter 8 discusses strategic planning in occupational health services.) The employee health service is a good venue for training, since hospitals present both a variety of hazards and surveillance measures, from which the new professional can learn and gain expertise. After experience in a hospital employee health service and with the service as a base, the provider can branch out into other industries and employment sectors. The hospital service provides a protected base for the new provider. Hospital committee participation is another key function for the OM physician, particularly the hospital's infection control committee, environment of care (safety) committee, and emergency management committee.

The hospital employee health service has sometimes been a foundation on which hospitals have developed occupational health services for local employers. Providing care to these two distinct employee groups, that is, the hospital and outside employers, leverages existing resources, amortizes overhead, and adds value and revenues. In addition, it allows a greater breadth of service and hence knowledge base for the ambitious occupational health care provider, making it a natural springboard into occupational health careers.

Recommended Reading and Resources

American College of Occupational and Environmental Medicine. Medical Center Occupational Health. Available at: http://www.acoem.org/medical_center_occ_health.aspx. Accessed January 20, 2011. Links to *Guidance and other documents*.

Barron BA, Beckett WS, Utell MJ (2005) Clinical activities in an academic hospital-based occupational health program. *J Occup Environ Med*, 47(6): 587–593.

Centers for Disease Control and Prevention. Influenza vaccine information for health care workers. Available at: http://www.cdc.gov/flu/healthcareworkers.htm. Accessed January 31, 2012.

Fell-Carlson D (2007) *Working Safely in Health Care: A Practical Guide.* Clifton Park NY, Thomson Delmar Learning. Written from the point of view of the health care worker.

Green-McKenzie J, Carusu G (2006) Health care workers crucial barriers. Occupational Health and Safety, April. Available at: http://ohsonline.com/articles/2006/04/health-care-workers-crucial-barriers.aspx Accessed 20 January 2012.

Green-McKenzie J, Pak V, Crawford G (2009) Thiuram allergy—a potential dermal allergy among health care workers. *AAOHN J*, 57(4): 139–141.

Green-McKenzie J, Watkins M, Shofer F (2012) Outcomes of a consultation program to emergency medicine clinicians for postexposure management of occupational bloodborne pathogen exposures. *Am J Inf Control,* In Press.

Guidotti TL (1984) Desirable characteristics of the teaching occupational medicine clinic. *J Occup Med*, 26: 105–109.

Horsburgh CR, Rubin E (2011) Latent tuberculosis infection in the United States. *N Engl J Med*, 364: 1441–1448.

Immunization of Health-Care Workers. Recommendations of the Advisory Committee on Immunization Practices (ACIP) and the Hospital Infection Control Practices Advisory Committee (HICPAC). Available at: http://www.cdc.gov/mmwr/preview/mmwrhtml/00050577.htm. Accessed January 4, 2012.

Knowles JH (1966) *The Teaching Hospital: Evolution and Contemporary Issues.* Cambridge MA, Harvard University Press. Of historical interest.

Konstantinos K, Crespo J (1998) Cost effective, hospital based occupational health programs. Successful program. *AAOHN J, 46(3): 127–131.*

Mazurek G, Jereb J, LoBue P, Lademarco F, Metchock B, Vernon A (2005) Guidelines for Using the QuantiFERON®-TB Gold Test for Detecting *Mycobacterium tuberculosis* Infection, United States MMWR Recommendations and Reports. December 16, 2005 / 54(RR15); 49–55.

McCunney RJ (1984) A hospital-based occupational health service. *J Occup Med*, 26(5): 375–380.

McCunney RJ (2001) Health and productivity: a role for occupational health professionals. *J Occup Environ Med*, 43(1): 30–35.

Mitchell, F (2002) *Instant Medical Surveillance.* Beverly Farms MA, OEM Press.

Rosenstock L (1984) Hospital-based, academically affiliated occupational medicine clinics. *Am J Industr Med*, 6(2): 155–168.

Summers M (2007–2008) The mixed-use clinic: occupational medicine + urgent care. *Occupational Health Tracker*, Winter, pp. 11–13. Available at: http://www.corporatehealthgroup.com/newsletters/pdf/mixed_use.pdf. Accessed January, 20 2012.

US Department of Health and Human Services. Centers for Medicare and Medicaid Services. Federal Register/Vol. 76, No. 205/Monday, October 24, 2011/Proposed Rules. 42 CFR Parts 482 and 485 [CMS–3244–P] RIN 0938–AQ89. Available at: https://www.cms.gov/CFCsAndCoPs/06_Hospitals.asp. Accessed January 20, 2011.

US Department of Health and Human Services. Centers for Medicare and Medicaid Services. Medicare and Medicaid Programs; Reform of Hospital and Critical Access Hospital Conditions of Participation. Available at: https://www.cms.gov/CFCsAndCoPs/Downloads/CMS3244P.pdf. Accessed on January 4, 2012.

Wright WE (2009) *Couturier's Occupational and Environmental Infectious Disease.* Beverly Farms MA, OEM Press.

10 Staffing and Personnel

Donna Lee Gardner and Karen O'Hara

An appropriate staff mix is essential to ensure efficient and profitable operations. Although it is certainly true that "people make the service," it is also indisputable that employing too many people can sink an occupational health service.

A considerable percentage of the total operating budget of an occupational health service (OH service) is consumed by salaries and benefits. It is helpful initially to have a "lean and mean" attitude toward staffing, although too few staff and customers complain about long waits and lack of attention to detail. Meanwhile, the occupational health service's own employees feel overwhelmed and unappreciated. Too many staff consuming too great a percentage of profits places the service's viability at stake, however. But when staffing is "just right," personnel consistently function at a high level of productivity and are able to handle even the busiest days with confidence, if not aplomb.

The principles of how to staff an occupational health service are well worked out from years of surveys and market research by organizations such as RYAN Associates and the National Association of Occupational Health Professionals. The same principles outlined in this chapter apply to any occupational health service provider model (see Chapter 1), whether community-based or on-site employer-sponsored, although it is written from the point of view of a free-standing community-based model (the "occupational medicine center," as in Chapter 19). Other provider models (see Chapter 1), particularly hospital-based or multispecialty group-affiliated occupational health services (see Chapter 9), may have an apparent advantage in having a large pool of experienced personnel already employed, because in theory staff can be readily reassigned to occupational health service internally, as needed. However, it is critical that the occupational health service control recruitment and assignment. Staff must have the required occupational health expertise and qualifications to deliver a quality service.

Developing a Staffing Model

Before accepting job applications and starting interviews for recruitment, one must first determine how many employees it will take to start up and then run the occupational health service. Initially, the service is not likely to require a fully-loaded staff. The staff mix must evolve as the clinic matures.

The development of an appropriate occupational health clinic staffing model is a multi-phased process. It begins with understanding the marketplace and establishing reasonable volume projections. Issues to consider include:

- clerical, clinical, and administrative requirements
- hours of operation
- population density
- client company demographics
- internal service capabilities (if embedded in a hospital or large medical group)
- potential use of ancillary departments and external vendors.

Work injury projections are the foundation of an optimal staffing model for an occupational health service. The first step is to identify the number of individuals working in the market to be served by conducting employer surveys and/or studying demographic data. For example, when using US census data and other sources to estimate the working population in a target market, one may assume 3.5 work-related injuries per 100 workers (per 2011 US Bureau of Labor Statistics data).

A reasonable percentage of these cases, or "market share," of total work-related injuries may then be assigned to the occupational health service, with the market spilt among all local providers providing services to employers. (In hospital network-sponsored occupational health services, this includes the hospital's own emergency room and sometimes urgent care facilities it controls.) In competitive markets one might estimate an initial share of only 10–15 percent of the total work injury market and assume the market share will grow over time. Conversely, in a market with minimal competition, a provider may assume a starting work injury market share as high as 40–50 percent. Market share is therefore a key piece of information which must be estimated as accurately as possible. (It is therefore important in starting a new service to know the politics of local hospital emergency rooms and their relationship to local employers, who may have a preference for one or another.)

Once initial injury volume is estimated from the occupational health service's anticipated market share of the total volume of cases, one can apply volume ratios that derive estimates of demand for other services from the number of new injury cases that come to the occupational health service. These volume ratios are based on national estimates for employer-related services such as drug screens and physical examinations using the following assumptions based on findings from the National Association of Occupational Health Professionals' survey of provider-based occupational health services:

- 1:13 preplacement evaluations to first injury visits (i.e. there is on average one preplacement evaluation for every 13 initial acute injury care encounters)
- five annual/executive physical evaluations per 100 employees at companies that conduct annual/executive physicals
- 43 examinations (Occupational Safety and Health Administration (OSHA)-mandated surveillance or fitness-for-duty, especially for firefighters and police) per 100 initial injury encounters
- other examinations (e.g. independent medical examinations (IMEs), return-to-work evaluations) average at 15 percent of initial injuries
- 152 revisits for every 100 initial injury visits
- three functional capacity evaluations for every 100 preplacement physical examinations (see Chapter 22)
- 20 functional capacity evaluations for every 100 post-injury physical therapy evaluation referrals (per national norm)

- 71.1 National Institute on Drug Abuse (Substance Abuse and Mental Health Services Administration, SAMHSA) drug tests per 100 preplacement exams (see Chapter 27)
- 91.7 non-National Institute on Drug Abuse drug tests per 100 preplacement exams
- 1:9 breath alcohol tests to drug screens
- 19 percent of evaluations (preplacement, medical surveillance, annual, and "other") require an audiogram
- 10 percent of evaluations (preplacement, medical surveillance, annual, and "other") require a lab test (primarily a complete blood count)
- 10 percent of non-injury evaluations (preplacement, medical surveillance, annual, and "other") require pulmonary function tests. (These are primarily done for periodic health surveillance such as OSHA-mandated asbestos surveillance or for respirator clearance; see Chapter 20.)
- 10 influenza vaccinations and other immunizations for every 100 preplacement physical examinations (per national norm).

The estimates of service volume form the basis for planning and marketing service lines (see Chapter 16) as well as staffing.

Staffing ratios are contingent on volumes, service mix, utilization of ancillaries, and hours of service. Table 10.1 assumes that all of these approach national norms, with a physician seeing an average of 28–32 patients per eight-hour day. Table 10.2 is a worksheet to assist with the development of appropriate staffing patterns. Hours of service requires close examination. The personnel overhead cost of staying open after usual business working hours may not be covered by revenue, but when care is given by local emergency rooms and urgent care centers, revenues will be lost for follow-up as well as initial care.

It is essential for efficiency, flexibility, and quality of care that qualified staff, including all licensed health care professionals, be cross-trained in those services that are most frequently provided: audiometry, vision screening, pulmonary function testing. Some job functions are combined or overlap in duties, such as nursing and audiometry or pulmonary function testing, so that special technicians are not required, but state and provincial practice acts determine who is allowed perform specific functions (e.g. take an X-ray, administer injections).

A staffing model that works well at one point in time is not necessarily going to be optimal at another. It is a moving target that requires constant adjustment to ensure that the right staff is on duty at the right time in order to deliver great service consistently.

Table 10.1 Staffing Ratios

	One physician	*Two physicians, or one physician + one OHN, PA or NP*
RC Clinical Supervisor	1	1
MA X-ray technician	1	2–3
Receptionists	1–2	3
Back office personnel	2	4
Office Manager	1	1

Key: PA = physician's assistant, OHN = occupational health nurse at COHN level, NP = nurse practitioner, RC = registered clinician, MA = medical assistant (who performs many functions)

Table 10.2 Worksheet for Staffing Patterns, Occupational Health Service

Parameter	Staffing Projection Assumptions	
Number of workers seen per day		
Average occupancy in waiting room		
Average care hours		
Description of unit (and capacity)		
Staffing Pattern	Projected FTEs (Number and sum of hours worked/week divided by 40)	
Director		FTEs
Administrative Assistant		FTEs
Nurse Practitioner/PA/COHN		FTEs
Nurse Clinicians I		FTEs
Nurse Clinicians II		FTEs
Licensed Practice Nurse		FTEs
Medical Technologist		FTEs
Account Service Representative (Sales and Marketing)		FTEs
Office Support		FTEs
Secretary/Receptionist		FTEs
TOTAL		FTEs
TOTAL Budgeted FTEs		FTEs

Nursing Support

Wherever possible and available, it is recommended to recruit trained and experienced occupational health nurses who have the skills and expertise to be major contributors to the success of the occupational health service, and to the health of the workers and the organization. Based in part on state regulations, in some cases it may be more appropriate to retain a licensed nurse (licensed vocational nurse (LVN) or licensed practice nurse (LPN)) to perform certain functions. In some regions, training in occupational health practice is available to LPNs, and should be encouraged and supported. A similar approach may be applied to technicians, depending on state regulations. For instance, some states allow certain kinds of nurses to complete an X-ray certification course.

Typically, a nurse and one additional person are needed to process patients. The second person may be a multi-modality technician or a certified nursing assistant. Two people assisting with patient care is all a clinic is likely to need when a physician, physician assistant, or nurse practitioner sees four or less patients an hour.

Rehabilitation Staff

A comprehensive staff model also includes rehabilitation professionals, either from an affiliated outpatient rehab department or by adding a physical therapist (or other qualified individual) to the occupational health staff. Depending on volumes, an exercise physiologist also is an excellent resource.

Rehabilitation services are usually offered in free-standing occupational health services through a contractor who occupies space at the facility or very nearby. In hospital-based or multispecialty group-based services, the in-house physical therapy service provides this. When the occupational health service is located within a hospital or multispecialty clinic, physical therapy is usually in the same facility. If it is set up as a satellite or outreach clinic, physical therapy is often at another location or at the network's main facility. This may not matter if it is convenient to where injured workers live but the staff may need training to be more sensitive to employer's expectations for return to work.

On-site Staffing Needs

On-site (formerly "in-plant") occupational health services at the employer's venue (see Chapter 1) can apply the same ratios and planning principles but the base injury rate on which projects are made will be for employees of the company in the service area, rather than in the community.

Increasingly, on-site medical clinics are providing primary care as well as occupational health services to employees. Occupational health services and multispecialty group practices are particularly well situated to provide internal employee health services as well as outreach to client companies. In such cases, staffing needs are dictated by the same principles of hours of operation, the types of services being provided, and the regulatory environment, for example medical surveillance. Most on-site clinics are open during regular business hours, but some provide extended or even 24/7 coverage.

Depending on stipulations in the practice Act of the state in which an employee health clinic operates, a nurse practitioner, or a certified occupational health nurse specialist (COHN-S, with advanced knowledge and training), or a physician assistant is typically the lead provider. Other staff may include a physician, an occupational health nurse, medical assistant, office support, and a certified wellness coach or exercise physiologist. The medical assistant role can be particularly flexible in this setting when the individual is trained to perform drug screens, collect initial patient history, perform registration, take vital signs, and conduct spirometry, audiometry, and breath-alcohol tests (if trained and certified).

Job Descriptions

Key positions in the occupational health service require written job descriptions. These job descriptions are the basis for recruitment, performance evaluation, and strategies for continuous improvement. There are many examples in the literature. Because occupational health care involves many screening and preventive services that can be provided by different licensed health care providers, it is less useful to think in terms of physicians and nurses than it is to identify executive functions within the occupational health service. Exhibits 10.1 through 10.5 at the end of this chapter provide a compilation of responsibilities by job title and provide guidance for key positions: Medical Director (Exhibit 10.1), Occupational Health Care Director (Exhibit 10.2), Account Services Representative (Exhibit 10.3, duties for which are expanded from sales executive), Senior Occupational Health Nurse or Physician Assistant (Exhibit 10.4), and Occupational Health Nurse Clinician (Exhibit 10.5).

Training

Well-trained staff are essential but training is not enough. Employees of the occupational health service must work well together. Their training and competency must also be documented. Exhibit 10.6 is a form for evaluating competency of the licensed health care providers on staff. These exhibits can be used for recruiting or policy development, by inserting the name of the facility where "[the occupational health service]" is entered in the Exhibit.

In order to demonstrate that the training is adequate, proper documentation of continuing competency as well as training and education has become increasingly important in occupational health. Exhibit 10.7 is a template for tracking the competency, skills performance, and certification of employees of the occupational health service, using as an example an occupational health nurse. The competencies are drawn from authoritative sources (competencies developed by the American Association of Occupational Health Nurses, the Canadian Occupational Health Nurses Association, and the Ontario Occupational Health Nurses Association). Similar competency documentation can be devised for other licensed health professionals and for technicians and clerks. Kept up to date at least annually (preferably in electronic format), it can be kept on an Excel or other spreadsheet and produced on short notice to employers, to OSHA, or to attorneys during discovery.

OSHA and the Department of Transportation (DOT) require medical technicians to undergo training to acquire certification demonstrating competency in the performance of certain procedures. (See Recommended Reading and Resources, at the end of this chapter, for the major requirements.) In addition, several states require phlebotomy certification for all staff. Certificates of completion may be posted in the screening room to demonstrate staff proficiency to patients and visitors.

In some cases, training and a certificate of completion is provided by the screening equipment manufacturer. This opportunity is one reason why it is so important to select product vendors carefully and to establish positive ongoing relationships with them.

Cross-training is essential to success in occupational health services, notwithstanding restrictions on qualifications imposed by practice regulation. Before employees can be evaluated, one must establish training and competency requirements for various staff members and recruit accordingly. Table 10.3 correlates services and functions with correspondingly responsible staff members.

Hiring

Creating the right attitude in the office is of paramount importance. Three key principles apply when hiring people to work in an occupational health clinic:

- Take time to hire the right person for the job.
- Be quick to get rid of a "toxic" employee who is not a team player.
- Hire people for their attitude first and for their skill set second.

A cooperative and motivated employee can be trained and gaps in knowledge and skill can be filled. A gap in attitude usually cannot be fixed.

Reassigning personnel from other parts of a hospital network or specialty group may work if the individual is motivated to learn of a new field of practice, is interested in the

Table 10.3 Competency Requirements of Staff Positions

Competency	Medical Assistant	X-ray Tech	Patient Care Tech	Billing Clerk	Receptionist	Clinic Supervisor	Clinic Manager
Audiogram	▓	▓	▓			▓	▓
Billing Accuracy				▓	▓	▓	▓
Billing Denials				▓	▓	▓	▓
Blood Pressure Check (manual)	▓	▓	▓				▓
Blood Pressure Check (Dinamap)	▓		▓				▓
Breath Alcohol	▓	▓	▓				▓
Chart Assembly	▓	▓	▓		▓		▓
Chart Hold	▓	▓	▓		▓		▓
Data Entry	▓	▓	▓				▓
Drug Screening – Collecting	▓	▓	▓				▓
Drug Screening – Resulting	▓	▓	▓				▓
Drug Screening – Shipping	▓	▓	▓				▓
Filing Dictation	▓	▓	▓		▓		▓
Foreign Body in Eye Assistance	▓	▓					▓
Glucometer	▓	▓					▓
Handwashing	▓	▓	▓			▓	▓
Injections	▓	▓	▓				▓
Laceration Repair Assist	▓		▓				▓
Medications	▓	▓	▓				▓
Morgan Lens	▓	▓	▓				▓
Phlebotomy	▓	▓	▓				▓

Random Blood Draws						
Record Release						
Resting EKG						
Saliva Alcohol						
Scheduling Appointments						
Spirometry						
Sterilization of Instruments						
Telephones						
Urinalysis Dip						
Vision Testing						
Vital Signs						
X-rays (receiving at front desk)						
X-rays						

differences between occupational health care and general patient care, and is not put off by the paperwork of workers' compensation. However, if the individual is more impressed with the similarities than the differences in care and considers the job to be equivalent to working in an urgent care center or emergency room, he or she may not be sensitive to the broader issues of workers' compensation, employer expectations, prompt notification of fitness for duty, the need for time efficiency in returning workers reporting for screening tests to their jobs, and early and safe return to work of injured workers. A probationary period should be considered for all new employees.

Supporting the Work Culture

It is incumbent on management to search for well-qualified individuals with appropriate certifications (see Chapter 14). However, a customer-service orientation is equally as important. When hiring, one should consider this question: "If I ran my occupational health service using only volunteers, what would I need to do to retain those volunteers?" The answer to that question correlates with the creation of a positive work environment.

Good morale is important in any service industry. Maintaining employee engagement and motivation can be particularly challenging in the occupational health sector of health care. Occupational health services are not like hospitals and family practices, where there is motivation and reward from directly helping families and children. It is not the same as specialty care, with the rewards of curing the desperately ill. Few patients express their undying gratitude for being saved. The very real intellectual rewards of solving difficult problems are enjoyed by the physicians and occupational health nurses, rarely the rest of the staff. There are enough hassles with workers' compensation carriers, problem patients, and resentful applicants whose workers' compensation claims have been denied to make working in an occupational health service hard on its office staff.

The key to staff engagement, motivation, and retention, and to maintaining a team work ethic is the presence of a strong work culture. The organization's "culture leaders," usually the managers and the top licensed health care professionals (physicians and occupational health nurses) must guide the development of motivation, morale, creativity, and ultimately marketplace success. They must live and believe the occupational health service's culture as well as articulate it. If they demonstrate a sincere and strong culture, employees will always be doing the right thing—because they will always be acting in the best interest of the worker, the employer, and the service providers.

The most detrimental thing the leaders of an occupational health service can do is to fail to create a culture of success. If that happens, providers will not be given the support they need, injured workers will not be given great care, employers will pick up on the lax attitude (even over the telephone), paperwork will seem like a chore and will be filed inaccurately and late, workers' compensation carriers will delay payment, a reputation for mediocrity will quickly circulate, and very soon the service will be in trouble. Neglect and a pervasive sense that quality does not matter and that the service's own employees are just going through the motions of their job may even lead to ethical or procedural violations that will cause embarrassment and further damage to the service's reputation.

It is critically important to create a culture in which the staff is excited to come to work and is excited to provide customers with amazing customer service. But how does one do this? The answer is to create something big, bigger than any individual on the team, with a mission that is bigger than the occupational health service and a vision of quality of care, helping injured workers and their families, and supporting economic growth and productivity.

The culture should be developed together in a team model. The senior leadership may have an idea of what type of culture they want in the service, clinic, or department. However, the staff of the occupational health service has to participate in creating the work culture if they are to "own" it. Otherwise, it will never become the strong work culture the occupational health service needs to do its job consistently and well.

The staff must not only get on board but feel that they are the crew on the boat. Even if it is something as simple as starting a tradition to recognize birthdays, sending postcards to the office while on vacation, or putting personal photos on their desk, the staff must feel like they contributed to and helped develop the culture. They must feel like they developed the culture, or it will never be what you want it to be. Take time together at team meetings to address the company culture.

It may be difficult to develop a distinct work culture if the culture in the parent organization is dysfunctional or highly dominant. For occupational health services that are part of a network, there may also be a corporate culture from their owner, and it is usually very strong and oriented toward hospital culture. For an on-site in-house department, the culture may be that of the employer and reflect the industry in which the employees work.

One way to start is by asking employees to think of past jobs, making a list of all the things they hated about those jobs. Then, the employees should list all the characteristics they think the perfect job should have. These are the things your team will and will not stand for. If everyone on the team understands these things—great. If not, the managers, professionals, and the team should take time to develop a culture together. It is well worth spending time at team meetings to address the work culture in the organization.

It is also important to remember that things that are not motivating to senior health care professionals and managers can be very motivating to staff and a source of inspiration. The team should therefore take time to develop a team motto that everyone agrees to work by and to hold each other accountable for.

The staff will be excited to come to work every day if:

1   *They feel like they are a part of something bigger than themselves.* Staff members should feel a sense of ownership in their job. If they feel that they can solve problems, impact the bottom line, and contribute to the success of the business, they will be more productive. Business owners in general tend to fear passing on more responsibility to employees. However, responsibility is often precisely what creates the feeling of ownership and belonging needed for employees to truly put forth their best effort. Managers tend to view the structure of companies as a pyramid, with the owners and administrative team at the top, and the employees at different levels on the bottom. Successful occupational health service managers realize the pyramid scheme is backwards. The employees should be at the top of the inverted pyramid, with the administrative team constantly asking them for input and advice on how the administrators can make the jobs of their employees more enjoyable and productive.

2   *They feel that their jobs are rewarding, challenging, and exciting.* The excitement that a new employee feels when they first join the staff comes from finding challenge in learning a new position. The constant feedback, especially rewards and praise, they get as they go through training help add to that excitement. But once the training period is complete, the excitement begins to fade. Less excitement leads to less outstanding customer service. To keep the team energized, leaders need to find new ways to challenge them. People, in general, love to be challenged. Younger employees like to show what they are capable of doing. Older employees like to solve problems using their experience and wisdom.

3   *The number one motivator for employees is not more money.* It is actually recognition. Everyone wants to be recognized for their achievements. They want to be noticed when they go above and beyond the call of duty. It is important that the occupational health service have ways of recognizing employees. Ideas for recognition can be as simple as giving someone a new title or selecting employees of the month, or more elaborate, like bonus occupational health services or extra vacation time for employees who go above and beyond. Unfortunately, too many accomplished professionals and managers do not appreciate that what may appear to them to be modest and inconsequential recognition is just as important to their employees as fellowships and professional awards are to them.

4   *They know what is expected of them.* The number one complaint that employees across the nation repeatedly give about their jobs may be surprising. Most employers think that the answer is that employees want better pay or a friendlier boss. Neither answer is correct. The number one thing employees continually hate about their job is not knowing what their supervisors expect of them. If employees walk into a monthly, quarterly, or yearly evaluation and are surprised by their performance review, the managers are doing something wrong. Evaluations should never be a surprise if the staff constantly knows what is expected of them. It is also important to realize and act quickly when there has been a mistake in hiring, and to get rid of that person before they ruin the attitudes of others. One bad apple can indeed ruin the whole barrel.

Recommended Reading and Resources

American Association of Occupational Health Nurses. Online Competencies and Self-Assessment Tool. Available at: https://www.aaohn.org/component/page,shop.product_details/flypage,shop. flypage/product_id,46/category_id,10/manufacturer_id,0/option,com_virtuemart/Itemid,414/. Accessed January, 8 2012.

American College of Occupational and Environmental Medicine. OEM Competencies. Available at: http://www.acoem.org/OEMCompetencies.aspx. Accessed January 8, 2012.

Guidotti TL (2010) *The Praeger Handbook of Occupational and Environmental Medicine.* Santa Barbara CA, Praeger ABC-Clio. See Chapter 20 on "Occupational Health Services."

Hart PA, Olson DK, Frederickson AL, McGovern P (2006) Competencies most valued by employers— implications for master's-prepared occupational health nurses. *AAOHN J,* 54(7): 327–335.

Moser R Jr. (2008) *Effective Management of Health and Safety Programs: A Practical Guide.* Beverly Farms MA, OEM Press, 3rd ed.

US Bureau of Labor. Labor statistics. Available at: http://www.bls.gov/iif/ Accessed January 20, 2012.

Federally Mandated Technician Qualifications

National Institute of Occupational Safety and Health (NIOSH) requires technicians to be certified after training in an approved spirometry course for conducting pulmonary function testing under the OSHA Cotton Dust Standard, 29 CFR 1910.1043 Subpart Z App D. The cotton dust standard outlines specifications for acceptable pulmonary function testing and for qualifications of technicians who perform the test. This is now the minimum standard applied to all pulmonary function tests mandated by OSHA (see Chapter 20), and courses are given frequently by many institutions and providers across the US. The cotton dust standard is available at: http://www.osha.gov/pls/oshaweb/owadisp.show_document?p_ id=10059&p_table=STANDARDS. Accessed January6, 2011. Information on NIOSH-approved spirometry training is available at: http://www.cdc.gov/niosh/topics/spirometry/ training.html. Accessed January 6, 2011.

The OSHA Asbestos Standard, 29 CFR 1910.1001(l)(1)(ii)(8). The asbestos standard requires that "persons other than licensed physicians, who administer the pulmonary function testing required by this section, shall complete a training course in spirometry sponsored by an appropriate academic or professional institution." Available at: http://www.osha.gov/pls/oshaweb/owadisp.show_document?p_table=standards&p_id=9995. Accessed January 6, 2011.

The OSHA Noise Standard, 29 CFR 1910.95(g)(3). The occupational noise standard requires that technicians are to be certified by the Council of Accreditation in Occupational Hearing Conservation, although "a technician who operates a microprocessor audiometer does not need to be certified." This is the type most "occupational health conservationists" (OHC) use, therefore the Medical Technician does not really need to be certified. Available at: http://www.osha.gov/pls/oshaweb/owadisp.show_document?p_table=standards&p_id=9735. Accessed January 6, 2011.

US Department of Transportation (DOT). DOT requires the Medical Technician to be trained as a designated Breath Alcohol Technician (BAT) as well as undergo training for urine collection. These are not OSHA mandates, but DOT. Available at: http://www.dot.gov/odapc/bat_stt.html. Accessed January 6, 2011.

Exhibit 10.1 Responsibilities of the Medical Director

1. Function as the supervising physician of record for the Nurse Practitioner/ Physician Assistant, and on an as needed basis. Review all cases seen as part of the provision of care by [the occupational health service]. The review includes:
    1.1. Injury Care—the history of the injury/medical problem(s) or the findings, diagnoses, treatment plan, limitations or restrictions, discharge, and follow-up. Open cases will be tagged and followed.
    1.2. Exams and Screenings—appropriate testing to meet individual company needs for functional tasks of the candidate, appropriate testing to meet OSHA guidelines, and appropriate screenings to meet drug-free workplace criteria.
2. Provide input regarding the development of medical and operational protocols used by Occupational Health staff and submit protocols, as requested, through appropriate medical staff process for approval.
3. Provide medical direction and consultation to the occupational health staff. Provide educational services in support of wellness and preventive health.
4. Meet at least weekly with the Occupational Health Care Director and staff.
5. Monitor referrals for appropriateness concerning both job-related and non-job related injuries and illnesses identified as a result of [the occupational health service] to physicians who are participating in referral panels.
6. Assist in the recruitment of physicians interested in participating in and advancing occupational health services.
7. Assume responsibility for medical direction of physicians conducting examinations, disability evaluations, return-to-work exams, etc. for [the occupational health service] and monitor the progress of employees referred to physicians. Hold referring physicians accountable for adhering to occupational health protocol and for their evaluation/treatment plans and ultimate outcomes.
8. Assume a leadership role in preventive medicine and encourage employees to seek care from their personal physicians for non-job related medical problems.
9. Provide regular contact with key company representatives, and make presentations to company executives in coordination with occupational health staff.
10. Advise occupational health staff on the content of physical exams and health screening appropriate to the industry setting. Assist in design of medical surveillance services based on safety data sheets and other company protocols. Assist in design of company occupational health services and strategies for promotion of wellness of employees.
11. Review and approve clinical outcome for injury and disability management and return-to-work services.
12. Maintain open communication between occupational health staff, administration, and the medical staff.
13. Provide an annual physician education in-service on occupational health.
14. Participate in case reviews of injured workers out of work for prolonged periods as a result of a work related injury.
15. Supervise staff providers regarding the use of guidelines as competency standards (see Exhibit 10.6):
    15.1. Provider performance criteria to be reviewed periodically and updated.
    15.2. Evaluate provider performance against criteria.

Exhibit 10.2 Responsibilities of the Director, Occupational Health Care

DUTIES

Under the direction of ___[Usually the Medical Director]_____perform a wide variety of, administrative, educational, clinical and supervisory duties within the occupational health service and serve as director [if an occupational health nurse], consultant, and advisor to the nursing staff. Assume responsibility for personnel and patient care within the occupational health service during operational hours. Responsible for the treatment, follow up and monitor of injured workers for client companies within the system.

RESPONSIBILITIES

1. Analyze the needs of the community and facilitate the establishment of expanded ambulatory services. Visit variety of area companies, and perform analysis and assessment; make recommendations, and implementat specific occupational health services in response to identified needs. Evaluate specific industries, within (market area), establish a product and/or service that the occupational health service could use in addressing those identified needs, within specific industries or clients.
2. Propose, develop, implement and cost out various new products to meet various community needs.
3. Perform continuing evaluation of the cost of various services provided in order to ensure appropriate pricing within a defined marketplace.
4. Serve as coordinator in assessing, proposing and developing various specific clinical and non-clinical occupational health services for client companies in [market area].
5. Review the specific work performed by any marketing consultants. Act as supervisor of any marketing consultant and their activities. Supervise other medical contracted vendors as assigned.
6. Develop, establish and maintain the best possible client relationships in marketing and servicing of the occupational health service within the (market area) involving: propose, develop, implement marketing strategies. Represent the (facility) in outside activities pertaining to the occupational health service. Make effective recommendations to applicable administration personnel regarding rate setting, fee schedules, etc., for occupational health service activities.
7. Work in cooperation with internal departments, client companies and contracted health care vendors, (e.g., physical therapy, occupational therapy, social services, emergency department, radiology imaging services, etc.), to propose, develop, and implement specific occupational health service activities pertinent to these individual departments and services.

ADMINISTRATIVE DUTIES AND RESPONSIBILITIES

1. Direct and supervise assigned personnel and activities within the occupational health service involving responsibility for employee performance evaluations, scheduling orientation and training. Make effective recommendations on assigned employee hiring, merit increase, promotion, separation, transfer and other similar personnel actions. Organize nursing regimens with physicians and other health care disciplines within area of responsibility. Prepare assigned employee performance evaluations. Resolve employee disciplinary problems within limits of own position responsibilities.
2. Monitor absence, tardiness and sick time for assigned personnel, counsel employees, and initiate other personnel actions as indicated. Plan and implement goals and objective for assigned areas. Assure assigned areas operate within budgets and responsible for preparation of annual budgets within assigned areas. Recommend improvement of facilities and purchase of new equipment. Recommend changes in staffing based on knowledge of needs, resources and current trends.
3. Maintain knowledge of performance testing on all special equipment, evaluating condition and initiating prompt action for repairs. Recommend changes in policies, procedures and occupational health services and submit to administration with adequate documentation to justify recommendations.

EDUCATIONAL DUTIES AND RESPONSIBILITIES

1. Identify the learning needs of the staff in providing superior occupational health service.
2. Propose, develop and implement educational presentations working in cooperation with the educational resources of the facility/community.
3. Identify appropriate training opportunities for key staff, balancing value against cost within budgetary constraints.
4. Participate in teaching health measures to patients and families in the occupational health service.
5. Participate in the orientation of newly assigned staff to policies and procedures and in their adjustment to new processes.
6. Participate in providing clinical experience for nursing students in the areas of occupational health services.
7. Foster an environment within the occupational health services for professional and personal development.
8. Maintain current knowledge of trends and developments, new products and procedures.

CLINICAL DUTIES AND RESPONSIBILITIES

1. Monitor and evaluate the quality of care in the occupational health service, analyze requirements and implement appropriate staffing patterns.
2. Develop and implement patient care presentations, insure proper documentation on charts is entered by assigned personnel in [the occupational health service].

OTHER DUTIES AND RESPONSIBILITIES

1. Plan, conduct, and document regular conferences to discuss departmental issues. Assist staff to develop and meet professional goals and objectives. Attend educational occupational health services as applicable to own position responsibilities.
2. Serve on various community and business/industrial committees and boards as they directly relate to position responsibilities.
3. Complete specific projects and studies as delegated by the facility administration.
4. Protect the confidentiality of information within areas of own position responsibilities by preventing unauthorized release, both verbally and/or in writing.
5. Assure conformity to all heath and safety requirements by assigned personnel.
6. Promote a continuous quality improvement effort to enhance the services provided to patients, their families, physicians and members of the staff by demonstrating positive attitudes and positive actions through a display of courtesy, congeniality, cooperation, sensitivity and professionalism
7. Perform other similar and related duties as required or directed.

BASIC KNOWLEDGE

Duties require intensive knowledge of a highly specialized field and broad knowledge of major functions or activities. Evidence of continuing education is also required. Broad marketing skills, i.e., sales/service with a business background are highly desirable. A business or related background is essential.

INDEPENDENT ACTION

Responsibilities include establishment of both short-range and long-range plans and objectives within scope of organization-wide policies and common goals. Consult with superior on specific matters only where clarification, interpretation, or exception to organization-wide policy may be required.

SUPERVISORY RESPONSIBILITIES

Duties include direct supervisory responsibility for personnel and activities of the occupational health services. Duties involve supervisory responsibilities for six subordinate personnel. Provide functional or technical supervision of multiple personnel from contracted vendors to [the occupational health service], physicians rendering care, occupational therapy, physical therapy, social service, laboratory, radiology, nursing, communication disorders as they participate in occupational health service, regarding client relations, quality of care, policy and procedures, issues making specific recommendations to those appropriate managers.

Exhibit 10.3 Responsibilities of the Account Services Representative

DUTIES

Under the direction of the Director of Occupational Health Care, perform diversified duties both within and in support of [the occupational health service]. Plan, organize, direct, control, and provide the leadership to achieve [the occupational health service]'s shortrange and longrange business development objectives in the regional product markets. Supervises sales and is responsible for sales management, sales, coordination with other departments, and marketing. Responds in the first instance to customer (i.e. employer) requests, complaints, and queries.

RESPONSIBILITIES

1. Market analysis: Analyze and define the market for product growth within the assigned product market segment. Maintain a served-market analysis defining the total market, company market share, competitor market share, and available market share by product line.
2. Forecast: Provide the data to prepare, update, and control forecasts covering projected newbusiness sales, contracts, proposal activity/costs, and retention of existing clients.
3. Marketing and business planning: Develops marketing plans, business plans, sales strategies, and action plans for identified targets of opportunity that clearly define objectives, goals, win strategies, schedules, and action assignments.
4. Training: Establish and maintain a professional, trained, and motivated staff through effective implementation of performance and career development, appropriate to occupational health services.
5. Appropriate care: Learn and understand which services are generally appropriate for marketing and which are not, and among those that are not appropriate which are illegal (e.g. genetic screening) and which are unethical (e.g. screening low back x-rays).
6. Confidentiality: Maintain high standards of confidentiality and ethics in all communications and interactions, respecting the privacy of patient and non-patient worker information, proprietary business information of clients, and discretion in dealing with the public.
7. Proposal management: Initiate, lead, and direct regional newbusiness proposal and proposal efforts.
8. Sales: Provide direction and leadership to all Account Service Representatives to implement regional sales strategy and tactics including:
   8.1. Develop sales goals and strategies,
   8.2. Responsible for written policies for marketing/sales operations,
   8.3. Hire and train sales personnel,
   8.4. Provide ongoing supervision of sales staff,
   8.5. Increase sales volume through direct sales efforts and by assisting sales reps,

8.6. Coordinate sales department in working toward common goals of the hospital,

8.7. Coordinate the sales team to develop an ongoing marketing effort.

BASIC KNOWLEDGE

Duties require intensive knowledge of highly specialized field and broad knowledge of marketing functions and sales. Masters in Business Administration in marketing and management is preferred. Excellent communication and interpersonal skills are necessary. Must demonstrate ability to coordinate a high level of activity under a variety of conditions and constraints. Direct sales experience with emphasis on major accounts and knowledge of the local area. Sales manager experience is required.

EXPERIENCE

Ten to fifteen years marketing experience in the health care industry is preferable.

INDEPENDENT ACTION

Responsibilities include establishment of both short- and long-range plans and objectives within the scope of organization-wide policies and common goals. Consult with director on specific matters only where clarification, interpretation, or exception to hospital-wide policy may be required.

SUPERVISORY RESPONSIBILITIES

Duties include direct supervisory responsibility for personnel and activities of [the occupational health service] team in marketing and sales.

Exhibit 10.4 Responsibilities of the Senior Occupational Health Nurse (COHN-S)/ Physician Assistant

DUTIES

Under the direction of the Medical Director and the Director of Occupational Health Services, perform a wide variety of duties both within and in support of [the occupational health service].

RESPONSIBILITIES

1. Assess the health status of employees by obtaining health histories, perform physical examinations, post injury examinations and establish treatment plans under the supervision of the Medical Director and the Director of Occupational Health Services.
2. Perform various specialized examinations (e.g., return-to-work evaluations, disability scar measurement evaluations and tonometric screenings).
3. Coordinate activities pertaining to preplacement examinations, working in cooperation with occupational health physician, nurse clinicians, employees, applicable client human resources staff, and client company personnel. Perform the monitoring of additional requested screenings (e.g., pulmonary function tests, urine drug screens and interpretation of results and appropriate follow up of abnormal findings).
4. Assess and refer employee health problems to applicable health care and related resources both within and outside the facility.
5. Support the Medical Director and/or designated physicians, in developing, implementing and maintaining [the occupational health service], but not limited to:
    5.1. Maintaining a current working knowledge of OSHA standards and requirements;
    5.2. Establishing personal contacts with both contracted and non-contracted area companies;
    5.3. Serving as a liaison and resource person between applicable area companies;
    5.4. Maintaining an accurate, professional and confidential medical record system;
    5.5. Consulting with area client companies in evaluating and recommending various preventive medical and educational occupational health services pertinent to their employee needs; and
    5.6. Providing the follow-through to problems and inquiries of client area companies.
6. Compile, prepare and present monthly statistics and reports as needed within the areas of position responsibilities to Medical Director and the Director of Occupational Health Care Director. Assist in budget preparation and monitoring for [the occupational health service] as well as for the contracted companies,

as requested. As necessary, assist in developing and revising policies related to occupational health.

7. Attend meetings, discussions, conferences, seminars and workshops, both within and outside [the occupational health service].

8. Protect the confidentiality of information within areas of position responsibilities by preventing unauthorized release, both verbally and/or in writing.

9. Promote a continuous effort in quality improvement, enhancing the services provided to patients, their families, physicians and members of the occupational health service staff by demonstrating positive attitudes and positive actions through a display of courtesy, congeniality, cooperation, sensitivity and professionalism.

10. Observe all health and safety requirements.

11. Perform other similar and related duties as required or directed.

12. [For hospitals and large specialty groups.] Work in cooperation with the [infection control department] regarding reporting, surveying, screening, and, as appropriate, implementing occupational health services pertaining to prevention or spread of infectious disease. Carry out and coordinate a variety of health care prevention measures for hospital employees including screening occupational health services, immunizations, skin tests, flu vaccinations, etc. in cooperation with occupational physicians.

BASIC KNOWLEDGE

Certification from a national accrediting body to practice as an Occupational Health Nurse Specialist (COHN-S) or a Nurse Practitioner with specific occupational health experience or a Physician Assistant with specific occupational health experience is required.

EXPERIENCE

Three to five years of experience is required.

INDEPENDENT ACTION

Incumbent functions independently within broad scope of departmental policies and practices; generally refers specific problems to supervisor only where clarification of departmental policies and procedures may be required.

SUPERVISORY RESPONSIBILITY

Not applicable

Exhibit 10.5 Responsibilities of the Occupational Health Nurse Clinician

DUTIES

Under direction of the Regional Clinical Manager [refers to satellite locations, if applicable] and the Director of Occupational Health Services, perform diversified duties both within and in support of [the occupational health service]. Perform all identified and specified duties and responsibilities commensurate with level at which appointed.

RESPONSIBILITIES

1. Participate in the development of and present educational occupational health services to the community and/or area client companies. (A minimum of two per year is required).
2. Participate in health screenings by developing goals, educational materials and be able to summarize population screened in report format. (A minimum of one per year is required).
3. Serve as a resource/consultant to client companies within areas of own position responsibilities by evaluating educational needs and providing in-service education to meet those needs. (A minimum of four per year is required).
4. Participate in quality assurance strategies for occupational health services by reporting and monitoring indicators, completing projects and submitting recommendations [to the Regional Clinical Manager or Occupational Health Care Director, whichever is applicable] relating to the indicators evaluated. (A minimum of two projects per year is required).
5. Participate in community health fairs by developing educational materials to address the needs of the fair. (A minimum of two per year is required).
6. Prescribe, delegate and coordinate nursing care.
7. Protect the confidentiality of information within areas of own position responsibilities by preventing unauthorized release, both verbal and/or in writing.
8. Promote a continuous quality improvement effort, to enhance services provided to workers, their families, physicians and members of the staff by demonstrating positive attitudes and positive actions through a display of courtesy, congeniality, cooperation, sensitivity and professionalism.
9. Observe health and safety requirements.
10. Support the theme of service excellence as part of job related activities.
11. Perform other similar and related duties as required or directed.

BASIC KNOWLEDGE

Duties require intensive knowledge of a highly specialized field or broad knowledge of major occupational health functions or activities equal to completion of four years of college. A Bachelor of Science Degree in Nursing or the equivalent is required. Current R.N. registration is required. Certification in Occupational Health

Nursing is preferred. Evidence of continuing education and current certification in Cardiopulmonary Resuscitation (CPR) is required.

EXPERIENCE

Four to five years of related work experience is required.

INDEPENDENT ACTION

Incumbent functions independently within broad scope of department policies and practices; generally refers specific problems to supervisor only where clarification of departmental policies and procedures may be required.

SUPERVISORY RESPONSIBILITY

Not applicable

Exhibit 10.6 Provider Performance Criteria

Each Provider shall:

1. Review each patient's medical history.
2. Perform history and physical exams on each client requiring a examination by a medical doctor.
3. Review abnormal findings and make recommendations regarding the same.
4. Act as a resource for patient questions and concerns.
5. Act as a medical consultant/advisor regarding the medical status of the clients presenting for physical examinations for the staff.
6. Provide work restrictions for those clients examined for return to work.
7. Provide medical evaluations for initial injury evaluations for employees as requested.
8. Complete the initial report of injury for all employees seen.
9. Identify causality for all injuries treated.
10. Coordinate evaluations for temporary and permanent disability.
11. Direct referrals for job-related injuries and illnesses identified as a result of the occupational healths service to physicians on the medical staff of the hospital who are participating in the occupational sealth service referral panels (if applicable).

Exhibit 10.7 Evaluation Form for Provider Competencies

Provider Competencies

Physician's Name: _____ Date:____

Manager's Name: _____

	Met	Partially met	Not met
A. General Responsibilities			
1.　Act professionally at all times			
2.　Arrive at office punctually			
3.　Act as gatekeeper for all patients presenting to the office for treatment and/or referral			
4.　Be responsible for all medical aspects of care in the office			
5.　Maintain patient satisfaction survey scores at or above threshold			
6.　Attend and contribute to provider meetings			
7.　Demonstrate willingness to treat urgent/emergent cases whenever they occur			
8.　Assume leadership role in the office			
9.　Communicate effectively with clients and staff			
10.　Communicate with subspecialists and case managers to promote resolution of case			
11.　Assign duty status of worker that is concordant with findings on physical examination			
12.　Keep cases heading towards cure or maximum medical improvement			
B. Computer Skills			
1.　Demonstrate ability to use EMR, enter results of history and physical examination, diagnosis, treatment plan and work restrictions for all patients evaluated. Demonstrate ability to navigate through medical records and chart box. Build and maintain injury and illness templates			
2.　Document findings of physical examinations in the EMR			
3.　Review and complete all forms related to injuries and exams in the EMR			
4.　Demonstrate competency to send/receive e-mail, view provider schedule			
C. Marketing			
1.　Maintain familiarity with employer contacts			
2.　Maintains telephonic contact with employer			
3.　Performs workplace walk-throughs			
4.　Attends sales calls when requested			
5.　Maintain familiarity with payers, insurers and TPAs			
6.　Identifies potential new clients to marketing staff			
D. Quality Assurance			
1.　Actively participate in QA program			
2.　Maintain quality standard at or above threshold level			
3.　Assist in development of new QA standards			
E. Clinical			
E1. Physical Examinations			
1.　Ability to perform and interpret complete history and physical examination results and document appropriately in the EMR			
2.　Be familiar with the regulatory guidelines for all types of physicals			
3.　Demonstrate expertise in evaluating drivers and other safety sensitive employees undergoing DOT examinations			

	Met	Partially met	Not met
4. Know the components of physical examinations requested by specific clients			
5. Advise clients of what components would be required for requested physical exams and laboratory tests need, based on type of work employee will perform			
E2. Soft Tissue Injury Treatment			
1. Demonstrate detailed knowledge of anatomy and physiology of the musculoskeletal system			
2. Perform a skillful, directed physical examination of the body part injured and arrive at an appropriate working diagnosis			
3. Analyze mechanism of injury and its causal relationship to the patient's complaints and physical findings			
4. Establish a treatment plan and then reevaluate the treatment plan and make appropriate adjustments when improvement does not occur as expected			
5. Appropriate use of home exercises and physical therapy			
6. Order appropriate diagnostic testing			
7. Make appropriate and timely referrals			
8. Perform aspirations and injections of joints and tendons			
9. Have working knowledge of durable medical equipment available and demonstrate ability to use these devices appropriately in the treatment and rehabilitation of injuries			
E3. Pulmonary Evaluations			
1. Ability to perform a complete examination of the respiratory system and apply the clinical findings to situations in the work place			
2. Treatment of acute and subacute inhalation injuries			
3. Have working knowledge of respiratory medications and their application to work related conditions			
4. Familiarity w/OSHA respiratory guidelines & questionnaire			
5. Perform respiratory clearances			
6. Ability to interpret PFT's and apply findings to work place situations			
E4. Cardiovascular Evaluations			
1. Ability to perform a complete cardiovascular examination			
2. Ability to interpret EKG tracings			
3. Familiarity with the indications for GETT & thallium stress tests			
4. Ability to interpret reports of cardiac tests and reports from cardiologist and apply the findings to workplace situations			
E5. Neurological Evaluations			
1. Evaluate, diagnose and treat injuries resulting in neurological symptoms			
2. Diagnose and treat concussions and post concussive syndromes			
3. Order appropriate neurological diagnostic testing			
4. Make referral to specialist when indicated			
E6. Radiology			
1. Order appropriate radiology tests for the evaluation and treatment of work related injuries and illnesses			
2. Perform preliminary review of the radiographs ordered and document in EMR			
3. Order special diagnostic testing (MRI, CT, bone scans, etc.) when indicated			

	Met	Partially met	Not met
4. Review reports of radiographs and special diagnostic tests, document in EMR and make appropriate changes in treatment plan and referrals, if needed, based on those results			
E7. Audiology			
1. Review audiograms and apply findings to work place noise levels			
2. Be familiar with OSHA guidelines for hearing conservation			
3. Be able to determine if significant threshold shifts have occurred when reviewing serial audiograms			
4. Know DOT regulations regarding hearing thresholds			
5. Make recommendations to employees regarding hearing conservation based on audiogram results			
E8. Visual Acuity and Eye Injuries			
1. Evaluate and diagnose work place eye injuries			
2. Demonstrate ability to use Wood's Lamp and slit lamp in the evaluation of eye injuries			
3. Ability to treat corneal abrasions and superficial foreign bodies in the eye			
4. Make appropriate ophthalmologic referrals when indicated			
5. Know DOT guidelines for visual acuity			
6. Have working knowledge of ophthmalogical medications for the treatment of work related eye injuries			
E9. Lacerations			
1. Evaluate lacerations in workers to determine the extent of the laceration			
2. Identify lacerations that require referral to specialist			
3. Demonstrate ability to repair simple and moderately complex lacerations with sterile technique and with appropriate techniques and suture material			
4. Ability to apply appropriate dressings to lacerations			
5. Ability to administer local anesthesia and digital blocks for the repair of lacerations			
6. Ability to use tissue adhesive for laceration repair when indicated			
7. Ability to remove sutures/staples from wounds			
8. Appropriate prescription of antibiotics for contaminated wounds			
9. Schedule appropriate follow up for wound checks and suture removal			
10. Review wound care with injured worker			
E10. Blood Borne Pathogen Exposure (BBPE)			
1. Evaluate workers with potential BBPE and determine if exposure has occurred			
2. Have working knowledge of BBPE protocol			
3. Order appropriate testing and prescribe medication according the BBPE protocol			
4. Assist in determining the donor's serological status			
5. Provide counseling to the exposed worker			
F. Medical Review Officer			
1. Obtain and maintain valid MRO certification			
2. Complete all recommended CME's for MRO			
3. Perform duties of MRO for validation of drug screen results			

Signature: _____Date: _____

Validated by: _____Date: _____

Exhibit 10.8 Competency Checklist – Occupational Health Nurse (COHN)

Function in OH Nursing	Reference / Certification Requirements	Continuing Education Relevant to Function	Date	How met*	Initials of reviewer	Recommendations if not met
Documents and codes patient visits						
Documents preplacement, periodic, and health surveillance visits						
a) health history						
b) occupational health history						
c) health risk appraisal (lifestyle)						
Conducts physical assessments						
a) preplacement						
b) periodic						
c) return to work						
d) retirement / workplace exit						
Conducts health education and counseling session						
Identifies potential work hazards and relationships to health						
Documents and refers FMLA requests						
Conduct, interprets and documents appropriate screening tests:						
a) audiometry (hearing)						
b) spirometry (respiratory)						
c) vision						
d) EKG						
Maintains competency and certification in Basic and/or Advanced Life Support						
Develops Nursing protocols and provides direct nursing care:						
a) vital signs						
b) injections						
c) phlebotomy						
d) test for occult blood						
e) minor surgical procedure assistance						
f) laceration repair assistance						
Conducts appropriate lab tests						
Maintains adequate knowledge and practice of blood-borne pathogens standard						
Performs triage correctly and quickly						
Performs appropriate respiratory fit testing						
Maintains accurate health records of workers, including strict confidentiality						
Analyses aggregate data (illness, injury, pharma) to identify trends						
Conducts case management in thorough and systematic manner						
Develops and implements worker education programs based on hazards and risks:						
a) needs assessment						
b) planning and implementation						
c) program evaluation						
Manages occupational health programs , including budgeting and cost containment						
Other						

* DO – direct observation (specify number of observations) ; D – documentation; SL   skills lab; E – Examination; VR – video review/test; O – other (describe separately)

11 Facilities and Equipment

Donna Lee Gardner and Frank H. Leone

This chapter applies to both on-site and external occupational health services' clinic facilities, including space considerations, recommended equipment, supplies and medications. Additional services, such as physical therapy, extensive health promotion activities, and associated industrial hygiene laboratories, are separate from and in addition to clinic needs.

Facility Design

Design needs can vary markedly from clinic to clinic. This chapter will focus on the general principles of space allocation and clinic design. Space projects are somewhat idealized. It is recognized that most occupational health services occupy space that has been made available to them or rented, not a building that has been purpose-built. However, whenever possible the space should be built out to accommodate the needs of the occupational health service.

Site selection is important. Occupational health services should be easily reached by automobile and close to where employees work, not necessarily where they live. In industries where the job site is large or the workforce is spread out or remote, the clinic should be near the traffic flow in and out of the area.

The building itself should be fully accessible to the disabled and should comply with the accessibility guidelines of the Americans with Disabilities Act (ADA). It is acceptable for the facility to be on an upper floor if access by elevator can be assured for disabled patients and injured workers can be brought downstairs to an ambulance directly and with reasonable privacy. There should be a key-controlled override system in the elevator so that patients can be brought down without stopping for other passengers, in an emergency. There should be a dedicated parking slot available for an ambulance next to an entrance and easily accessible to the elevator. Otherwise, the clinic is best positioned on the ground floor for easy access.

Space is money. Clinic design should be streamlined and clustered by modules so that the assessment area and the initial testing areas are separate from the examination pods. If electronic health records (EHRs) are used, entry can be done in the examination room and the size of the nurse's station and file room can be much smaller.

A well-designed clinic should include:

- a central receiving and triage area for injured workers or well employees
- a barrier-free and sufficiently wide entrance
- examination rooms equipped for minor surgery and stabilization of trauma cases
- a curtain and stool for patients when undressing
- a toilet and shower in the clinic area

- a separate toilet for staff
- an administrative area
- offices for professional staff
- areas for interviews and individualized or small group health education programs
- record-keeping areas and files in hard copy
- special rooms for audiometric testing (including a sound-proof booth)
- procedure room equipped with slit lamp for eye injury examination
- a small dispensing pharmacy
- modern interior fixtures
- a bright, comfortable waiting area
- examination rooms with table, wall-mounted oto- and ophthalmoscopes, vision charts, wall-mounted sphygmomanometers, overhead lighting, sinks, and scales
- a surgery room with overhead adjustable lamps, an adjustable table, resuscitation equipment, and stools
- a small writing desk and a prominent wall clock in each room in which a patient is likely to be interviewed
- locks on all rooms or cabinets containing instruments, syringes, or drugs.

Clinic configuration can be enhanced by estimating the appropriate space needs per provider. Table 11.1 provides a prototype space assessment for a one-provider clinic staff. Provider space allocations must be adapted to the number of providers. Table 11.2 provides an overview of an appropriate space allocation for non-provider space of a prototype occupational health clinic. The best floor plan for a particular facility will depend on the space available, anticipated patient volume, staffing, and services to be provided. Traffic flow is particularly critical; paths to be taken by different types of patients should be traced and areas where paths cross and where patients are likely to stand waiting should be identified and separated. Privacy is essential; the interior of examination rooms should never be visible from the waiting area.

A small, quiet room for ill employees to lie down is very desirable for on-site occupational health services.

Equipment

Although there is some variation among occupational health clinics, most clinics require a basic core of equipment. Box 11.1 is a list of standard equipment required for examination rooms and clinic areas, emphasizing diagnosis and treatment. Table 11.3 provides a list of equipment used for screening and diagnosis, with the cost estimated for each item in 2011 in US dollars.

Table 11.4 provides a list of office equipment needed for each fully-furnished, enclosed professional office with the estimated cost for each item in 2011 in US dollars. The senior occupational health professionals, such as the Medical Officer and Occupational Health Care Director (see Chapter 10), usually have an enclosed office so that highly confidential documents can be worked on in private. Some facilities have spartan working offices or cubicles for providers but a well-furnished, traditional "presentation office" that can be used as needed for meeting with clients and visitors.

The advisability of having a crash cart in an occupational health facility requires careful consideration. The presence of a crash cart in the office requires that staff must at all times be able to handle a code, training must be kept up to date and documented, and the clinic liability is increased. For services that share space in a hospital or medical group, this presents no problem. In facilities that also perform trauma care or that perform stress testing or allergy

Table 11.1 Space per Provider

Position	Location	#	Square Feet	Square Meters
Center Manager	Front Office	1	100	9.5
Receptionist	Front Office	1	Included in reception area	0
Patient Registrars	Front Office	1	Included in reception area	0
Account Exec	Front Office	1	Included in bookkeeping	0
Medical Director	Back office	1	120	11
Add Medical Doctor or Physician's Assistant	Back office	0	110	10
Medical assistants	Exam Bay	2	150 back to back stations	14
X-Ray Tech	Exam Bay	1	Included in radiology	0
Subtotal		9	480	44.5

This is a subtotal for provider space only. Total space requirements will depend on services provided, space allocated to prevention and educational services, storage, and space allocation per Table 11.2. Total space requirements are the sum of 11.1 and 11.2.

Table 11.2 Non-Provider Clinic Space Allocation

Support Space	#	Square Feet	Square Meters*	Comments
Registration Area	1	495	46.0	Waiting and registration
Reception/Charting	1	270	25.0	
Bookkeeping/Admin	1	145	13.5	
File room	1	100	9.5	
Drug Screening	2	150	14.0	2 toilets for urine samples
Procedure rooms	1	140	13.0	
Audio	1	65	6.0	
Breath Alcohol Test	1	65	6.0	May be enlarged for exam room
Pulmonary Function Test	1	65	6.0	
Central Supply	1	115	10.5	Shelving on both sides
Exam Rooms	3	100	9.5	
Lab	1	120	11.0	
Lab storage	1	60	6.0	
Radiology	1	120	11.0	
Dark room	1	45	4.5	Omit with digital films
Employee Lounge	1	140	13.0	
Conference Room	1	170	16.0	May double as library with shelving
Storage	1	200	19.0	
Patient Toilet	1	65	6.0	Not for drug testing
Employee Toilet	1	65	6.0	
Janitorial closet	1	40	4.0	
Electrical/Phone room	1	65	6.0	
Subtotal		3085	287.0	

This is a subtotal for shared operational space only and does not include clinical space for individual providers, given in 11.1. Total space requirements are the sum of 11.1 and 11.2."

Total Net Square Footage Area = 3605 is the total with the addition of about 30% for circulation area (corridors, door clearance, passageways, etc.).

* Rounded up.

Box 11.1 Recommended Equipment for Occupational Health Services

Office furnishings
- Bookcases
- Storage cabinets with locks
- Clocks
- Tables
- Writing boards
- Wastebaskets
- In/out baskets
- Desk lamps
- Bulletin boards
- Calculators

Clinic furnishings
- Adjustable stools with back, height appropriate to counter
- Chart-holders, with priority and occupancy indicators not needed if EMR
- X-ray view boxes – not needed with digital films
- Sinks with surgical handles on faucets, towel racks
- Exam tables
- Chairs
- Medication cabinet, with locks
- Pedal-operated wastebaskets with lid and liners
- Medical records filing cabinets
- Opaque movable screens or curtains
- Instrument trays
- Autoclave
- Cold sterilizer
- Refrigerator

Major Instruments
- Wall mounted oto-/ophthalmoscope
- Wall mounted sphygmomanometer (blood pressure cuff)
- Scales
- Electrocardiograph
- Audiometer
- Vision screening apparatus
- Spirometer, recording
- Suction apparatus
- Slit lamp

Hand Held Instruments
- Canes and crutches
- Ear casettes
- Clamps (Halsted, Kelly, vascular, mosquito)
- Automatic external defibrillators (AED)*
- Crash cart*
- Dental mirror
- Dynamometer (grip strength meter)
- Flashlights
- Laceration repair kits
- Laryngoscope (in crash cart)
- Magnifying lens
- Percussion hammer
- Stethoscope
- Tape measures
- Thermometers
- Tuning forks
- Vision chart, color

Disposable Supplies
- Syringes
- Needles
- Gloves
- Vacutainers
- Blood-draining apparatus
- Tongue depressors
- Cotton swabs
- Gauze pads
- Dressings
- Suture material
- Needles
- Specimen containers
- Elastic bandages
- Cold packs
- Cervical collars
- Surgical masks
- Surgical hoods and drapes
- Eye patches
- Eye pads
- Cotton
- Inflatable splints
- Finger splints
- Wrist splints

Patient/staff education aids
- Videocasette player
- Monitor
- Tape recorder and player
- Patient education material

---

* The necessity for an AED or crash cart in a free-standing occupational medicine clinic and the associated liability if one is present is controversial. See text for discussion.

Table 11.3 Additional Recommended Equipment

Item	#	Unit Cost	Total cost
Pulmonary function	1	3,000	3,000
Breathalyzer	1	2,500	2,500
Audiometric booth	1	2,000	2,000
Visionoter	1	1,500	1,500
Centrifuge	1	800	800
Lab chair with arm	1	225	225
Lab refrigerator	1	125	125
Slit lamp	1	4,500	4,500
Scale	1	200	200
Stethoscope, sphygmomanometer	4	500	2000
Exam tables – straight	3	800	800
Exam tables – gyn	1	1,500	1,500
Exam chair stools	4	100	400
Medical waste bins	8	40	320
Procedure room exam light	2	1,100	2,200
Mayo stands	2	80	160
Drug disposable boxes	4	20	80
Medication refrigerator with lock	1	250	250
Eye chart, patient education tools (spine, arm, etc.)		4,000	4,000
X-Ray	1	50,000	50,000
Portable EKG	1	825	825
			$77,385

desensitization, and for remote locations, a crash cart is required. However, if there are no nurses or physicians in the center during part of the day, during which it may be staffed by medical technicians, a crash cart becomes a liability, not an asset. A free-standing occupational health center that does not provide high-risk services or emergency care would not be liable if there is not a crash cart in the center, unless they perform services. In the absence of a crash cart, the occupational health center would only be held to the standard of a physician's office.

Automatic external defibrillators (AEDs) have become nearly ubiquitous in airports, public spaces, and in many industrial workplaces as well as health care facilities. Although many states do not require them to be in physician's office, they are required in other states and are expected by employers and patients who are aware of them. Recent studies have suggested that they are less effective than once thought but their absence would still be difficult to explain. Having AEDs in the occupational health service facility requires that they be maintained, appropriately programmed, and that the staff be trained, drilled in their use, and covered by written standard operating procedures and policies.

Table 11.5 provides a list of information technology (IT) equipment needs by provider workstation.

Table 11.4 Recommended Equipment

Office Equipment		#	Cost per Unit	Total Cost
Desks, chair, file cabinet	Staff	4	1,000	4,000
Desks, chair, file cabinet	Medical Director	1	1,500	1,500
Chairs	Reception	8	75	600
Television w/ VCR	Reception	1	250	250
Plants	Reception	5	30	150
Artwork	Various	6	50	300
Microwave	Staff Room	1	100	100
Coffee pot	Staff Room	1	50	50
Fax machines	Reception Billing	2	150	300
Copier		1	n/a	Lease
Lockers	Staff Room	1	200	200
Coat rack	Reception	1	100	100
Refrigerator	Staff Room	1	150	150
Phone system	Various	1	2,000	2,000
Miscellaneous office	Various	1	500	500
Minimum for staff of 4 and 1 medcal director				$10,200

Table 11.5 Hardware and software requirements

Hardware and Software		#	Cost per Unit	Total Cost
Center Manager	Computer	1	1,000	1,000
Receptionist	Computer	1	1,000	1,000
Patient Registrars	Computer	1	1,000	1,000
Account Exec	Laptop	1	1,500	1,500
Medical Director	Computer	1	1,000	1,000
Network	Server	1	4,000	4,000
Printers	Billing	2	500	1,000
Office Practice	Software	1	20,000	20,000
Sales Management	Software	1	500	500
Minimum to accommodate staffing assumptions; additional providers will require individual or shared access depending on need and schedule.		10		$31,000

Pharmacy

It should not be necessary for an injured worker to take valuable time to obtain a common drug from a pharmacy, whether it is under the same roof as the occupational health service or not. To expedite care and to ensure patient education by the treating provider, a limited formulary should be available for dispensing on site at the time of the visit. Dispensing pharmacy needs are often met by commercial services that maintain stocks for the clinic, so that inventory is not required.

Medications that should be available for dispensing by the providers in the facility are listed in Box 11.2. Opiates and other major drugs of abuse should never be kept in stock, under any circumstances. Injuries that involve such severe pain that morphine would be required and that would require major analgesics to be dispensed on site should be triaged to an emergency room. Today there is widespread overprescribing of opioids, and an increase in deaths of injured workers on opioids for chronic pain, estimated to be at least 200 per year in the US and probably much more, given evidence for considerable underreporting. (The American College of Occupational and Environmental Medicine has developed guidelines for chronic use of opioids.) In addition, the presence of opioids on the premises leads to avoidable security issues with clinical facilities. Synthetic (non-opiate) opioids for pain relief during stabilization for transfer or short-term use might be kept in stock, depending on the preference of the medical staff, but only in a double-locked, secure facility. They can always be prescribed if a pharmacy is nearby, at the cost of modest inconvenience to the patient.

If an occupational medicine service has several facilities within a reasonable distance, the most central or largest should be designated as a travel center and central dispensary to maintain a limited stock of more expensive but uncommonly used drugs, vaccines, and immunoglobulin (hepatitis B immunoglobulin, immune globulin). It is much more cost-effective for a clinic staff person to drive it to another location or to send the dose as needed by courier than to maintain stocks of expensive, perishable, and seldom-used medications at every location.

Design and Decor

Interior fixtures should be those appropriate to a modern clinic. The waiting area should be bright, comfortable, and relaxing. All surfaces should be easily cleaned and light-colored, with a minimum of nooks and crannies. Locks should be on all rooms or cabinets containing instruments, syringes, and drugs, even if constantly attended, and should be used after hours, even if the main clinic door is secured. Whenever possible, built-in fixtures and indirect lighting are preferred for convenience, appearance, and functionality, since they can be mounted above cabinets to conserve space and reduce clutter.

Interior decor serves many functions. One of the functions is communication. An occupational health service that looks like a modern medical facility will inspire confidence. It will reinforce the impression that the occupational health staff is serious and dedicated. An on-site clinic that looks shabby will convey the impression that the health of employees is a low priority in the organization. Bold primary colors are fine for accent but are visually disconcerting when overused. Reds and yellows may even make people uncomfortable because they are colors used in warning signs in the workplace. The color combinations used should be soft and warm. Pastels, on the other hand, are not preferred in a predominantly masculine workforce. A bright decor, preferably with some natural lighting, will lend a more cheerful aspect to the clinic. Clinics should not experiment with their decor, which should be familiar and reassuring, neither overly trendy nor bland.

Another function of decor is orientation. Even workers who are well and reporting only for screening or preventive services are often anxious on entering a medical facility. The anxiety is even greater among new employees and among the injured or ill. Nonverbal cues help to orient a person. Color-coded rooms and lines on the wall (not on the floor, because the patient has to look down to see them and misses other cues) as well as snappy graphics help to orient the patient and thereby reduce anxiety, as well as increasing efficiency.

Box 11.2 Recommended Dispensing and Treatment Pharmacy for an Occupational Health Service

1. Antibiotics: keep one for intravenous (IV) administration on hand and several oral alternatives
   1.1. Rocephin™ (good choice for IV- also covers everything you would use penicillin (PCN) for)
   1.2. amoxicillin
   1.3. amoxicillin/clavulanate (Augmentin™)
   1.4. cephalaxin
   1.5. erythromycin (could consider azithromycin)

2. Analgesics: keep one for IM administration on hand and multiple oral
   2.1. ketorolac for IM
   2.2. acetemenophen
   2.3. ibuprofen, naproxen, and another 1-2 NSAID of provider choice
   2.4. tramadol
   2.5. Non-opiate opioids (If synthetic opioid pain medication is allowed, consider hydrocodone/acetaminophen (Vicodin™) and or oxycodone/acetaminophen (Percocet™)

3. Muscle relaxants
   3.1. cyclobenzaprine
   3.2. skelaxin
   3.3. valium

4. Steroids: IV and po
   4.1. methylprednisolone IM
   4.2. Medrol™ dose pack
   4.3. Prednisone™ (Some providers are very reluctant to prescribe steroids and do not even keep prednisone in stock)

5. Eye drops
   5.1. sulfacetamide opthalmologic
   5.2. gentamycin opthalmologic
   5.3. tobramycin opthalmologic
   5.4. combined product (Controversial. Provider may elect to use eye antibiotic with steroid such as TobraDex™. However, one must be very sure of the eye examination before dispensing, because administering steroid in a herpetic infection can lead to severe consequences. If an injured eye requires steroid, the patient should probably be referred to an ophthalmologist.)

6. Artificial tears

7. Antihistamines: 1 IM and several oral
   7.1. diphenehydramine, as Benadryl™ IM
   7.2. Benadryl™ po
   7.3. non-sedating antihistamine. Providers choice: fexofenadine (Allegra™), loratadine (Claritin™).

8. Topical creams
   8.1. Silvadene
   8.2. Topical antibiotic
   8.3. Topical analgesic (Such as pramoxine/zinc (Caladryl™ clear, for poison ivy dermatitis)

9. Vaccines
   9.1. Tetanus and diphtheria (Td)
   9.2. Influenza
   9.3. Hepatitis B
   9.4. If a designated travel medicine center, will need many more.

10. Epinephrine - or EpiPen™

11. Immunoglobulins
    11.1 Hepatitis B immunoglobulin (HBIG)
    11.2 Other immunoglobulins specific to the practice. (Inventory can only be justified if the likelihood of need is high, otherwise stocks will expire before use.)

Recommended Reading and Resources

American College of Occupational and Environmental Medicine. Guidelines for the Chronic Use of Opioids. Available at: http://www.acoem.org/Guidelines_Opioids.aspx. Accessed January 25, 2011.

Harnett T. Create a standard of emergency care in the office to protect against legal liability. *Medscape News*. Available at: http://www.medscape.com/viewarticle/545432. Accessed January 11, 2012.

Miller RL, Swensson ES (2002) *Hospital and Healthcare Facility Design*. New York, W. W. Norton.

National Institute of Building Sciences. Whole Building Design Guide: Clinic / Health Unit. Available at: http://www.wbdg.org/design/clinic_health.php. Accessed January 9, 2012.

Rousmaniere P. How many injured workers die from opioids? Conventional claims operations have helped sweep the opioid issue under the rug. *Risk & Insurance*. January 24, 2012. Available at: http://www.riskandinsurance.com/story.jsp?storyId=533344681. Accessed April 12, 2012.

US Access Board. ADA Accessibility Guidelines for Buildings and Facilities. Available at: http://www.access-board.gov/adaag/html/adaag.htm. Accessed January 9, 2012. The Access Board is a joint standards-setting body of the US government, involving the Department of Justice and the Department of Transportation.

12 Office Procedures

Donna Gardner and Karen O'Hara

Office procedures and workflow processes that expedite patient care are critical to occupational health service operations. Rapid and responsive service, efficient and accurate handling of workers' compensation information, timely reporting, familiarity with specialized vocabulary and procedures, and minimizing downtime for the worker are all hallmarks of a successful occupational health service and the keys to adding value and making it competitive on cost with other health care providers.

The objective is to optimize the use of space, protect privacy, and streamline the manner in which both patients and workers who present for screening and preventive services progress through the clinic from reception to discharge. This chapter applies to all models of occupational health services that handle a moderate to high volume, whether community-based (see Chapters 1, 9, and 19) or employer-based (see Chapters 1 and 6).

Optimally, clinic workflow is supported by a computerized information management system equipped with a dedicated occupational health software program and electronic medical record capabilities. There are several proprietary occupational health systems on the market. It is essential that one of them be used, because software designed for hospitals, outpatient clinics, or primary care work poorly and the occupational health service that uses them risks losing competitive advantage, making mistakes in processing critical information, and using incorrect and possibly prejudicial terminology in reports. Using a dedicated occupational health-related software program, receptionists may also easily access client company information such as physical exam requirements, laboratories used for drug screening, post-injury specialty testing, contact names for results reporting, and billing information for workers' compensation and employer-paid services.

Smooth workflow in an occupational health setting depends on a clearly defined documentation and tracking process. Using specially-designed occupational health care software, registration may be performed with a minimal amount of effort, because the software stores client contact information, company protocols, examination components, and other screening criteria for post-offer, post-accident, and return-to-work physicals. Proper software also triggers scheduling for periodic health surveillance and generates detailed reports for employee groups as well as longitudinal data for individuals. Because the medical director and other clinical staff are responsible for patient care, they should be consulted when screening forms, treatment templates, and other patient documentation processes are developed or new software is implemented. Time spent in the development phase results in a more comprehensive patient record and less time spent correcting problems in the implementation phase.

Upkeep of the client (employer) database is another critical component. This can be done routinely when a worker presents for injury care or other services, by making periodic phone calls to client companies, and by conducting annual client satisfaction surveys that request current contact information. Surveys can also be done using paper questionnaires (which are likely to have a low return rate), by telephone (which has the advantage of allowing discussion and capturing comments), email, or a web-based survey instrument (generally preferred these days).

Scheduling

As in all health care operations, scheduling helps to even the workflow through the day. However, occupational health services cannot expect all or even most visits to be scheduled well in advance. Community-based services, especially, rely on walk-ins. It is only practical to schedule follow-up appointments and screening or preventive services. Table 12.1 provides estimates of the amount of time required for common functions in an occupational health service.

In addition to occasional emergencies that need to be triaged to an emergency room, occupational injuries occur unpredictably and require that the injured worker proceed promptly to the occupational health service for evaluation, documentation (to initiate the process of workers' compensation or to determine whether the case is entered into the Occupational Safety and Health Administration (OSHA) 300 log as a lost-time injury), and disposition (treatment, referral, return-to-work determination, scheduling follow-up). It is somewhat helpful to encourage employers to telephone the occupational health service to notify the provider that a patient is coming, but many supervisors will not bother, especially when the injury is minor.

Because of the costs involved in having a worker off the job, employers are very conscious of time and efficiency. Seasonal downtime can be anticipated and planned for. When the workplace is unexpectedly slow, however (for example if there is downtime, unanticipated repairs or maintenance, or a delivery problem of needed parts), employers should be encouraged to send their workers for screening (periodic health surveillance) and preventive services early, so as to take advantage of the time.

Table 12.1 Scheduling Policies

Occupational health patients will be scheduled for initial and return appointments. Recommended time for appointments are as follows.

Type of Appointment	Time (minutes)
1. Preplacement evaluation	
1.1 Brief	15
1.2 Moderate	20
1.3 Comprehensive	40
2. Initial visit for injury	30
3. Follow-up visit for injury	
3.1 Standard	15
3.2 Brief follow-up	10

Adequate initial appraisal and/or treatment and/or advice must be offered to all employees who are scheduled. Any scheduled patient who presents himself or who is presented to the service by those claiming responsibility for the patient is eligible for care. No patient may be refused care for financial, religious, social, or socioeconomic reasons.

Registration

The registration process is the cornerstone of the operation. "Reception" is often on the firing lines of patient complaints, for example long waits, patient in pain, etc. A customer-service orientation is essential, as well as a proactive approach to address any concerns before they escalate. Employees who are sent to a clinic by their employer, rather than going there by choice (see Chapter 2), may be particularly sensitive and may overreact to a less than stellar customer service experience.

Registration procedures for employer-related services typically require the patient's name, the name of their employer, and the department in which they work. Picture identification in the form of a driver's license or legal identification card is recommended, in order to validate the identity of the patient. This can be scanned into the electronic medical record or copied into the paper chart. The occupational health service has no reason to and should not involve itself with issues of citizenship, immigration status, or legal residence.

Candidates presenting for preplacement, post-offer fitness-for-duty evaluations (see Chapters 22 and 23) and other screening functions need to complete health, medications, and occupational history forms; these workers are not "patients" because there is no treatment planned, and they should be considered to be "subjects," with a different status and a different relationship to the health care provider (see Chapter 3). Figure 12.1, later in this chapter, demonstrates the flow for these subjects. These workers are subject to different procedures and rules. For example, the family history (because it is construed as "genetic information" and falls under the Genetic Information Nondiscrimination Act in the US) cannot be obtained or recorded in the medical record. There is also no defined provider–patient relationship for such subjects (see Chapter 3).

Workers become patients when they are injured, and diagnosis and treatment is contemplated. There are also specific workers' compensation and medical forms providers need patients to complete when evaluating an injury. Patients should be asked to describe the nature and cause of their injury as part of the examination process. Forms may need to be translated from English to other languages, which is also facilitated by computer. Many clinics now use kiosk-based electronic processes rather than paper forms to obtain initial information from patients. Figure 12.2, later in this chapter, demonstrates the flow for these patients.

It is advisable to have all staff members who interact with subjects and patients at the front desk, even if only occasionally or to fill in, to practice by conducting mock registrations to ensure they understand the process for all patient visit types. It may even be worthwhile taking the time to simulate adverse situations, such as an angry patient or impatient worker, using someone the staff member does not know, so that front-office staff will gain some insight into managing fraught situations.

Front-office staff should be trained in phone etiquette—with scripts provided—and well-versed in the information management system adopted by the occupational health service. Receptionists must be familiar with client-company protocols, all paperwork and procedures associated with initial and follow-up patient encounters, and federal patient privacy provisions under the Health Insurance Portability and Accountability Act (HIPAA) (see

Chapter 13). While it is true that HIPAA does not strictly apply to workers' compensation or to confidentiality of records in occupational health, it would be a serious mistake to confuse staff and to risk a misunderstanding and reputational damage by treating non-HIPAA covered records differently (see Chapter 3).

Triage

Triage is an important function of the reception staff, who should be instructed when to give priority to an obviously injured patient or to call one of the licensed health professionals to triage patients with certain signs, symptoms, and conditions such as lacerations, broken bones, inability to walk unassisted, eye injuries, toxic exposures, difficulty breathing, and complaints of chest or arm pain requiring emergency transport to a hospital. The provider has a duty to call an ambulance for patients and visitors who require emergency care (including walk-ins who may have come into the nearest medical office for personal health problems). In situations where a patient or visitor who is impaired or in apparent distress declines an ambulance and states an intention to drive, the provider must be firm and persuasive in talking them out of it and should immediately document their efforts for the record.

At the same time as care is being given to a priority patient or an emergency is being triaged, workers who present as subjects for scheduled screening services or preventive services should not be sidetracked, and should enter a second line of flow so that their care is not delayed by an acute emergency (see Chapter 19). One reason that employers prefer committed occupational health services is that their workers are not kept waiting by primary care patients who assume a higher priority.

The role of an occupational health service in triage is not always either to provide definitive treatment or to refer the patient to an emergency room. There are many situations in which partial care at the level required may be provided at the time for definitive management by another provider at a more convenient time. For example, a ruptured tendon in the hand or a spiral fracture of the ankle are generally not a surgical emergency requiring immediate operation, and if they present after hours the emergency room physician may only confirm the diagnosis and schedule treatment for the next day or later. In such situations it is an inadvertent disservice to the patient to refer the injured worker to a crowded emergency room for a long wait that is unnecessary. The licensed health care providers in the occupational health service should be able to recognize these situations, stabilize injuries, provide pain relief (without opiates), and make follow-up appointments with an appropriate specialist, most often an orthopedic surgeon.

Pre-Examination

Many clinics have a "registration area" (no longer called a "waiting room") and have set aside a separate space within it where medical technicians can take vital signs and prepare patients for their evaluation. Within their scope of training and certification, the medical technician may perform all the screening tests required by the employer. This process is more efficient than if the clinic has a screening room set aside behind the registration area, with multiple testing stations. Audiometry, spirometry, height/weight and vitals, special vision testing, blood draw, and electrocardiogram (screened and out of sight) all may be performed in this space. A private, secure area for breath-alcohol and urine drug screening (see Chapter 27) is also required.

Policies and procedures for each testing procedure are retained electronically in a clinical care manual. This includes tables or checklists containing each component of the screening process. The medical technician is responsible for documenting all tests completed before the patient is "roomed" (placed in an examination room) for the examiner.

Scheduling is used to maximize utilization of staff and available space. With multiple stations, the staff can circulate patients through the screenings quickly, preferably with automatic uploading of test results. Practice management software is used to document results for each screening test, to identify trends over time for the worker, to identify trends on a group basis that may signal a problem in the workplace, and to ensure that data are accurate and complete.

Examination

Once screening is completed, the medical technician escorts the patient to the "exam room."

Prior to HIPAA most occupational health services (like many emergency departments in hospitals) used a whiteboard in the medical provider area to alert medical providers that a subject or patient is ready to be seen. Posting the patient's last name, the type of exam, and the time placed in the room allowed the medical providers to triage patients by condition and arrival time. After HIPAA, with its demands for stringent confidentiality, many occupational health services have transferred this information to either their electronic information system, or paper that is covered to prevent the accidental release of information.

The simplest method of signaling that a patient is ready to be seen is to mount a file holder on the door and to put the chart in it when the patient is ready. In larger occupational health services the dedicated occupational health nurse or lead medical technician may function as triage officer and direct the medical providers to the next patient.

Some occupational health services use a flag system, either electronic with colored lights, or mechanical with plastic flaps. The main drawback of the use of flag systems occurs if the medical providers cannot see the room flags from their workstation. Multiple flags can be used as notification to alert support staff for the need to provide ancillary services such as X-ray, splinting, gait training, discharge, etc.

The paper chart or electronic medical record provides clinical documentation for the examiner. Templates for specific exams are contained in the clinic software. Many organizations find it works best to keep patients in exam rooms until they are ready for discharge in order to expedite workflow. The medical technician escorts the patient to the discharge processing area.

Discharge

The discharge process also must be HIPAA compliant. Discharge staff provide a summary of the visit to patients undergoing post-offer exams and initiate the process for reporting results to the prospective employer.

If the patient has suffered an injury, the process includes a review of specific instructions for aftercare, including an explanation of any restrictions on work or home activities, and follow-up appointments, as necessary. Additionally, a process must be established to provide the employer information to facilitate the return-to-work process. In some clinics the physician/provider calls the client company with the initial injury report and others fax a work status report to the employer. Email is generally not used because of the risk of a breach in confidentiality, unless the message can be encrypted, the arrangement of which with the employer is more trouble than faxing.

It is important that the information sent to the employer contain only the return-to-work status ("fit," "unfit," and "fit with accommodation," specifying the restriction and accommodation needed; see Chapter 22) and follow-up appointment dates. The diagnosis

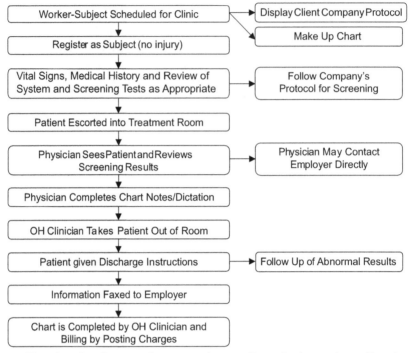

Figure 12.1 Flow chart for office procedures: screening tests (fitness for duty and surveillance)

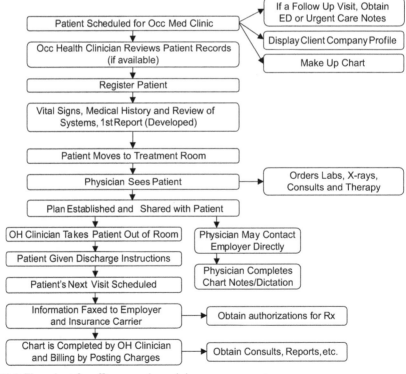

Figure 12.2 Flow chart for office procedures: injury management

and other confidential medical information should never be sent directly to the employer unless the patient signs a release (see Chapter 3).

Information sent to the workers' compensation insurer must be complete and accurate and must be accompanied by the physician's detailed examination and "SOAP" notes (subjective symptoms, objective signs and findings, assessment, plan) for each appointment.

When a patient requires additional treatment or follow-up care by a specialist (most often an orthopedist, pulmonary specialist, neurologist, or rehabilitation medicine specialist), it is extremely important to provide the specialist with a copy of the medical evaluation and any other pertinent information that may be relevant to the treatment and outcome for the patient. Patients must sign two "release of information" (ROI) forms, one of them "From–To" and the other "To–From," to ensure that the information can go both ways. In addition, the occupational health services should request a copy of the results from the specialist and from physical therapy, and any follow-up information required until the patient is completely discharged from their care and subsequently from the occupational health service.

The employer should remain fully advised as to the work status of the patient until he/she is returned to work with no restrictions or if fully discharged from care with continuing work restrictions. It is extremely important that the return to work plan and any work restrictions are understood by and communicated to both the patient and the employer contact in a consistent manner, as misunderstandings over what was meant can be difficult to reconcile.

Billing and Accounts Receivable

The billing process starts at registration and upon discharge involves documentation of specific medical procedures and tests performed, and any supplies used during the visit. The provider is responsible for coding the level of care provided during the evaluation and management process as defined in the Current Procedural Terminology (CPT) coding manual. The provider also is responsible for determining the diagnosis. Accurate documentation and coding is critical in order for the provider to receive appropriate reimbursement from the employer or insurer.

Occupational health services that are part of a larger network may be required to use the billing office of their owner or the larger facility, instead of maintaining a separate operation. There should at least be a core staff of billing personnel who are trained and expert in workers' compensation and its special features, who are able to transmit or at least track clinical reports together with billing information, and who are given authority to make telephone calls to resolve billing problems promptly.

Billing procedures are specific to the software in use, but in general it is the provider who identifies the codes and the registration clerk who reconciles charts at day's end to ensure that all necessary documentation is complete before all documentation is sent to the billing department. This finalizes the billing information.

The process for monitoring the payment cycle is triggered once the bill is finalized. Typically, employer bills for exams and screenings are sent monthly. Bills for injury treatment are sent to workers' compensation insurance carriers and self-insured companies as soon as they are ready, and not later than three days post-treatment.

Private insurance bills generated by clinics that provide episodic care for employees at contracted companies are sent immediately after the visit. Insurance billing follows a more structured format than billing to employers. Insurers follow a specific process, and if they do not receive adequate documentation for the services provided, they will not pay the bill. To avoid denials, it is important to monitor breakdowns in the documentation process and take necessary corrective action.

Billing procedures have been standardized in the US largely through the influence of Medicare reimbursement. All facility bills must be in UB 04 format. All outpatient provider and physician bills must be in HCFA 1500 format. CPT/Health Care Common Procedure Coding System (HCPCS) codes must be entered and complete. Any competent billing agent will know what these are. Table 12.2 defines the most common codes used for clinic encounters for patient care.

Table 12.2 Important CPT/HCPCS Coding Definitions for Occupational Health Services

Coded Service	Required Three Components and Level of Severity*	Definition
99201. Office or other outpatient visit for the evaluation and management of a new patient	Minimal severity 1 Problem-focused history 2 A problem-focused examination 3 Straightforward medical decision making.	Counseling and/or coordination of care with other providers or agencies are provided consistent with the nature of the problem(s) and the patient's and/or family's needs Usually, the presenting problems are self-limited or minor.
99202. Office or other outpatient visit for the evaluation and management of a new patient	Low severity 1 An expanded problem-focused history 2 An expanded problem-focused examination 3 Straightforward medical decision making.	Counseling and/or coordination of care with other providers or agencies are provided consistent with the nature of the problem(s) and the patient's and/or family's needs. Usually, the presenting problem(s) are of low to moderate severity.
99203. Office or other outpatient visit for the evaluation and management of a new patient	Moderate severity 1 A detailed history 2 A detailed examination 3 Medical decision making of low complexity	Counseling and/or coordination of care with other providers or agencies are provided consistent with the nature of the problem(s) and the patient's and/or family's needs. Usually, the presenting problem(s) are of moderate severity.
99204. Office or other outpatient visit for the evaluation and management of a new patient	High severity 1 A comprehensive history 2 A comprehensive examination 3 Medical decision making of moderate complexity	Counseling and/or coordination of care with other providers or agencies are provided consistent with the nature of the problem(s) and the patient's and/or family's needs. Usually, the presenting problem(s) are of moderate to high severity.

* Definitions of levels of severity:
- Minimal: A problem that may not require the presence of the physician, but service is provided under the physician's supervision.
- Self-limited or minor: A problem that runs a definite and prescribed course, is transient in nature, and is either not likely to permanently alter health status or has a good prognosis with management/compliance.
- Low severity: A problem where the risk of morbidity without treatment is low; there is little to no risk of mortality without treatment; full recovery without functional impairment is expected.
- Moderate severity: A problem where the risk of morbidity without treatment is moderate; there is moderate risk of mortality without treatment; either uncertain prognosis or increased probability of prolonged functional impairment.
- High severity: A problem where the risk of morbidity without treatment is high to extreme; either there is a moderate to high risk of mortality without treatment or a high probability of severe, prolonged functional impairment.

There is a supplemental code (S9088) that is recognized by many payers (for example, workers' compensation in Colorado) for unscheduled walk-in urgent cases outside of regular business hours. This one of the "S codes" that define the nature of certain services and are not allowed for billing to Medicare. (Medicare is only very rarely a payer for occupational health services, for example in a consultation for diagnosis of a disorder with a toxic etiology, and never for workers' compensation. However, Medicare already carries a huge burden of recognized occupational disease and complications of disability, and may be more responsive in the future to disability management and prevention services as the workforce ages.)

Obtaining timely payment on accounts receivable is less often a problem in workers' compensation than with general health insurance and often more than makes up for more modest allowable fees. Bills for employer-paid services, on the other hand, must be carefully monitored in order to avoid extended days in accounts receivable or providing services to a client that has fallen behind on payment. The rule of thumb for employer-paid services is a maximum of 45 days in accounts receivable, and for injury care, 75 days, although this varies widely by state in the US. The billing department provides the manager with a list of delinquent client companies. Collections calls typically are handled internally. This task may fall to one or more clerical/billing trained staff, and, in the case of a major client, possibly the manager him- or herself. A discrete call may be all that is needed to determine if there is an oversight or if the client wishes to make arrangements for installment payments.

In Canada, billings for services are reimbursed through the provincial health care insurance plan, with later inter-fund transfers from the workers' compensation board to the health plan for qualifying cases.

Documentation

Documentation in workers' compensation cases is usually more detailed and complete than for other injuries. This is because it is necessary to establish the grounds for determining causation and work relationship and to provide for case management and monitoring by the carrier.

Quality assurance depends in part on the completeness of records, which should be reviewed periodically as the basis for continuous quality improvement, process efficiency, provider performance evaluation, resolution of problems and complaints, audits, and random quality assurance monitoring. (See Chapter 17 for a discussion of process improvement and performance indicators.)

Exhibits 12.1 through 12.3 are a series of criteria for the completeness of records, which can be used as documentation quality standards. They cover initial visits for injury (Exhibit 12.1), follow-up visits (Exhibit 12.2), and discharge visits (Exhibit 12.3).

In a busy, high-volume service most notes are dictated. Exhibit 12.4 provides a template for organizing dictation that is consistent with the criteria used to review the record for completeness.

In order to enforce good practices in documentation and quality assurance, there should be a written policy for documentation in the occupational health service that applies to all providers, even for small operations. Exhibit 12.5 is a concise policy that can be adopted for the purpose for small operations that still use paper charts. It recognizes the differences between the worker as patient, with an injury, and as a subject, for screening and preventive services. In the age of the electronic medical record, however, the use of paper predominantly or exclusively is to be discouraged.

Tracking the progress of a case is essential for injured workers, in order to optimize care and ensure early but safe return to work when they are able. Working with the case manager at the workers' compensation carrier, the occupational health service representative can expedite care, ensure adherence to treatment, and closely monitor recovery. The point at which the permanently impaired injured worker reaches "maximum medical recovery" can also be identified more readily, for the purposes of impairment assessment and disability evaluation (see Chapter 26). Exhibit 12.6 is a template for tracking injury cases that can be used in paper format for case management.

Recommended Reading and Resources

American College of Occupational and Environmental Medicine (ACOEM) (2004) *Occupational Medicine Practice Guidelines*. Chicago, ACOEM, 3rd ed., as updated. Purchase includes one-year subscription to online version and regular updates. Available at: http://www.acoem.org/practiceguidelines.aspx. Accessed January 6, 2011.

Moser R Jr. (2008) *Effective Management of Health and Safety Programs: A Practical Guide*. Beverly Farms MA, OEM Press, 3rd ed.

Stern D. Practice Velocity Urgent Care Solutions. Available at: http://www.practicevelocity.com/urgent_care/coding/S9088.php. Accessed January 11, 2012. Because of the similarity between occupational health services and urgent care, the practice management literature on urgent care often applies to occupational health. Dr. Stern writes a column on "Codes and Coding" in the *Journal of Urgent Care Medicine*, the topic of which for this one is the S9088 code.

Exhibit 12.1 Criteria for Documentation Review: Initial Visit for Injury

Sample scripts are provided in italics to illustrate the criteria and can be used verbatim in dictation. Elements of the documentation given below in capital and lower case letters can be used as headings in the record, dictated note, and review document, to keep documents consistent.

- Review of History must include reference to past medical, social, family and occupational histories and any contributing factors that would affect this injury/illness, such as comorbidities and states of susceptibility. Possible script might read: *"Past Medical History, allergies to medications, and current medical treatments were obtained and reviewed. Occupational, social and family histories were obtained and reviewed. All the above stated information is documented in the confidential medical record."*
- Review of Systems must be documented and the systems identified as below in the medical record, but only those pertinent to the injury treatment should be discussed in the worker's compensation note. Possible script: *"Information regarding vital signs and review of systems documented in the confidential medical record".*
- A minimum data set for the Review of Systems may be:

Review of System (Circle Positive)	Review of System (Circle Positive)
Systemic: *fever, chills, weight loss, weakness*	MSK: *new bone or joint pain, back problems, swollen, hot*
Eyes: *acuity changes, tearing, photosensitivity, pain*	Skin: *skin lesions, rash*
ENT: *hearing loss, earache, nasal drainage, sore throat, tinnitus, vertigo*	Neurological: *syncope, focal weakness, HA, seizure, dizziness, loc*
Respiratory: *shortness of breath, cough, sputum, wheezing*	Psychiatric and behavioral: *prior psych history, depression, anxiety*
Cardiovascular: *chest pain, palpitations, paroxysdmal nocturnal dyspnea, orthopnea, ankle edema*	Endocrine: *polyuria, polydipsia*
Gastrointestinal: *nausea, vomiting, diarrhea, pain, melana, hematochezia*	Blood/Lymphatics: *bruising, adenopathy*
Genitourinary: *dysuria, urgency, frequency, nocturia, hematuria*	Allergic/Immunologu: *urticaria, hay fever*

- Physical Exam includes the actual findings and relate to the degree of functional impairment relating to the injury/illness. Documentation of the examination dictated in terms of inspection, palpation, motion, function (Motor, Sensory, Vascular), and special tests: straight leg raising (SLR), Neer's sign for rotator cuff impingment, Tinel's sign, Waddell's signs, estimation of validity, etc.
- Vital Signs should be interpreted, not included unless there is a pertinent connection to the injury care. (VS's normal except for slight elevation in BP, referred to primary care provider). Pain Scale findings are part of the vital signs and this "fifth vital sign" needs to be included in the dictation (notwithstanding objections from many practitioners who believe that it is not helpful in workers' compensation cases because pain estimates are often inflated when minor and minimized by the stoic when great).
- General Observations are an important factor and should include how the patient looked, acted, moved, if there was consistency in actions, guarding, etc.
- Records and Laboratory Findings reviewed are described with prominent mention of important results, overall interpretation for x-rays, lab, physical therapy, history forms, ER reports, specialists reports, etc.
- Assessment includes diagnosis with descriptors for severity, stability, etc.
- Discussion includes provider's reasoning, conclusions, interactions, issues with work accommodations, and other pertinent issues regarding the employee, employer, and insurance company.
- Diagnostic work-up needs to be identified and the diagnosis documented in full.
- Causality is defined, with explicit description of the mechanism of injury and any reasons why the patient might have been unusually susceptible.
- Work Relatedness requires the examiner to determine if the injury/illness is a direct result of job tasks with an explicit statement of the determination of work-relationship: "work related" or "non-work related."
- Plan clearly documented to include treatment, referrals to and for what with goals defined, potential length of treatment, estimated time to full duty, restrictions documented (in most clinics a reference to the Work Status Report/Form is sufficient), pain management, and any reports pending and the patient disposition. Plan includes:
  - Meds – list medications (e.g. Naproxen 550 mg, 1 bid with food. #60 Rx1; DCM 1 q4h prn # 20, NR)
  - Tests – tests ordered, records requested
  - Referrals – requested, specialists, rehabilitation, etc.
  - Work Status documented and reference made to the form used.
  - Follow Up Plan – length of time to regular work, estimated maximum medical imporovement, special needs for the future.
- Patient Instructions, impression of patient understanding and, if appropriate, patient's demonstration of understanding, completed to the provider's satisfaction. Script: *"Discussed Diagnosis, Rx, Work Status, and F-U, patient verbalized understanding of all of the above." Note whether verbalization of understanding was in English or through an interpreter.*
- Employer contact documented and describe what information was shared.

Exhibit 12.2 Review Criteria for Documentation Review: Follow-up Visit for Injury

Sample scripts are provided in italics to illustrate the criteria and can be used verbatim in dictation. Elements of the documentation given below in capital and lower case letters can be used as headings in the record, dictated note, and review document, to keep documents consistent.

- Status from last visit: Has the patient had any issues with increase symptoms, difficulty with functional job tasks?
- Subjective: How does the patient feel?
- Pain Scale Rating as compared to last visit
- Objective Findings: as compared to last visit
- Impression: same or change in diagnosis
- Treatment Plan: patient status to original goals
- Duty Status: changes
- Return Visit: if necessary
- Patient Education and Understanding should be documented per ACOEM Practice Guidelines (see Readings and Resources at end of chapter)
- Educate and reassure patient about treatment and expected duration of symptoms
- Consider the following sample script:
  "Discussed the diagnosis, treatment plan, follow up (if needed), and work restrictions with the patient. The patient verbalized understanding of all."
- Company Contact: Document that contact was made with the employer and by what method. Script: *"Provided employer with patient's work status report via fax to [designated company contact on file]."*

Exhibit 12.3 Criteria for Documentation Review: Discharge Visit for Injury

- Status compared to last visit:
- Subjective: Review of injury causality, initial evaluation, diagnostic findings, course of treatment, rehabilitation, functional results.
- Medications: on discharge
- Objective: data
- Impression: final diagnosis
- Outcomes: Work injury on _[date]_ resulting in _X_ lost work days, _X_restricted duty days, ___X___clinic visits, ___X___rehabilitation visits
- Maximum Medical Improvement as of __[date]__
- Work Status on discharge
- Maintenance Care if needed
- Patient Education and Understanding: as in Exhibit 12.2
- Company Contact: Document contact made and what method. Script:
  "Provided employer with patient's work status and discharge from care. Reported via fax to [designated company contact] on file."

Exhibit 12.4 Template for Dictation

Demographic

Patient:	Medical Record Number:
Soc Sec #:	Account #:
DOB:	
Employer:	
Job Title:	
Insurance:	Claim #:

Initial Evaluation

Date of Service:

Date of Injury:

Chief Complaint:

Subjective:

Job/Employment History:

Review of Systems:

Past Medical History:

Past Worker's Compensation History:

Family History:

Social History:

Current medications: if pertinent

Allergies:

Immunizations: if pertinent

Vital Signs: Stable/Abnormal   Pain Scale:

Physical Examination:

Diagnostic Testing:

Impression:

Causation:

Work relatedness:

Treatment Plan:

Work/Duty Status:

Return Visit:

Patient Education and Understanding:

Company Contact and Transmittal of Information:

Follow Up

Date of Service:

Status from last visit:

Subjective:

Pain Scale Rating as compared to last visit:

Objective Findings:

Impression:

Treatment Plan: patient status compared to original goals

continued ...

Exhibit 12.4 *continued*

Duty Status:
Return Visit:
Patient Education and
Understanding:
Company Contact and Transmittal of Information:
Discharge Summary
Date of Service:
Status compared to last visit:
Subjective: Review of injury causality, initial evaluation, diagnostic findings, course
of treatment, rehabilitation, functional results.
Medications:
Objective:
Impression: Work injury on _____resulting in _____ lost work days , _____
restricted duty days, _____clinic visits, _____rehabilitation visits.
Maximum Medical Improvement: as of [date]
Work Status:
Maintenance Care:
Patient Education and Understanding:
Company Contact and Transmittal of Information:

Exhibit 12.5 Model Policy for Documentation for an Occupational Health Service

1. All patients (injured workers) will have a chart or individual electronic record:
    1.1. All workers initially presenting for injury will have a complete record/chart
          assembled that includes all parts/chart dividers.
    1.2. Preplacement evaluations will have a basic record/chart assembled with no
          dividers. No family history of genetic information is allowed in this chart.
    1.3. In the event that an employee sustains an on-the-job injury then record
          divisions or chart dividers will be inserted to the established chart.
    1.4. Employee wellness and preventive services will have a basic record/chart
          assembled with no divisions or dividers.
2. Separate records and reporting practices (with a firewall or physical separation)
    will be maintained for the following:
    2.1. Medical records for personal medical care will not be combined with records
          for occupational health services.
    2.2. Reports of screening tests for preplacement evaluation will not contain the
          family history ("genetic information" protected under GINA) and will have
          no field in which it can be entered.
    2.3. Drug and alcohol testing will be kept separate from the rest of the medical
          record and reporting system.

Exhibit 12.6. Template for the Care Management and Injury Tracking Log

	Mon	Tue	Wed	Thu	Fri	Result/Outcome
Name: *Dorothy Gofarios* Phone#: *555-7654* Patient: *Esteban Fernandez* Employer: *City Connection, Shelbyville* RE: *Physical Therapy*			(Wed)			*C 10:30 am* *W Renewal of authorization for physical therapy*
Notes:						
Name: Phone#: Patient: Employer: RE:	Mon	Tue	Wed	Thu	Fri	Result/Outcome
Notes:						
Name: Phone#: Patient: Employer: RE:	Mon	Tue	Wed	Thu	Fri	Result/Outcome
Notes:						

C = Called   **FU** = Follow-up   **F** = FAX   **W** = Waiting for Information

13 Records

Donna Lee Gardner

"If you didn't document it, it didn't happen." While this is an old saying, in occupational health—where information is king and electronic record-keeping is rapidly becoming standard practice—it is truer than ever.

Record-keeping permeates all facets of an occupational health operation, from injury and illness documentation, coding, and billing; to clinic and worksite-based administrative activities; to screening exam results reporting; to individual and population health risk assessment data collection and reporting. Accurate medical record-keeping is necessary for providers to perform case management, track and publish outcomes, and obtain appropriate reimbursement from workers' compensation insurance carriers, self-insured employers, and other payers.

The Occupational Health and Safety Administration (OSHA) regulates the length of time that records must be retained (for at least 30 years after the employee has left the job) and lost-time injury record-keeping (OSHA 300 Log). The Americans with Disabilities Act of 1990 (ADA), 42 U.S.C. §12112(d)(3)(B)–(C) (see Chapter 23) generally requires employers to keep employee medical information confidential. Equal Employment Opportunity Commission (EEOC) standards, however, do not prohibit employers from making the disclosures required by the OSHA's medical access standard (see Chapters 3 and 4).

Electronic Health Records

Similarly to a paper record, an electronic health record (EHR) contains health information about individual patients as well as populations. Records in digital format can be shared across different health care settings via enterprise-wide information systems, thus supporting better coordinated, more expedient, and higher-quality patient care.

Computerized storage permits automatic and rapid retrieval of data in any combination and desired sequence. This is invaluable not only for worker health evaluation but for health program operations and audit. However, computers require special measures to ensure secure control of access to recorded personal health information. Access to computerized records must be strictly controlled and policed. Optimally, EHRs are stored on a password-protected server or in a cloud computing environment.

In an occupational setting, an EHR can be used by providers as an investigative tool to evaluate the source of a patient's injury or illness and to identify health issues in work teams or larger workforce populations. According the National Institute for Occupational Safety and Health (NIOSH), improved care and improved surveillance of occupational injuries and illnesses will only be realized if occupational information is included in the EHR. Consequently, NIOSH supports sustained collaborative efforts to address challenges such as constructing a case for "meaningful use" of data as defined by law, developing standards for data capture, and initiating pilot tests for EHR systems in clinical settings. At NIOSH's request, the Institute of Medicine is conducting a study to examine the rationale and feasibility of incorporating work history information into patient EHRs by 2015.

Transitioning

Most occupational health practices either already have or are preparing to make the transition to EHRs. Smaller practices with fewer resources are expected to be slower to adapt because of the cost of systems, confusion about federal incentives for using them, and fears about practice disruption.

The Certification Commission for Health Information Technology (CCHIT®) is a nonprofit, 501(c)3 organization with the public mission of accelerating the adoption of health information technology (IT) in the US. CCHIT® certifies EHRs in response to provisions contained in the American Recovery and Reinvestment Act (ARRA) and the Health Information Technology for Economic and Clinical Health (HITECH) Act, which allows practices to receive up to US$44,000 per physician over five years from Medicare or nearly US$64,000 over six years from Medicaid if they show "meaningful use." Payments began in 2011. The criteria for meaningful use are based on a series of specific objectives, each of which is tied to a measure that allows practitioners and hospitals to demonstrate that they are meaningful users of certified EHR technology.

CCHIT® certification includes a rigorous inspection of an EHR's integrated functionality, interoperability, and security. EHR products are tested against criteria developed by the commission. The program is intended to serve health care providers looking for greater assurance that a product will meet their complex needs.

The best way to keep records is in the simplest manner possible. Electronic forms and templates are particularly useful. Coding of illness and injury should be in accordance with the International Classification of Diseases, ICD), which has recently undergone its tenth major revision: ICD-10. ICD-10 is really a coding system, rather than a list of diagnoses. The Clinical Modification to ICD-10 (ICD-10-CM) is used for diagnosis coding and the International Classification of Diseases, 10th Revision, Procedural Coding System (ICD-10-PCS) for inpatient hospital procedures. Version 5010 Transaction Standards (including ASC X12 Version 5010, NCPDP Telecom D.0, and NCPDP Medicaid Subrogation 3.0.) are now required for eligibility for many insurance purposes, risk miscoding violation penalties, and claim status requests. Competent billing and coding personnel will know this.

Documentation standards are essential when implementing a program. Defined policies and procedures as well as forms and guidelines for form completion assist the practitioners in meeting compliance standards (see Chapter 12). Using paper or an electronic record requires the same attention to detail in the documentation process.

For the new occupational health service considering the possibility of recording specific information or ceasing to record it, the following questions should be asked:

1   Is this information required by regulation?
2   Will this information actually be used?
3   Will its use justify the cost of maintaining it?
4   Can the information be obtained easily and with accuracy?
5   Will the process of obtaining the information contravene or compromise legislated human rights?

Only then should issues of format and warehousing be considered.

Individually Identifiable Health Records

A good occupational health record allows the reader to piece together a clear and coherent picture of a worker's exposures on the job, health status, treatments, job assignment, and identity and to do so for at least 30 years after the fact, under the OSHA Records Retention Standard. Many epidemiological associations between chronic diseases and occupational exposures have been made using such records and they are always important legal documents.

The term "personal health record" is commonly used in the literature to refer to individually identifiable health records. However, "personal health record" has now become a term of art referring specifically to individually maintained and controlled EHRs, either those supplied by a third party (e.g. Google, Microsoft) or accessible via a portal to the individual's EHR maintained by a health care provider. It is therefore necessary to use the longer formulation "individually identifiable health record", in order to respect the proper legal use of the other term.

Individually identifiable health records in an occupational health setting inevitably contain personal, privileged information that must be protected from unlawful distribution to third parties. Significant constraints are placed on medical professionals with regard to the release of personal health information, especially when sharing information with an employer. These obligations also apply to the maintenance and internal use of company-initiated individually identifiable health records.

The physical record is normally the property of the employer or, in the case of an occupational health service serving many employers, whoever originated the record. However, with certain exceptions under the law, only the worker can authorize release of health information from his or her individually identifiable health record.

The employer's access to patient information is generally restricted to narrow determinations of fitness for duty and job accommodation. In the case of drug screen results, the employer may be informed of a positive or negative finding.

For maximum accuracy and medicolegal reliability, entries should be made in the health record chronologically as the worker is seen, and each should be signed by the person making the entry. Each entry should concisely and accurately reflect the care given and actions taken on the employee's behalf.

Because a worker's individually identifiable health record only reflects his or her health status insofar as it applies to the job, the content may vary considerably. Box 13.1 lists information usually contained in the record.

Privacy and Confidentiality

Occupational health clinics and hospital-affiliated programs are subject in the US to the Health Insurance Portability and Accountability Act (HIPAA) and the HITECH Act. The HITECH Act was signed into law on February 17, 2009 in order to promote the use of electronic medical records; Subtitle D addresses the privacy and security concerns associated with the electronic transmission of personal health information, in part through several provisions that strengthen civil and criminal enforcement of HIPAA rules.

The EHR requires the appropriate designation of access and passwords to ensure confidentiality. The paper chart requires attention to locked storage of all records with sufficient space to contain the records in a secured and safe environment for at least 30 years beyond the worker's employment, to comply with OSHA standards.

The HIPAA Privacy Rule (45 CFR 164.512(l)) permits covered health care providers to disclose health information for workers' compensation purposes without individual

Box 13.1 Content of Medical Records

1. Demographic information
2. Personal identifiers
3. Ethnicity
4. Present illness, history
5. Past and present medical history
6. Medication
7. Allergies
8. Physical examination results
9. Laboratory reports (including electrocardiogram, pulmonary function results, audiograms)
10. Imaging reports
11. Acute care entries and progress notes (an additional separate "Acute Care Register" is often also kept)
12. Record of immunizations
13. Occupational and exposure history
14. Hazard exposure record
15. Health programs participation record
16. Informed consent forms and authorizations for release of information
17. Documentation of refusals to undergo examination, testing, and program participation
18. Workers' compensation and insurance medical records
19. Fitness-for-duty determinations
20. Progress notes for rehabilitation
21. Consultant reports

authorization. Universal application of the Act is recommended in occupational health programs for all services, even those that are not clinical, to ensure consistency and to minimize the possibility of a breach.

The HIPAA Privacy Rule allows covered health care providers to share protected health information for treatment purposes without patient authorization, as long as they use reasonable safeguards when doing so. These treatment communications may occur orally or in writing, by phone, fax (generally the most secure), email (if secure), or otherwise. This provision allows laboratories to communicate results to providers, physicians to talk with nurses, two treating physicians to discuss the patient, and referral to specialists and consultations and back without hindrance.

The Privacy Rule requires that covered health care providers apply reasonable safeguards when making these communications, in order to protect information from inappropriate use or disclosure. These safeguards may vary depending on the mode of communication used. For example, when faxing protected health information to a telephone number that is not regularly used, a reasonable safeguard a provider might take is first confirming the validity of the fax number with the intended recipient. Similarly, a covered entity may pre-program frequently used numbers directly into the fax machine to avoid misdirecting the information. When discussing patient health information orally with another provider in proximity of others, a doctor may be able to reasonably safeguard the information by lowering his or her voice.

Meanwhile, a public health provision in the rule permits covered health care providers to disclose an individual's protected health information to the individual's employer without the employee's authorization in certain limited circumstances:

- The covered health care provider is providing the health care service to the individual at the request of the individual's employer or as a member of the employer's workforce.
- The health care service provided relates to the medical surveillance of the workplace or an evaluation to determine whether the individual has a work-related illness or injury (see Chapter 20).
- The health care service provided relates to findings concerning a work-related illness or injury, including workers' compensation.
- The employer has a duty under the OSHA, the Mine Safety and Health Administration (MSHA), or the requirements of a similar state law, to keep records on or to act on such information.
- For workers' compensation.

For example, OSHA requires employers to monitor employees' exposures to certain substances and to take specific actions when an employee's exposure level exceeds a specified limit, for example a blood lead determination. A covered entity that tests an individual for such an exposure level at the request of the individual's employer may disclose that test result to the employer without authorization. The language that applies to occupational health is provided in Box 13.2. This language is quite clear and should be closely and narrowly followed. Just because the Privacy Rule permits some disclosure without the individuals' consent or authorization does not mean that sharing health information with an employer would be legal or represent sound, ethical practice.

When a health care service does not meet the above requirements, covered entities may not disclose an individual's protected health information to the individual's employer without an authorization, unless the disclosure is otherwise permitted without authorization by other provisions of the rule. However, nothing in the rule prohibits an employer from conditioning employment on an individual providing an authorization for the disclosure of such information.

OSHA Record-Keeping

OSHA record-keeping has been very contentious among employers, who are required to comply with OSHA record-keeping (OSHA 300 Log) and record retention rules (29 CFR 1894). OSHA has attempted to simplify its system for tracking workplace injuries and illnesses. The required record-keeping log now uses a question-and-answer format, and the revised regulation answers questions about recording occupational injuries and illnesses, and explains how to classify particular cases. Flowcharts and checklists make it easier to follow the record-keeping requirements.

All employers covered by the Occupational Safety and Health Act of 1970 (P.L. 91-596) must report to OSHA within eight hours of any workplace incident resulting in a fatality or the in-patient hospitalization of three or more employees. If a company has ten or fewer employees during all of the last calendar year or is classified as a low-hazard retail, service, finance, insurance, or real estate industry, it does not have to keep injury and illness records unless the Bureau of Labor Statistics or OSHA demands otherwise. OSHA uses the employer's North American Industrial Classification System (NAICS) code to determine which establishments must keep records.

Box 13.2 Provisions of the HIPAA Privacy Rule (45 CFR 164.512(b)) that Apply to Occupational Health Care

The HIPAA Privacy Rule (45 CFR 164.512(b)) permits a covered entity to disclose protected health information for the purpose of public health activities. This includes (1) "a public health authority authorized by law to collect or receive such information for the purpose of preventing or controlling disease, injury, or disability, including but not limited to, the reporting of disease, injury, vital events such as birth or death, and the conduct of public health surveillance, public health investigations…", to public health agencies for control of communicable disease, and for the activities of the Food and Drug Administration. Elsewhere (45 CFR 164.212(d– g)) the rule permits disclosure for the purposes of government enforcement, adjudication of public benefits programs, demonstration of compliance with government programs, in the investigation of criminal conduct, and for judicial or administrative proceedings, as under subpoena or discovery, with the caveat that if the request is not covered by subpoena or court order the covered entity should receive assurance that the party requesting the information has made reasonable efforts to give notice to the individual.

It also states that the covered entity may allow employer access to individually identifiable health information to be provided to an employer, about an individual who is a member of the workforce of the employer, in the following circumstances (45 CFR 164.512(b)(v):

- The covered entity is a covered health care provider who is a member of the workforce of such employer or who provides health care to the individual at the request of the employer:
1.   To conduct an evaluation relating to medical surveillance in the workplace; or
2.   To evaluate whether the individual has a work-related illness or injury.
- The protected health information that is disclosed consists of findings concerning a work-related illness or injury or a workplace-related medical surveillance.
- The employer needs such findings in order to comply with its obligations under 29 CFR 1904 –1928, 30 CFR parts 50–90, or under state law having a similar purpose, to record such illness or injury or to carry out responsibilities for workplace medical surveillance.
- The covered health care provider provides written notice to the individual that protected health information relating to the medical surveillance of the workplace and work-related illnesses and injuries is disclosed to the employer:
1.   By giving a copy of the notice to the individual at the time the health care is provided; or
2.   If the health care is provided on the work site of the employer, by posting the notice in a prominent place at the location where the health care is provided.

Employers use the Log of Work-Related Injuries and Illnesses (Form 300) to list injuries and illnesses and track lost work days, restricted duty, or job transfers. They use the Injury and Illness Report (Form 301) to record supplementary information about recordable cases. Employers are allowed to use a workers' compensation or insurance form in lieu of the 301 record if it contains the same information. A summary form (300A) shows the totals for the year in each category and must be posted in a conspicuous place from February 1 to April 30 of each year.

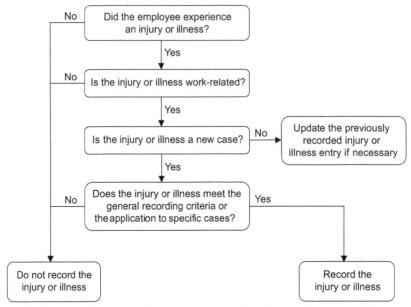

Figure 13.1 Decision tree for determining whether to record work-related injuries and illnesses

Work-relatedness is presumed for injuries and illnesses resulting from events or exposures occurring in the work environment, unless an exception in §1904.5(b)(2) specifically applies. The employer must also consider an injury or illness to be work-related if an event or exposure in the work environment either caused or contributed to the resulting condition or significantly aggravated a pre-existing injury or illness. Figure 13.1 is a decision tree for determining whether to record work-related injuries and illnesses. Table 13.1 lists the valid reasons why an employer may not be required to record an injury and illness.

Preexisting injury or illness

An injury or illness is a preexisting condition if it resulted solely from a non-work-related event or exposure that occurred outside the work environment. An injury or illness is considered to be a "new case" if the employee has not previously experienced a recorded injury or illness of the same type that affects the same part of the body, or the employee previously experienced a recorded injury or illness of the same type that affected the same part of the body but had recovered completely (all signs and symptoms had disappeared) from the previous injury or illness and an event or exposure in the work environment caused the signs or symptoms to reappear.

A preexisting injury or illness that has been significantly aggravated is work-related, for the purposes of OSHA injury and illness record-keeping, when an event or exposure in the work environment results in any of the following:

- Death, provided that the preexisting injury or illness would likely not have resulted in death but for the occupational event or exposure.
- Loss of consciousness, provided that the preexisting injury or illness would likely not have resulted in loss of consciousness but for the occupational event or exposure.

Table 13.1 Valid Exemptions from Reporting an Injury or Illness

An injury or illness occurring in the work environment that falls under one of the following exceptions is not considered work-related, and therefore is not recordable. Roman numerals in the left column refer to relevant parts of the OSHA record-keeping standard.

1904.5(b)(2)	Employers are not required to record injuries and illnesses if . . .
(i)	At the time of the injury or illness, the employee was present in the work environment as a member of the general public rather than as an employee.
(ii)	The injury or illness involves signs or symptoms that surface at work but result solely from a non-work-related event or exposure that occurs outside the work environment.
(iii)	The injury or illness results solely from voluntary participation in a wellness program or in a medical, fitness, or recreational activity such as blood donation, physical examination, flu shot, exercise class, racquetball, or baseball.
(iv)	The injury or illness is solely the result of an employee eating, drinking, or preparing food or drink for personal consumption (whether bought on the employer's premises or brought in). For example, if the employee is injured by choking on a sandwich while in the employer's establishment, the case would not be considered work-related. Note: If the employee is made ill by ingesting food contaminated by workplace contaminants (such as lead), or gets food poisoning from food supplied by the employer, the case would be considered work-related.
(v)	The injury or illness is solely the result of an employee doing personal tasks (unrelated to their employment) at the establishment outside of the employee's assigned working hours.
(vi)	The injury or illness is solely the result of personal grooming, self-medication for a non-work-related condition, or is intentionally self-inflicted.
(vii)	The injury or illness is caused by a motor vehicle accident and occurs on a company parking lot or company access road while the employee is commuting to or from work.
(viii)	The illness is the common cold or flu. Note: Contagious diseases such as tuberculosis, brucellosis, hepatitis A, or plague are considered work-related if the employee is infected at work.
(ix)	The illness is a mental illness. Mental illness will not be considered work-related unless the employee voluntarily provides the employer with an opinion from a physician or other licensed health care professional with appropriate training and experience (psychiatrist, psychologist, psychiatric nurse practitioner, etc.) stating that the employee has a mental illness that is work-related.

- One or more days away from work, or days of restricted work, or days of job transfer that otherwise would not have occurred but for the occupational event or exposure.
- Medical treatment in a case where no medical treatment was needed for the injury or illness before the workplace event or exposure, or a change in medical treatment was necessitated by the workplace event or exposure.

If an injury or illness does not involve one of these situations, the employer may check the box on the OSHA 300 form for cases indicating the employee received medical treatment but remained at work and was not transferred or restricted. In such cases, "medical treatment" means the management and care of a patient to treat disease or disorder. It does not include visits to a physician or other licensed health care professional solely for observation or counseling or the conduct of diagnostic procedures, such as X-rays and blood tests, including the administration of prescription medications used solely for diagnostic purposes (e.g. eye drops to dilate pupils) or first aid.

First aid

The occupational health center or clinic should keep a record of all first aid treatment it provides. First aid records are sometimes mandated by government regulation and are always important to the assessment of compensation claims. They are the responsibility of designated first aid or operations personnel. First aid records also provide data vital to the assessment of the company's safety and injury prevention program.

"First aid" is defined for the purposes of OSHA record-keeping as:

- Using a non-prescription medication at non-prescription strength (for medications available in both prescription and non-prescription form, a recommendation by a physician or other licensed health care professional to use a non-prescription medication at prescription strength is considered medical treatment for record-keeping purposes).
- Administering tetanus immunizations (other immunizations, such as hepatitis B vaccine or rabies vaccine, are considered medical treatment).
- Cleaning, flushing or soaking wounds on the surface of the skin.
- Using wound coverings such as bandages, Band-Aids™, gauze pads, etc., or using butterfly bandages or Steri-StripsTM (other wound closing devices such as sutures, staples, etc., are considered medical treatment).
- Using hot or cold therapy.
- Using any non-rigid means of support, such as elastic bandages, wraps, non-rigid back belts, etc. (devices with rigid stays or other systems designed to immobilize parts of the body are considered medical treatment for record-keeping purposes).
- Using temporary immobilization devices while transporting an accident victim (e.g. splints, slings, neck collars, back boards, etc.).
- Drilling of a fingernail or toenail to relieve pressure from a subungual hematoma, or draining fluid from a blister.
- Using eye patches.
- Removing foreign bodies from the eye using only irrigation or a cotton swab.
- Removing splinters or foreign material from areas other than the eye by irrigation, tweezers, cotton swabs, or other simple means.
- Using finger guards.
- Using massages (physical therapy or chiropractic treatment are considered medical treatment for record-keeping purposes).
- Drinking fluids for relief of heat stress.

First aid records are often kept at the first aid station at each worksite rather than in a centralized occupational health clinic. This permits minor traumatic injuries to be recorded at the worksites where they occur, thus eliminating the need for an employee with a trivial injury to leave work and go to the clinic simply to record the occurrence.

Unfortunately, in recent years there has been frequent and sometimes strong pressure placed on providers to provide only services that can be construed as "first aid" and to return injured workers to their jobs the same day so that they will not be counted as lost-time injuries and to avoid entering them on the OSHA 300 Log. This should be resisted.

Needlestick and sharps injuries

Recording criteria for needlestick and sharps injuries are laid out in a special section of the OSHA regulations, 29 CFR 1904.8. Cuts, lacerations, punctures, and scratches are only recorded under this provision if they are work-related and involve contamination with another person's blood or other potentially infectious material.

Medical providers and other covered entities must record all work-related needlestick injuries and cuts from sharp objects that are contaminated with another person's blood or other potentially infectious material (as defined by 29 CFR 1910.1030). The incident must be noted on the OSHA 300 Log as an injury. To protect the employee's privacy, however, the employee's name is not entered on the OSHA 300 Log (1904.29(b)(6)–1904.29(b)(9)).

Medical Removal

Medical removal occurs when an employee has to be removed from a certain exposure in the workplace for a period of time because the individual has had a physiological response to the exposure in excess of the relevant OSHA standard. (It is most common with lead exposure and elevated blood lead levels.) Recording criteria for cases involving medical removal under OSHA standards are covered in 29 CFR 1904.9.

If an employee is medically removed under the medical surveillance requirements of an OSHA standard, this must be recorded on the OSHA 300 Log.

Records Retention

OSHA regulations require that employee exposure records must be retained for 30 years and that medical records must be retained for the duration of employment plus 30 years (under 29 CFR §1910.1020). This must be observed by all occupational health services, as well as other providers who treat injured workers. Employers do not have to retain the records of employees who have worked there for less than one year but must give the record to the employee.

In addition to the OSHA record retention requirement, the majority of states have specific retention requirements for medical records and for their state-operated health insurance plans (Medicaid). In the absence of specific state requirements for record retention, the provider should keep health information for at least the period specified by the state's statutes of limitations or for a sufficient length of time to prove compliance with laws and regulations. If the patient was a minor, the provider should retain health information until the patient reaches the age of majority (as defined by state law) plus the period of the statute of limitations, unless otherwise provided by state law. A longer retention period is prudent, since the statute may not begin until the potential plaintiff learns of the causal relationship between an injury and the care received. As a practical matter, the OSHA record retention standard is longer than any of these state requirements and so occupational health services that also provide other types of care are advised to manage all records under the OSHA rule, for consistency and guaranteed compliance.

The American Health Information Management Institute (www.ahima.org) generally advises a retention time of ten years after the patient was last seen and permanent retention of patient registries. However, some state programs require as short a retention period as three years.

The documentation should be retained according to applicable federal (principally OSHA) and state law and regulations, and must be maintained for a sufficient length of time to ensure their availability to prove compliance with laws and regulations. The organization's legal counsel should review policy for the retention of compliance documentation.

Occupational health services should establish written policies to address the retention of all types of documentation, covering clinical and medical records, health records, claims documentation, and compliance documentation. Compliance documentation includes all records necessary to protect the integrity of the compliance process and confirm the effectiveness of the program, including employee training documentation, results of internal investigations, results of auditing and monitoring, modifications to the compliance program, and self-disclosures.

Each health care provider should ensure that patient health information is available to meet the needs of continued patient care, legal requirements, research, education, and other legitimate uses. For occupational health services, this is particularly important because occupational exposure and health records are heavily used in workers' compensation, OSHA investigation, epidemiological investigations, and litigation.

The provider should develop a retention schedule for patient health information that meets the needs of its patients, physicians, researchers, and other legitimate users, and complies with legal, regulatory, and accreditation requirements. The retention schedule should include guidelines that specify what information should be kept, the time period for which it should be kept, and the storage medium, along with documentation on the format and access. Old paper and microfilm records may not be worth converting to searchable formats until there is a need. Electronic formats, including optical disk and magnetic tape, should be converted as better technology becomes available.

If the employer of the occupational health service goes out of business, there are several options. Preferably, employers should transfer all records subject to this standard to the successor employer (for example, in a merger or acquisition). If there is no successor, the employer should notify current employees at least three months before the business closes of their right to access their records. Employers without a successor must then either transfer the records required to be preserved under this standard to NIOSH or notify the Director of NIOSH in writing of the employer's intent to dispose of the records three months in advance. Likewise, the occupational health service and its successor, if another provider takes over the practice, may retain the records indefinitely, if it is willing or stays in business. If not, the occupational health service should consider availing itself of the NIOSH option.

Special Issues

Environmental Hazard Records

Environmental hazard records include site visit reports, hazard monitoring results, worksite health and safety committee reports and accident investigation files (see Chapter 21). These records are normally produced and maintained by the employer's safety or industrial hygiene staff, but in a small company they may be the responsibility of designated operations personnel. Personal health data should not be included in any of these records. Access is controlled only by individual company policy and applicable legal requirements.

On-Site Surveillance and Screening

On-site occupational health services and providers who perform services on site (such as mobile audiometry) must implement a medical record system that meets OSHA as well as HIPAA criteria for confidentiality and regulatory compliance.

The occupational health service providing on-site surveillance, other screening, and prevention services faces a challenge if it does not have an EMR. In such circumstances, records are usually kept in one file under the client company name.

With an EHR, it is recommended that each employee be registered during the screening and the information be copied to their individual medical record. This avoids fragmentation and ensures that all pertinent health data is contained in the individual patient record.

Training Programs

Programs provided to the employees of client companies regarding training for regulatory as well as safety topics should document the training program content, objectives of the training, what regulatory compliance the training is meeting, duration, credentials of the trainer, and an individually signed attendance sheet documenting the date, time, topic, name of the presenter, participants, and their departments. Some programs require demonstration of competency. This should be included and the format for competency identified as well as those participants that successfully completed the training and demonstrated competency.

These programs should be filed under the client company and the date of training. Examples of such training might be first aid, cardiopulmonary resuscitation (CPR), blood borne pathogens standard compliance, lock out-tag out, substance abuse recognition, defensive driving.

Wellness Fairs

Wellness fairs have historically provided health stations where the client company employees and sometimes their families could have screening tests and testing for health risk appraisal while being educated in a fun environment. Very little record-keeping was done because the information was typically shared only with the participant. With the advent of the EHR it is possible to register the patient and follow them through the health stations, documenting pertinent health information in a confidential manner. The data could then be collated and the employee provided with a report card of their health status and actions to take to improve it.

Miscellaneous Records

In addition to administrative records common to all organizations, the occupational health service keeps additional records and generates reports for specific purposes:

- Daily log of the number of workers seen and services performed. (The EHR system should be able to generate this easily.)
- Health program records and reports. (These are for the evaluation of ongoing programs such as hearing conservation, environmental monitoring, and employee assistance. See Chapter 17, on performance indicators.)
- Drug register. (This is a mandatory record of medications held and dispensed to workers by the service.)
- Hazardous materials record and safety data sheet files. (Essential for on-site services, highly useful for community-based services for regular clients. Safety data sheets for most products can be obtained from the Canadian Centre for Occupational Safety and Health inexpensively. Commercial services are available to manage access to safety data sheets but these are expensive.)

Worker Right to Know

Workers have a right to access relevant exposure and medical records, as do their heirs if they are deceased. Current and former employees have the right to examine and copy medical and exposure records and also analyses based on these records, when they concern the worker's employment. An employer must comply and permit employees or their representative with written authorization (such as a lawyer or a union representative) to access exposure and medical records relevant to the employee, free of charge, within a reasonable period of time. The right of access to exposure records for employees and their designated representatives, such as unions, is protected under the OSHA Standard on Access to Employee Exposure and Medical Records (1910.1020). Such records include:

- Exposure records:
  - Monitoring results from industrial hygiene surveys and other measurements.
  - Biological monitoring results, such as blood and urine test results.
  - Safety data sheets with information about a substance's hazards to human health.
- Employee medical records:
  - Medical and employment questionnaires or histories.
  - Results of medical examinations and laboratory tests.
  - Medical opinions, diagnoses, progress notes, and recommendations.
  - First aid records.
  - Descriptions of treatments and prescriptions.
  - Employee medical complaints.
- Analyses (compilations of data or statistical studies of employee medical and exposure records that concern the worker's working conditions or workplace, without information that identifies other employees).

Exposure records and analyses can also be accessed without individual worker consent by union representatives recognized in a collective bargaining agreement.

Some types of information are excluded from this standard, if they are not kept together with medical records. They include insurance records, documents created for litigation that are privileged from discovery, employee assistance program records (see Chapter 28), and proprietary business information on ingredients or proportions in exposure records. If individual records are not available for the worker, the employer is required to produce exposure, but not medical, records of other employees (with personal identifiers removed) with similar duties or working conditions.

This standard imposes an obligation on the employer, and therefore the occupational health service, to do the following:

- Preserve and maintain accurate medical and exposure records for each employee.
- Inform workers of the existence, location, and availability of those medical and exposure records.
- Give employees any informational material regarding this standard that OSHA makes available to you.
- Make records available to employees, their designated representatives, and to OSHA, as required.

Recommended Reading and Resources

Canadian Centre for Occupational Safety and Health. MSDS Search. Available at: http://ccinfoweb. ccohs.ca/msds/search.html. Accessed January 7, 2012.

US Department of Health and Human Services. Summary of the HIPAA Privacy Rule. Available at: http://www.hhs.gov/ocr/privacy/hipaa/understanding/summary/index.html. Accessed January 25, 2012.

US Government Printing Office. 45 CFR 164.512 164.512. available at: http://edocket.access.gpo. gov/cfr_2004/octqtr/pdf/45cfr164.512.pdf. Accessed January 25, 2012.

US Occupational Safety and Health Administration. North American Industrial Classification System. Available at: http://www.osha.gov/oshstats/naics-manual.html. Accessed January 7, 2012.

US Occupational Safety and Health Administration. OSHA Injury and Illness Record-Keeping. Available at: http://www.osha.gov/recordkeeping/index.html. Accessed January 7, 2012.

US Occupational Safety and Health Administration. Recording and Reporting Occupational Illness and Injuries – 29 CFR 1904. Available at: http://www.osha.gov/doc/outreachtraining/htmlfiles/ record.html. Accessed January 7, 2012.

14 Professional Preparation and Training

M. Suzanne Arnold and Tee L. Guidotti

The supply of trained occupational health professionals falls far short of demand and always has. The demand for occupational licensed health care professionals (physicians and nurses) is now as strong as it has been in 20 or 30 years, and cannot possibly be satisfied by the few specialty training programs that exist. This creates a career opportunity for health care professionals who are willing to enter the field and learn what they need to know to become occupational health care providers. Relatively few practicing occupational physicians or nurses have formal specialized credentials in occupational health, despite the availability of academic training and credentialing. Many more nurses have certification in occupational health nursing than physicians have board certification in occupational medicine. Most industrial hygienists have some formal credentials but relatively few safety professionals do.

Occupational health clinics now rely on board-certified occupational medicine specialists, certified occupational health nurses, and other qualified occupational health professionals, when they are available, primarily for leadership and quality assurance, and for oversight of primary care providers, who still provide most occupational health care. That will not change in the foreseeable future.

Occupational health professionals require rapid and uncomplicated access to the information they need to deal with new situations or unfamiliar hazards. Regardless of what on-line resources are available, it is useful and advisable to set up a small library in the occupational health service facility where providers can look up what they need quickly, without logging on, and browse for the purpose of self-education when the pace of work allows. Appendix 2 provides a recommended bookshelf of textbooks and references that have been found useful

The Transition to Occupational Health Care

Health professionals who approach occupational health practice in a spirit of inquiry and discipline find many opportunities for a satisfying and demanding practice, particularly in group practice settings. The key to success in this effort, however, is a willingness to learn the principles and technical content of occupational health practice and to recognize the existing structure and institutions in the field. Those who are prepared to do so and who are committed to the field will find it challenging and rewarding. This is especially true for physicians in acute-care primary specialties and nurses in medical–surgical practice. This section describes the transition from primary care to occupational medicine from the health professional's point of view.

The world of occupational health is different from most other health care specialties. Rarely does an occupational physician admit a patient to the hospital, for example. The practice of occupational health can be very disconcerting to physicians and nurses who are oriented to traditional primary care; teamwork, administrative ability, and versatility in handling different types of complaints play a greater role here. Just as a surgeon relies on an operating room team, the occupational health professional soon finds that he or she depends heavily on professionals in allied disciplines, such as occupational health physicians, occupational health nurses, safety engineers, and industrial hygienists, each with its own training, certification, and licensing arrangements. Physicians are not necessarily the "leaders of the team." Just as often, the initiative and authority lies with industrial hygienists who are investigating hazards, safety professionals who have a detailed personal knowledge of the facility, occupational health nurses who are managing occupational health services at the plant site, nurse case managers, and the human resources department. Community-based practitioners, especially, may find that they have been very much out of the loop with respect to developments in the workplace when asked to address situations in which their expertise is required.

The new occupational health professional, especially the physician, faces some challenges, none of which are insurmountable:

* *Lack of appreciation for value added.* Employers and their insurers were not always sold on the value of prevention and the need for quality in occupational health services in the past, but this is changing.
* *Lack of institutional support.* In too many cases, when an occupational health service is based in an organization such as a hospital, medical group, or managed care organization, management will set it up for their own marketing or strategic purposes, often based on faulty assumptions, and do not think through the requirements for it to succeed as a provider in its own right.
* *Labor–management relations.* The position of the occupational health professional, standing between the worker and management, complicates some issues. Political attitudes toward unions or employers need to be checked at the door.
* *Administrative burden.* Physicians and nurses who do not like to fill out forms and prefer to write short, telegraphic progress notes will probably not do well in this field. Those who appreciate the value of accurate documentation and who like to write long, thoughtful reports like they did in medical or nursing school will enjoy it.
* *Frequent involvement in litigation.* Many physicians do not wish to become involved in cases that may require extensive medicolegal involvement. Others, however, seek it out for the intellectual challenge and learn to serve as effective expert witnesses.
* *Frequent ethical dilemmas.* (This subject is discussed in detail in Chapter 5.)
* *Infrequent recognition and external rewards.* Occupational health practice is singularly devoid of professional recognition, emotional displays of appreciation by families and grateful patients, and awards, so the provider has to be highly self-motivated and intellectually curious about the field.
* *Disproportionate weight played by marketing, rather than performance and quality of health services, as a factor in success.*

The complexities of occupational health practice are further complicated by strong economic, political, and social pressures, including workers' compensation, disability claims, law suits, government regulations, labor–management relations, budgeting, and other issues far removed from primary care practice. The single biggest obstacle for many years was that employers did not recognize or accept the need for specialized expertise in occupational health. This was due in part to the scarcity of trained personnel and in part to the tradition of recruiting the company's medical director from personal contacts, such as the chief executive officer's own physician, a golfing buddy, or a prominent local physician who had visibility in the community but limited experience in the workplace setting. Occupational health nurses also suffered from the perception that "a nurse is a nurse" without recognition of the value of specialty training in the field. The result was usually ad hoc and inconsistent policies and practices, often to the detriment of the employer.

Physicians and nurses who are not occupational medicine specialists or occupational health nurses but who choose to enter into this type of practice have an essential role to play and stand to benefit from the relative openness of occupational health as compared to other areas of practice. This opportunity comes with a responsibility to learn, understand, and ultimately to apply the same professional commitment and standards to occupational health as in any other practice of medicine or nursing.

Every occupational health professional seeking to enter occupational health practice from another practice domain should, at a minimum, do the following:

- Become knowledgeable through systematic training. (Most organizations in the field sponsor courses at their annual meetings for new entrants into the field.)
- Use continuing medical education (CME) credit opportunities and conference allowances to master the new field. (There is often a tendency to cling to one's previous professional identity and to use conference benefits as an opportunity to keep up with the old area of practice or to see old friends. This is ultimately both unsatisfying and not helpful to engaging in a new field.)
- Become thoroughly familiar with the ethical framework of occupational health (see Chapter 5).
- Separate personal or political beliefs (for example, against unions or against employers) from professional practice with respect to individual patients.
- Begin regularly using and reviewing the major clinical practice guidelines sources appropriate to the relevant profession. (In medicine, this is the *ACOEM Practice Guidelines*. In nursing, it is the *AAOHN Standards of Practice for Occupational Health Nursing*.)
- Join at least one of the major professional organizations in the field of occupational medicine or nursing. (Do not rely on committees or sections of the state or local medical or nursing associations, as they will always focus on narrower issues of the moment and not the broad, overarching issues of the field.)
- Become involved in a professional community or network in the local area. (This is important for professionalism and to hear about issues, local professional politics for self-defense, and new opportunities. An isolated occupational health professional is vulnerable to pressure regarding his or her decisions and to uncertainty regarding effective ethical practice.)
- Read, or at least scan, at least one major journal in the field from cover to cover for at least two years, including letters to the editor, author's affiliations, article references, and advertisements. (This is important not just to keep up with the literature but to learn where the literature in fact is: where is important work published and referenced, who are the prominent names, what are the major institutions, and what are the big questions that keep coming up.)

- Register with the online "Occupational Environmental Medicine List" (Occ-Env-Med-L, http://occhealthnews.net/). (All other social media sites in occupational health are optional: this one is essential.)
- Become highly knowledgeable and skilled in the occupational health issues (fitness-for duty requirements, hazards, health risks, and local politics) of at least four broad occupational categories, three of which should be public safety personnel (police and firefighters, who are ubiquitous and the key to winning municipal government contracts) and health care workers (also ubiquitous, familiar, and often a "starter" opportunity for moving into occupational health; see Chapter 9), and commercial drivers (interstate bus and truck drivers, who are subject in the US to Department of Transportation regulations). The fourth should be an occupation important in the local area (for example welding, mining, or, in rural areas, farming, as there are abundant hazards in agriculture). (Such specialization positions the practitioner to be a local expert, opens practice opportunities, and builds credibility.)
- Identify two or more mentors who will welcome the opportunity to give advice and talk the new occupational health professional through difficult problems. (Ideally, one should be in the immediate area and know the state or local situation well, and another should know the big picture across the country.)

Practitioners of most health professions cluster together and are linked by affiliation to a hospital or clinic where they have privileges. There, they have a natural peer group and the support of a professional community. It is easy to talk about cases in the corridor or over lunch. Occupational health professionals tend to be much more isolated and dispersed, with few others close by to talk to, even in major cities. The specialized management problems that occupational health providers deal with day to day are different from the clinical challenges that occupy their professional colleagues. There is a risk of losing one's bearings on what constitutes good practice. In order to stay focused on occupational health, to resist being unduly influenced by local and often ill-informed opinion or bias, and to benchmark best practices, it is essential for occupational health professionals to be part of a network of peers dealing with similar issues.

Visits to well-reputed occupational health clinics are always, without exception, worthwhile learning experiences. Plant tours and visits to industrial sites should be made at every opportunity in as many industries and employers as possible, in order to follow changing conditions in the workplace, to observe different industries, and to compare and benchmark. One may learn a lot about workers and employers as well, because conversations are likely to be more candid the further away from one's own workplace.

Staying current requires reading at least two major textbooks in the field. (For example, *The Praeger Handbook of Occupational and Environmental Medicine*, written by one of the authors of this book, is recommended for all physicians entering the field, plus one other title to get a contrasting point of view.) Occupational health nurses should have a textbook on occupational diseases (such as *The Praeger Handbook*) in their professional reference library, and an occupational health nursing textbook (such as *Occupational and Environmental Health Nursing: Concepts and Practice*). Every occupational health professional should then follow the journal literature appropriate to their profession: the *Journal of Occupational and Environmental Medicine*, the *American Journal of Industrial Medicine* (the use of "industrial medicine" in the title is historical), *Workplace Health & Safety: Promoting Environments Conducive to Well-Being and Productivity* (formerly the *American Association of Occupational Health Nurses Journal* (AAOHN Journal)), the *Ontario Occupational Health Nurses Association Journal* (OOHNA Journal), the

Journal of Occupational and Environmental Hygiene; Professional Safety: Journal of the American Society of Safety Engineers, and others.

Professional Preparation

The various occupational health professions have developed credentialing systems that recognize systematically prepared and evaluated practitioners. Familiarity with these credentials and the agencies that certify them is helpful in recruitment, career planning, and marketing to employers.

Occupational Medicine

Occupational medicine is the official name of the specialty of medicine that identifies, treats, and particularly seeks to prevent disorders related to work, and that promotes measures to improve the health and fitness of the working population. Occupational medicine specialists are also experts in certain fields, such as toxicology, that equip them with specialized knowledge and certain skills of practice that help them understand both the workplace and the environment generally. Hence, the preferred name for the modern specialty is actually "occupational and environmental medicine," although the certifying board still calls it "occupational medicine."

The gap between supply and demand is particularly acute for physicians. Over the years, many more physicians and surgeons have entered practice in the field of occupational medicine in the middle of their careers through informal preparation than have qualified formally as residency-trained, board-certified specialists. This trend is certain to continue in the future, because formal qualification is simply not practical under the current system for most physicians with an interest in the field. Occupational health care practice attracts emergency physicians, internal and family medicine practitioners, physiatrists, and others only after they discover its advantages and have an opportunity in the local community, usually in mid-career and not in medical school, where the field is essentially invisible. This is not really a problem for the field of practice, since these people bring life experience and valuable skills to the practice of occupational medicine and strengthen its community ties. Although these primary care physicians may not consider themselves occupational medicine specialists, they are practicing occupational medicine and their services are essential to meeting demand. The challenge is simply for these practitioners to prepare properly and to be willing to adapt and to some degree rethink their medical approach.

This creates opportunities for physicians in compatible specialties (such as internal medicine, family medicine, and emergency medicine) to move laterally into the field with relative ease, assuming that they have board certification in their first field and are willing to learn. The paltry numbers of qualified and trained specialists formally qualified in occupational health disciplines mean that for many years to come, occupational health practitioners will continue to be drawn largely from primary care practice and other allied health care fields. This is only a problem insofar as the complexities and technicalities of advanced occupational health practice and care delivery are concerned. For the most part, the primary care level of occupational health can certainly be delivered by practitioners without special qualification if the systems are in place to support quality occupational health care and the practitioner is clear on what is required (see Chapter 1).

The American College of Occupational and Environmental Medicine (ACOEM) and the Occupational and Environmental Medical Association of Canada (OEMAC) both sponsor continuing education programs designed to facilitate the transition of already good physicians into the field.

In the US, training in the specialty of occupational medicine is formally undertaken through a residency program, with a minimum three-year commitment for eligibility for board certification by the American Board of Preventive Medicine (ABPM). ABPM (established 1949) is one of the 24 medical specialty boards (representing about 145 medical specialties) recognized by the American Board of Medical Specialties (ABMS), which is the umbrella organization for specialty certification in the US. (There are around 180 self-designated "boards" that are not recognized by ABMS, some of which are entirely legitimate and others are highly questionable. One such organization relevant to occupational and environmental medicine is the American Board of Independent Medical Examiners, which is not actually a specialty board but provides legitimate certification for mastery of a particular skill set described in Chapters 25 and 26.)

As a practical matter, five years of training is really required for board certification in occupational medicine because few if any contemporary occupational medicine residency programs take candidates who are not already fully trained in another, preferably primary care, specialty. (In the past, this has disappointed some non-boarded physicians who mistakenly identified occupational medicine as an "easy" board certification for credentialing to satisfy their hospitals, only to find that there is no easy route. There is no path to certification in the US that does not require a physician to do further residency training.)

The required training period is five years for specialists in Canada, in preparation for the fellowship of the Royal College of Physicians of Canada (FRCPC), where occupational medicine is a subspecialty of internal medicine. In Canada there is also an alternate pathway to recognition through continuing education, experience, and examination, through the Canadian Board of Occupational Medicine (CBOM), which recognizes three levels of accomplishment. The CBOM has been the subject of much discussion as a potential model for the US, because it provides an employer-recognized credential of added competency for practitioners without competing with established specialty certification.

Occupational medicine has a very long history, with precursors dating to ancient times, and was codified into a coherent body of knowledge in 1700 AD by the brilliant Italian physician–scholar Bernardino Ramazzini. The field of "industrial medicine and surgery" (there was no specialty at the time) became critically important during the Industrial Revolution in England, France, and the US, particularly for railroads, and with the rise of workers' compensation (see Chapter 2). The national organization, ACOEM, dates to 1916. The term "occupational medicine" began to replace "industrial medicine" in the 1950s, when the field became a recognized medical specialty. In 1992 the leading organizations adopted the name "occupational and environmental medicine" to reflect the growing importance of environmental health risk in practice and management responsibilities, as well as the workplace environment.

Occupational Health Nursing

Although the formal certified specialty (Certified Occupational Health Nurse, COHN) is not a large nursing specialty by standards of the profession, it is very attractive to nurses because it offers more autonomy and leadership potential than most hospital-based nursing careers and so tends to attract highly motivated practitioners. The nursing specialty is much larger than occupational medicine, roughly twice the size in the US. Even so, experienced COHN-qualified nurses are still uncommon and in demand by employers.

Table 14.1 Roles, Functions and Qualifications of Occupational Health Nurses at Benchmark Professional Levels

General Description / Qualifications	Functions
Level 1 Provides occupational health (OH) nursing care to all employees, including treatment of illness and injury, worker health promotion and education. Qualifications: • Has 3–5 years occupational health experience. • Has participated in courses and/or conferences relating to occupational health nursing practice.	• Provides OH services to workers. • Implements primary care in the treatment of illness and injury. • Presents health promotion programs and education to workers. • Maintains appropriate records, incorporating confidentiality. • Counsels workers and refers as appropriate to medical/community resources. • Evaluates programs and services for effectiveness.
Level 2 Requires Level 1 plus Provides occupational health nursing care to all employees, including health assessments, appropriate record-keeping, and legislation compliance. Includes some supervisory and/or administrative responsibilities. Qualifications: • Has a minimum 5 years experience in occupational health. • Has completed a Certificate or Diploma in occupational health nursing. • Is eligible for national certification in occupational health nursing (COHN).	• Conducts health assessments (preplacement, periodic). • Implements care plans. • Develops an appropriate record-keeping system, including maintenance of confidentiality. • Acts as a resource in maintaining a safe work environment. • Interprets government legislation relevant to health, safety, and environment. • Applies critical thinking in the application of nursing principles and social skills.
Level 3 Requires Level 2 plus Supervises and is responsible for a multi-nurse unit in the development, administration, co-ordination, and implementation of activities within an OH service. Qualifications: • Has 5–7 years experience in occupational health including incremental roles at supervisory and management level. • Has undergraduate degree in Nursing or equivalent. • Has Certificate or Diploma in occupational health nursing. • Has national certification (COHN), or CCOHN(C), or equivalent. • Safety designation is an asset. • Management, business skills are additional assets.	• Supervises OH programs such as preplacement, periodic health assessments, immunizations, etc. • Ensures the maintenance of confidential the record system. • Prepares annual budget for OH department. • Selects, supervises and evaluates staff. • Develops and promotes professional development for staff. • Works collaboratively with other occupational health and safety (OH&S) disciplines on common issues. • Implements and monitors disability management and safe return to work strategies. • Interacts with management to ensure that OH&S programs articulate with corporate goals and policies.

Level 4

Requires Level 3 plus

- Manages and is responsible for at least two types of Health/Safety professionals.
- Oversees development, administration, and evaluation of the total OH service.

Qualifications:

- Has minimum seven years of experience in occupational health, with advanced responsibilities for program management and supervision of professional staff.
- Has undergraduate degree in Nursing or equivalent.
- Has Certificate or Diploma in occupational health nursing (OHN).
- Has national certification (COHN), or CCOHN(C), or equivalent.
- Safety designation is an asset.

- Represents OH service to management, workers, and community agencies.
- Acts as consultant in OH to departments within the organization, supporting programs and health initiatives.
- Prepares and coordinates annual budgets for full department.
- Assists in recruitment of staff, and maintains personnel performance appraisals.
- Prepares evaluation reports and develops plans for future requirements.
- Participates as active member of company management team.

Level 5

Requires Level 4 plus

- May be an employee in a senior capacity or may practice as an outside consultant for evaluating and developing employee health services.
- Can provide OH services in administration or health education as well as develop and implement appropriate and relevant Health and Safety programs.
- May be self-employed, employed by an organization, or a representative of an OH services provider.

Qualifications:

- Has a minimum of 7 10 years experience in OH including supervisory or managerial responsibilities.
- Has a Certificate or Diploma in Occupational Health Nursing and national certification as an OHN specialist (COHNS).
- It is recommended that graduate school preparation as clinical Nurse Specialist, or Nurse Practitioner be considered. Graduate (Masters) degree may also be in education, business administration, health sciences, or occupational and environmental health.

- Advises clients on the recommended scope and content of employee health service based on needs assessment and analysis.
- Promotes interdisciplinary health management of hazards and risks in the workplace.
- Serves as a resource for case management of employees through knowledge of relevant government legislation and disability management process.
- Participates in the OH program through various activities, for example development of training programs based on needs assessment, evaluation of hazards and risks in workplace, implementation of health surveillance programs, physical demands analysis, worker health assessments, health promotion.

Source: Ontario Occupational Health Nurses Association (2005), Benchmark Position Descriptions for Occupational Health Nurses. Available at www.oohna.on.ca.

Occupational health nurses are registered nurses trained and certified in this specialization of nursing, which provides care for injuries and acute illness in the workplace, monitors the health of workers, and promotes wellness. A number of universities in the US, including Harvard, Johns Hopkins, and the University of North Carolina at Chapel Hill, offer graduate programs in Occupational Health Nursing to qualified candidates. The American Association of Occupational Health Nurses (AAOHN) has prepared a document outlining a basic education curriculum for occupational health nurses. The AAOHN offers courses and programs in a variety of modalities, including conferences, webinars, online interactive learning, and traditional distance education formats. The American Board for Occupational Health Nurses (ABOHN) is the nursing specialty certification board, with over 12,000 active certified nurses working today. The core credential is the COHN. This credential is offered to registered nurses (RNs) and is focused primarily on direct clinical practice, with some content relating to program coordination and case management. The Certified Occupational Health Nurse-Specialist (COHN-S) credential may be earned by registered nurses with a Bachelor's degree and/or graduate degrees. In addition to the elements of the COHN certification examination, the COHN-S certification adds the roles of the occupational health nurse in management, education, and consultation. Eligibility requirements of the certification process require a combination of experience in the field and continuing professional education in occupational health nursing. In Canada, the Canadian Nurses Association examines and certifies occupational health nurses (CCOHN(C)), using similar eligibility criteria to those in the US.

Occupational health nurses are recognized at five levels of capacity. The roles, qualifications, and functions appropriate for each level are summarized in Table 14.1.

The AAOHN, as well the Canadian Occupational Health Nurses Association (COHNA) and the Ontario Occupational Health Nurses Association (OOHNA), offer continuing education opportunities for nurses, in the form of online courses, webinars, and educational conferences specific to occupational health practice.

The evolution of occupational health nursing, originally called "industrial nursing," dates back to the late 1880s and was grounded in the recognition that many of the illnesses and injuries in the workplace were preventable. The first industrial nurses based their practice on a prevention and public health nursing model, providing care to workers in their workplaces, and to the workers' families in their homes. In the early 1900s the growth of industrial nursing was influenced by the development of workers' compensation legislation, World War I, and the focus on prevention of communicable diseases, particularly tuberculosis. During the Great Depression, economic growth ceased, unemployment increased, and workers' health and safety issues became less important to employers and government. As a result, the number of practicing industrial nurses decreased. Well into the 1940s, industrial nurses worked in isolation from their peers, without standardized nursing procedures and with limited specialized training available. The need to keep workers healthy and productive for the war effort of World War II resulted in a resurgence in industrial nursing. Concurrent with this new growth in the field, a number of colleges and universities in the US began offering industrial nursing courses at the baccalaureate level, and later at the graduate level. The industrial nurses, through their professional association, the American Association of Industrial Nurses (AAIN), also developed their own practice standards: "Qualifications of Nurses in Industry." However, educational opportunities for industrial nurses, including specialty certification, continued to ebb and flow through the 1960s.

By the early 1970s, the Occupational Health and Safety Act (1970) provided the impetus for graduate level training and continuing education for nurses working in industry, and, in

1977, the AAIN changed its name to the American Association of Occupational Health Nurses (AAOHN) and the term "industrial nurse" was replaced with "occupational health nurse," to reflect the expanded clinical and preventive scope of practice. In the 1980s the roles and responsibilities of the occupational health nurse grew to include more senior roles in management and policy development, in cost containment, in regulatory compliance, and in health promotion and research. In the early part of the 21st century, occupational health nursing added the element of environmental concerns to its mandate and changed its name once again to "occupational and environmental health nursing." Occupational and environmental health nurses continue to promote, protect, and preserve the health of workers in all sectors of the economy.

Industrial Hygiene

Industrial hygiene is the term in the US for an engineering- and chemistry-based profession of specialists who anticipate, recognize, evaluate, and control exposure in the workplace, principally chemical hazards. (In Canada and most of the rest of the world the preferred term is "occupational hygienist.") Training in occupational hygiene includes extensive study in ventilation, analytical chemistry, mathematics, and toxicology. Most industrial or occupational hygienists work for major employers, on contract, or as consultants. Individuals wishing to enter the field of industrial hygiene must have completed a baccalaureate degree in basic sciences, preferably with a focus on biology, chemistry, chemical engineering, and/or physics. The American Board of Industrial Hygiene (ABIH) examines and certifies industrial hygienists in the US. Candidates seeking certification must meet the basic academic requirements of an undergraduate degree in science and additional coursework specific to industrial hygiene; they must submit proof of workplace experience in industrial hygiene; they must currently be practicing industrial hygiene; and they must successfully challenge the examination. The Canadian Registration Board of Occupational Hygienists (CRBOH) examines and certifies occupational hygienists in Canada, using the same basic criteria for eligibility to challenge the examination. Additionally the CRBOH offers a certification for occupational hygiene technologists which does not require an undergraduate degree, but which does demand relevant academic preparation and experience in the field, prior to sitting the examination specific to this sub-specialty.

Health Physics and Radiation Safety

Health physics, or radiation safety, is a profession similar to industrial hygiene but devoted to radiation, primarily but not exclusively ionizing. Although a relatively small occupational health profession, health physics is highly visible because of the work of medical health physicists in hospitals and clinics and is central to occupational health in the nuclear industry. Health physicists, also known as radiation safety officers, monitor exposure to radiation and the adequacy of protection. Health physicists are trained in university programs at the bachelor's and graduate levels. Health physics technicians are trained at the two-year associate's degree level and mostly do monitoring. National certification is by examination and is provided by the American Board of Health Physics (ABHP) and National Registry of Radiation Protection Technologists (NRRPT), respectively. The professional organization in North America is the Health Physics Society.

Safety

Safety professionals (sometimes called "safety officers" or "safety engineers," although most are not trained engineers) are professionals with specific training in the recognition and control of safety hazards. Safety education is usually not at the graduate level; most safety professionals move into their positions through experience and have obtained their training in short-term, intensive institutes or seminars. A few still learn on the job. The American Society of Safety Engineers (ASSE) offers several levels of professional certification through examination. Certification credentials include: Associate Safety Professional (ASP), Certified Safety Professional (CSP), Occupational Health and Safety Technologist (OHST), and others. Eligibility to challenge the examination is based on a combination of academic preparation and/or professional development and workplace experience in the field. The Board of the Canadian Registered Safety Professionals manages credentialing in Canada. The American Society of Safety Engineers and the National Safety Council are the principal organizations in the US; in Canada their counterparts are the Canadian Society of Safety Engineers and the Canada Safety Council.

A number of programs, courses, and other educational opportunities in occupational health are offered by distance learning modalities. Some academic programs, such as the Master's degree in Occupational Health Sciences at McGill University (Montreal, Canada), integrate students from the various disciplines in occupational health, resulting in dynamic interactions and a focus on the independent and interdependent roles of occupational health professionals in the workplace.

Audiology

Audiologists are engaged in the evaluation of hearing disorders. Within audiology is a professional category devoted to the identification of noise-induced hearing loss in the workplace, the "occupational hearing conservationist." These professionals possess certification from the Council on Accreditation in Occupational Hearing Conservation, which attests to skill in performing audiometric evaluations of workers exposed to noise.

Loss Prevention

Risk, loss, or liability control officers are usually found in a large corporation or public agency and are responsible for keeping to a minimum the likelihood of injury, property damage or loss, exposure to litigation, the amount of the workers' compensation assessment paid by the company, and often the exposure of the company to uncontrolled employee health care costs. They are rarely part of the occupational health team but are often in management positions relating to occupational health. Sometimes they are in a position to influence the occupational health exposure (liability) of their client employers by steering them to occupational health services or requiring them to correct problems as a condition of coverage.

Many of these business professionals entered their positions from personnel management or from the insurance industry. The insurance industry itself has established an elaborate system of professional education designed to assure uniformity and equity in claims processing. The Insurance Institute of America and the Insurance Institute of Canada maintain countrywide systems of classes, self-study courses, and examinations leading to the degree of Associate in Loss Control Management, which includes an introduction to safety, industrial hygiene, and occupational medicine, and which may lead to the standard advanced credential in the insurance industry, Chartered Property Casualty Underwriter. These individuals investigate insurance claims and evaluate employers for workers' compensation coverage.

Work Evaluation or Rehabilitation Counseling

The work evaluation or rehabilitation counselor is trained at the bachelor's or master's level to assess the work skills, physical tolerances, specialized training, and motivation of the worker. This assessment is used in judging disability in workers' compensation cases. Most practitioners have training up to a master's degree. The Commission on Rehabilitation Counselor Certification (CRCC) grants certification to counselors on the basis of educational requirements and an examination, leading to Certified Rehabilitation Counselor (CRC) in the US or CCRC in Canada.

Recommended Reading and Resources

American Association of Occupational Health Nurses. Available at: https://www.aaohn.org/. Accessed December 22, 2011.

American Board of Industrial Hygiene. Available at: http://www.abih.org/. Accessed December 22, 2011.

American Board of Occupational Health Nurses. Available at: http://www.abohn.org/. Accessed December 22, 2011.

American Board of Preventive Medicine. Available at: http://www.abprevmed.org. Accessed December 22, 2011. (Note that www.abpm.org brings up the American Board of Pain Medicine, a non-ABMS specialty board.)

American College of Occupational and Environmental Medicine. *Occupational Medicine Practice Guidelines*. Chicago, ACOEM, 2004, 3rd ed. in hard copy, one-year access to APG-1 online version included in purchase. APG-1 is revised frequently and is also available as a free-standing application.

American Conference of Governmental Industrial Hygienists. Available at: http://www.acgih.org/. Accessed December 22, 2011.

American Society of Safety Engineers. Available at: http://www.asse.org/. Accessed December 22, 2011.

Board of Certified Safety Professionals. Available at: http://www.bcsp.org/. Accessed December 22, 2011.

Board of the Canadian Registered Safety Professionals. Available at: http://www.bcrsp.ca/index.html. Accessed December 22, 2011.

Canadian Council of Occupational Hygiene. Available at: http://www.ccoh.ca/ccoh.htm. Accessed December 22, 2011.

Canadian Nurses Association, Certification information, available at: http://www.cna-nurses.ca/CNA/nursing/certification/default_e.aspx. Accessed December 22, 2011.

Canadian Occupational Health Nurses Association. Available at: http://www.cohna-aciist.ca/pages/default.asp. Accessed December 22, 2011.

Canadian Registration Board of Occupational Hygienists. Available at: http://www.crboh.ca/page.cfm?onumber=1. Accessed December 22, 2011.

Guidotti TL (2010) *The Praeger Handbook of Occupational and Environmental Medicine*. Santa Barbara CA, Praeger/ABC-Clio. See Chapter 1, on "Occupational and Environmental Medicine."

Ontario Occupational Health Nurses Association. Available at: http://www.oohna.on.ca/. Accessed December 22, 2011.

Rogers B. (2003) *Occupational and Environmental Health Nursing: Concepts and Practice*. Philadelphia, Saunders, 2nd ed.

Rogers B, Randolph S, Mastroiani K (2008) *Occupational Health Nursing Guidelines for Primary Clinical Conditions*. Beverly Farms MA, OEM Press, 4th ed.

15 Marketing

Frank H. Leone

"Marketing" refers to the strategies and tactics used to introduce services and products to the market and in turn to learn and to respond to what the market wants. Marketing works both ways, which is why the sales officer of an occupational health service should properly be called the "Account Services Representative" and why this is not a euphemism (see Chapter 10). This person is not only responsible for promoting what the service has to offer potential users, but as the primary contact between the client and the provider is in the best position to resolve problems and to learn what clients need, and to understand how their attitudes shape their needs into wants. Marketing is different from "advertising," which is commonly understood as the commercial use of media to persuade people to obtain a product or purchase a service, with little feedback or interaction. Advertising plays a less significant role in the modern technologically-oriented era where social media predominate and customers search for what they want, and is now best understood as one tool used for marketing outreach, and a diminishing one at that. Marketing is vastly different from "sales," which involves considerable consumer education, generally more intense persuasion, and typically addresses an individual or small group directly.

Effective marketing reaches out to as many potential users of a program's services as possible, reinforces the program's identity in the public eye, explains why their product or service is the preferred option, and motivates the client to choose them from among the alternatives. Marketing is the framework, strategy, and route that one takes to achieve these goals.

Marketing Strategy

Marketing occupational health services requires different strategies in different situations. Free-standing occupational health centers that work directly with employers to provide services to their workforce primarily need to raise awareness of themselves and secondarily to build their reputation as the preferred provider for the provision of high-quality occupational health care services. Multispecialty group practices and hospital-affiliated occupational health services usually seek to leverage their reputation for quality care into a dominant position in the occupational health care market as part of a broader community marketing strategy; their occupational health services must often fight within the organization for their special marketing needs to be addressed and not to be subsumed as one more item under a more general advertising campaign. Corporate-based occupational health services and on-site providers would seem to have a captive patient base, but they need to market themselves to justify their position within their own company and to keep

Box 15.1 Factors in a Marketing Strategy

These factors are critical in determining a marketing strategy for occupational health services:

- *Market size.* Use different strategies for major metropolitan areas, mid-sized communities, and small and rural markets.
- *Industrial mix.* Erie PA (manufacturing), Bakersfield CA (agriculture), Pittsburgh (no longer manufacturing but today dominated by services), and Las Vegas (gaming/ hospitality, therefore highly service-oriented) are demonstrably different markets that require different strategies.
- *Position in the market.* Is the provider the market leader, a market challenger, a new-market entry, or an established market plod-along? Each scenario is likely to suggest a different approach to marketing. Hospitals and multispecialty groups will require different internal business plans to support expansion into occupational health services, depending on their position.
- *Nature of your team.* Not everyone is comfortable expanding services into wellness or biomonitoring. Some people love the contentious realm of medicolegal work and others don't want any part of it. Providers should adapt to the personality and strengths of the existing staff, but only up to a point, and not be afraid to bring on new personnel with other strengths or to form business relationships with other businesses, such as industrial hygienists.
- *Your persona.* Avoid trying to fit the proverbial round peg through a square hole. Socrates said "Know thyself." The prime leader (usually the founder) or leaders of the occupational health service should incorporate their personal strengths into marketing tactics and not be afraid to use their own reputation to build "brand identity." However, if they are introverted or do not like marketing, they should not, because their discomfort will come across.

their reputation high. Individual practitioners or consultants that contract directly with one or more employers need to ensure that they are meeting the needs of their clients and must continually remind their clients that they are doing so.

The provider should consider the variables in Box 15.1 in devising a marketing strategy. These factors should be thoroughly understood, thought through, discussed with the team, and researched until they are part of the team's thought process.

Marketing Plans

Once the overall strategy is identified, the tactics used to achieve the marketing goals should be identified and combined into a coordinated program or campaign through a marketing plan. The providers may need to get professional help by involving people outside their business to explore potential marketing tactics but at the beginning can get started by coming up with a broad list of potential tactics through brainstorming. Some tactics may seem silly, but even the silliest idea can provide a kernel for a more interesting approach. Think, create a "laundry list," and whittle the list down until only one or two tactics remain.

Which tactics take priority? Prioritization usually comes down to return on investment. The best tactics offer the provider the greatest opportunity for financial return for the lowest investment in human and financial capital. Providers should judge the merit of a strategy by a reasonable estimate of both its impact and cost.

Great marketing is great marketing, no matter the product, service, or even a political campaign. On the whole, occupational health marketing as a whole would seldom be mistaken for great marketing. Both the senior manager and whoever is responsible for marketing should keep an eye on what marketers are doing in other health care sectors, in completely unrelated service industries (particularly the dominant industries in the community), and in other communities. A political campaign is a good place to observe fundamental principles because it features the basic tenets of effective marketing and communication: remain on message, keep the message simple, and keep repeating the message.

The marketing plan is a blueprint, not a manual. Marketing plans often break down because they are lengthy and verbose, too general, uninspired, or forgettable. A written plan is the foundation of any business endeavor; it is the master document intended to keep you moving forward and on track. However, it is probably better written as a PowerPoint business presentation than as a fleshed-out lengthy memo, because its application will require flexibility, response to the unexpected, and the capacity to respond to targets of opportunity.

There are eight steps to developing the marketing plan:

1   *State your mission.* If applicable, elaborate by stating how that mission relates to the larger mission of the parent organization or network, such as the employer (for an on-site service) or a hospital or multispecialty group. (This obviously does not apply to free-standing community-based occupational medicine centers.) This elaboration should involve input from the senior management of the network, which also is useful to educate them.

2   *State your financial goals.* For community-based occupational health services, this may be "to grow profit by 10 percent during the coming year," and should be based on a single parameter—gross revenue. The financial goal for an employer-based, in-house service (but not necessarily an on-site contract service), may be "to reduce direct workers' compensation costs by 10 percent." Avoid mixing apples with oranges when stating a financial goal. For example, increasing injury management revenue by 12 percent and discretionary services revenue by 15 percent represent two potentially competing goals and are more specific than necessary: keep it simple.

3   *Examine the service's inherent strengths and challenges.* Identify value in each strength and offer solutions to any barriers you may identify. A "SWOT analysis" (strengths, weaknesses, opportunities, threats) is a standard business tool for this process. It is critical to be very honest about shortcomings and modest about strengths.

4   *Define your competitive advantage.* "Why are your services the best option for most employers in your market?" If the provider is unable to provide a concise, supportable answer to this question, the success of the marketing effort is in doubt. A competitive advantage statement should be:
    • Short (one or two sentences) and to the point.
    • Measurable (see Chapter 17).
    • Unique.
    • Legitimate.

5   *List your marketing tactics in priority order.* Embrace the communications technology revolution by using email, voice mail blasts, virtual (online) and actual clinic tours,

worker education, and social networking as core outreach tools. Do not be self-serving about it but share expertise: use education as a calling card.

6   *Program marketing tactics.* Place marketing tactics and the discrete steps to execute each tactic on a master calendar, update it through the year as needed, and follow the plan meticulously.

7   *Continually review prospects.* Build a large and up-to-date prospect universe. Maintenance is just as important as building the file in the first place: in an era in which perhaps 20 percent of the labor force turns over every year, yesterday's pristine mailing list is today's inaccurate one.

8   *Keep the level of activity high.* More is better. Marketing is largely a numbers game. Twice as many sales calls results in twice as much business. Touch twice as many employers with a marketing tactic and clinics are likely to get twice as much walk-in business. More up front usually means more at the end.

Defining the competitive advantages requires further discussion. Key characteristics that will resonate with employers are trust, past success (implied by longevity in business), demonstrable cost reduction and value added (see Chapter 18), and positive business. These days, the quality of care for routine injuries is widely assumed, rightly or wrongly, to be at least adequate for any contemporary health care facility in North America, and so comparative quality is not a selling feature. A higher level of care than what is (perceived to be) needed suggests increased expense. Therefore employers are more likely to respond to the message that the provider promises better outcomes than to a message that the provider is superior in terms of expert care, advanced technology, or specialization. Consider the "pitch" developed by "Healthworks" (an anonymous example):

- "Workplace health and wellness since 1982." (Longevity implies client satisfaction.)
- "Better access," not described in words but accompanied by a picture of the facility, within sight of a construction site at an airport, and an accompanying map. (Allows the prospective client to visualize how easy it is to get there.)
- "Reduce costs," with examples of employer's experiences in reducing lost-time injuries. (These are even more convincing if published.)
- "Improve productivity through a healthier workforce." (Employers are bombarded by messages from vendors promising to improve quality; it is important to tell them how this will be done.)

The other side to aggressive marketing of performance, however, is that it is not advisable to set a target as part of a compensation formula, for example by risk-sharing through capitation or performance-related fee adjustments. Plans that tie the fee schedule to reductions in absence or lost-time injuries are almost never advisable. ("Never" is too strong only because there may be models where it is possible if the workforce covered is very large and actuarial principles can be applied.) For individual clients, risk-sharing can be dangerous for the provider. This is not a failure of confidence in the effectiveness of the approaches in this book. It is that there are entirely too many factors outside the control of service providers for them to share risk without unacceptable exposure. One year of moderately severe influenza in the community, or a failure of the client to document productivity correctly (for which the client may have little incentive if they expect to get money back), or a single bad safety-related incident will not only cost the provider but will generate ill will and reputational damage.

Implementing the Marketing Plan

The first principle of implementation is to understand the client. Fortunately, this is much easier today than in the past, because of the wealth of information available on the internet. It is now easy to find a prospective client's line of business and often the North American Industrial Classification System (NAICS) code (see Chapter 13), which is the key to determining whether Occupational Safety and Health Administration (OSHA) considers it to be high risk, and to determine their locations, size of workforce (approximately), senior officers, and recent history. This information is invaluable in approaching the client and shows not only an interest in the employer as a purchaser of services but an interest in the business and responsiveness to its needs. This information finds a second use when the client begins using the occupational health service for screening services, treatment referrals, and eventually business-sensitive support services.

Implementation of the marketing plan is fundamentally about communicating with as many prospective clients as possible as efficiently and briefly as possible while individualizing the message and making each prospect feel special. Some people, mostly natural extraverts, are able to do this effectively and even sincerely. Most, including most health care professionals, are not, which is why a specially-hired staff is almost always required for good sales performance.

When devising strategy to market occupational health services, one should follow certain principles, outlined below:

- *Emphasize consumer education.* Marketing occupational health services requires that the provider educate the audience of potential clients. Occupational health, at its best, is an integrated, systematic series of services that represents more of a relationship than a commodity. Educate clients by making them understand that a comprehensive, integrated approach to workplace health and safety works best and to establish easy to understand, measurable value for every aspect of the provider's service.
- *Embrace the new technologies.* The "good old days" of health care marketing through paid advertising, printed newsletters, live seminars, big fat bulky folders containing information, and various plastic trinkets, are largely in the past. As the world has rapidly advanced technologically, so has marketing. In the past a brochure had to be informative and provide all the information needed for the client to make a decision. Nowadays, a website can be more visual and therefore exciting and much less wordy, because a click of the mouse can link to more detail on other pages. The marketing world now centers around search engines, email blasts, interactive websites, educational webinars, virtual clinic tours, robo-calls, blogs, and social networking. Social networking, in particular, offers a glimpse into the occupational health marketing world of tomorrow. LinkedIn is a particularly compelling example of a social networking venue for professionals and is easy to use.
- *Update regularly.* Information on websites must be updated and refreshed frequently to maintain the loyalty of current and interest of prospective clients. It is useful to think of website viewers as a community with which the provider is hoping to interact, not as an audience for disseminating information. Features that are actually useful and interesting will draw more traffic, repeat viewers, and return visits from customers, which builds affinity. These might include updates on health issues (such as immunization schedules), blogs, health tips, and provider-related news. Within limits of protecting the confidentiality of provider staff, personal items (such as congratulations

on non-work-related achievements or births or marriages) help to personalize the staff and generate a sense of relationship, while professional items convey a message of competence and quality.

- *Develop a good relationship with a client or prospect through a link with that person.* If prospects or clients are not involved or familiar with LinkedIn, one should encourage their participation and send them an invitation to link in order to get the ball rolling. Over time, anyone who cultivates LinkedIn will be linked to scores, if not hundreds, of local decision makers, and will have access to everyone who is linked to them, expanding the virtual network to thousands.

- *Solicit testimonials and recommendations.* LinkedIn raises testimonials to another level by offering an easy path for any of a provider's linkages to write a short recommendation about that provider. Recommendations on the provider's LinkedIn page are readily accessible to visitors.

- *Push out news and information.* LinkedIn (and also Facebook, which is less often used for business) makes it easy to announce just about anything to everyone with whom a provider is linked: a new product, a new colleague, a new achievement (such as an award), a lecture a staff member recently gave, or a clinic open house. It is an expedient way to spread information and a welcome adjunct to email blasts and other communication modes.

- *Be timely.* One should present the message in a manner and at a time when there is minimal competition for a prospect's attention. If one sends an email message to an employer at virtually any time of the day, it will sit with scores of other promotional messages that are usually ignored. An automatic update notification email from a social media site will be more likely to be isolated from other emails.

- *Be brief.* Marketers vie for attention in an information-saturated world. Virtually everyone feels overwhelmed and protective of their time. Avoid conceptual clutter. Keep the message simple, short, and focused. Every extra word takes a proportionate amount of attention away from the words that describe the core message.

- *Be innovative.* Use marketing tactics that are different than the mode du jour. Choosing a promising marketing tactic is akin to buying an undervalued stock low and selling it high. Resist the temptation to react to yesterday's good news or the last big thing. Innovation does not necessarily mean original or inventive. Innovative providers may introduce services that are new to their communities, such as wellness, or may distinguish themselves by making innovative improvements and efficiencies in an old process, such as highly efficient handling of workers' compensation paperwork.

- *Be original.* Avoid jumping on the "what's hot" bandwagon and repeating message, clichés or stock phrases. It is tempting to presume that if a marketing tactic worked before, or currently works for another organization, it will work for you. Given the absence of marketing innovation in today's occupational health environment, the easy way out is to do the "same ole', same ole'." The outcome will be the "same ole'" results and stagnation for a long time, until it stops. Suddenly things change and "same ole'" doesn't work anymore, but when that will happen is never announced in advance.

- *Be agile.* Marketing is an art, not a science. Some people view marketing as if it were a technology, expecting and using one-size-fits-all marketing strategies and tactics. Marketing is actually more about being different. Providers must be agile and willing to devise strategies that reflect unique circumstances. If their circumstances are not unique, they have a problem in a competitive environment—and need to think hard about market differentiation.

- *Be essential.* One of the most important dimensions of marketing and selling occupational health services is relationship building. This can be time-consuming and may take several months to years to achieve solid relationships built on mutual trust and benefits. However, it is most important, particularly in an area with growing competition. A good, strong relationship with the employer's decision maker is vital to maintaining business over the long term as well as resisting competitors. Remember to allow for "entertainment" expenses within your marketing budget.

These are the essential principles of effective marketing. Like any field, however, marketing has its own received wisdom of tips based on long experience of skilled practitioners. Box 15.2 summarizes some of these tips.

Market Differentiation

In a competitive market for health care services, small differences in location, cost, and service hours may matter greatly. Big differences, however, can create a new market by allowing a more agile service to compete on price or to carve out a new service area, so that what used to be one market is now two. Where there are special needs and the industry is highly specialized, such as the oil and gas industry or aviation, preparation, special training, and diligent learning from every experience may allow the provider to forge a much deeper relationship with employers based on need and mutual reliance.

Most employers probably do not perceive much difference in quality of care between a well-managed modern occupational health service and other providers, such as a hospital emergency room or urgent care center. For them, the decision is based on (1) convenience, not value, which saves time and therefore money; (2) cost, which is why hospital services are often not competitive; and (3) added value. If the added value is in accuracy and efficiency in reporting on fitness for duty and in managing workers' compensation documentation, then the occupational health service will have the advantage. If the added value is in social or business relationships, for example if the chief executive officer (CEO) or the responsible manager of a company knows a group practice manager from meetings at the chamber of commerce or favors a local physician as a golfing partner, then the decision will not be made on those considerations. The occupational health service has to be situated as conveniently as possible, provide services at reasonable cost, demonstrate that the quality of its care is at least up to community standard, and then must compete on added value.

The provider should always consider, honestly, what makes their occupational health service different from the competition: Why should the provider be considered the best option in the market?

Even astute marketing professionals have a difficult time identifying what makes them different. It is easy to focus on unsubstantiated platitudes, for example "We offer the best customer service." That sort of empty argument is no longer persuasive. Today, the provider in a competitive environment needs to frame the most compelling competitive advantages in quantitative terms. If a particular occupational health service is the most experienced program in your community, say so: "We have treated more than 30,000 work-related conditions since 1995 and are more likely to correctly diagnose and manage a work-related injury, thereby saving your company time and money." Such a statement is accurate, quantifiable, and sets the provider apart from others.

Whenever possible, the provider should tie the marketing argument or "value proposition" (a popular business term that providers should use freely) into the ability to save employers

Box 15.2 Occupational Health Sales: Tactics and Tips

- *Do not over-promise.* Most employers feel that their workplaces are unique and want customized services, which increases cost. A few ask for bending the rules on OSHA reporting or confidentiality. Sales professionals should not be "yes men," agreeing to every prospect's wish list. Learn how to deal with these requests diplomatically, create "win–win" scenarios, and substitute the phrase "we will try" for "we will" when employers ask for too much.
- *Maintain a full prospect pipeline.* Have a full pipeline with prospects at various stages of development in the sales cycle (e.g. initial contact, first meeting, follow-up meeting, closing activity). At some point you will have a good feel for how many new contacts you need each week in order to keep the pipeline full and how many new companies can be added to the pipeline every week.
- *Maintain an accurate database.* The sales process will grind to a near halt if the contact database is filled with outdated or incorrect information. In an age in which perhaps 20 percent of the workforce changes employers every year, it does not take long for a previously flawless contact base to become obsolete. Proactively update your contact base at frequent intervals, as described in Chapter 12.
- *Hire the "right" sales professional.* The ideal sales professional should have a genuine sales persona, direct sales experience *in some* industry, and be able to relate to an employer's typical view of their own world. Sales experience with hospitals and insurance is not necessarily an advantage; occupational health sales is more like pharmaceutical detail work, where the provider's representative educates, cultivates longer-term relationships, and functions less as a salesperson and more as an account service representative.
- *Ensure Accountability.* This applies both to the occupational health sales professional and the person supervising him or her. An occupational health sales professional is rarely held appropriately accountable for their performance and long periods go by when they are not seen if they are making calls. They should be rewarded for increasing gross revenues and held accountable for making promises that cause ethical problems or reputational injury to the provider.
- *Ensure accountability of the person supervising the OH sales provider.* Occupational health sales professionals are used to playing the game with both hands tied behind their back, with no rules for the road, minimal coaching, and little or no guidance from within their organization, followed by abrupt firing when things do not go right. The person in charge of sales at the management level should be held accountable for guidance.
- *Provide performance incentives.* Any sales force is motivated by incentives and competition. Providing appropriate financial incentives to occupational health sales professionals results in a stronger, more focused performance.
- *Develop the necessary tools.* Occupational health sales professionals are usually sent out without a full or appropriate tool kit.
  - *Create an electronic library.* Avoid leaving a heavy stack of printed materials. Out of courtesy to the potential client, leave a CD or flash drive and promise customized follow-up materials later, as appropriate. Include pages

that describe each service line (see Chapter 16), being certain to emphasize the value and benefit to the buyer rather than merely describe the services.

- *Maintain client reference sheets and testimonials.* Electronic libraries can feature many elements. Maintain specialized client reference sheets and testimonial letters that may be sent to prospects that are looking for certain attributes.

- *Support the logistics of sales.* A sales professional should not go into the sales zone without a connection to home base, a contact person (such as the secretary of his or her supervisor) to facilitate communication, and a full complement of supporting tools and materials. At a minimum the sales professional should have:

  - A company car or appropriate compensation per mile driven for work-related travel.
  - A laptop computer with protected files that summarize relevant services and your complete sales universe database.
  - A PDA, tablet, iPad, or smart phone with email capability.

money in the long run. However, this value proposition should be real, not rhetorical. Employers are good at weighing value—it is the essence of being in business. They will kick the proverbial tires.

Examples of market differentiation and the chain of logic that appeals to employers include:

- *More locations* = less lost work time = saves employer money. However, satellite locations that combine occupational health services with family medicine or urgent care may not be good selling points if the mildly injured worker or the worker presenting for a screening test will have to sit in a waiting room with coughing children, crying babies, and patients with urgent problems, who will always take priority in primary care.
- *More experience* = superior diagnosis and patient management = saves employer money. However, this only applies to relevant experience. A hospital that has been in business for a century may be a novice at providing occupational health services and still has to demonstrate that it can get workers' compensation paperwork right.
- *Excellent care management software* = manage cases more appropriately and expeditiously = saves employers money. However, the software has to facilitate occupational health care for this to make sense. A specialty group-wide electronic health record may be great for coordinating diabetic care, but if it does not track periodic health surveillance outcomes on a group as well as individual basis and labels post-offer, pre-hire screening tests as "pre-employment" rather than preplacement, it is useless to the occupational health service.

Monitoring the client list

The core of the book of business for the occupational health program is its client (company) list. Careful attention is needed to keep the list current for contact, marketing, billing, and communication needs. This task is usually assigned to an account services representative (see Chapter 10), a sales representative, or the sales team. Periodic review of the list is important in understanding the provider's market and to identify those that have left the area.

Individual clients should be contacted at least annually, more often for the top 20 clients. Many occupational health programs use the time in updating client data as an "up selling" opportunity, to expand the scope of services provided. The call might be scheduled in July or August, when volumes of patients are down and business is usually slower.

Developing a script for the use of all making these calls ensures a standard approach to the companies. The staff calling need not be limited to sales staff. Calls can be made by temporarily underutilized clinical staff as well, as long as the scripts are in place and frequently-asked questions are anticipated and addressed in a supplement to the script before the calls are made.

Occupational Health Sales

"Occupational health sales" is the process of dealing directly with individuals or small groups to secure some or all of their business. Occupational health sales is largely about educating the potential client (the employer is the consumer in this situation) and attaching legitimate value to the provider's services, then demonstrating that the provider solves a need that the client feels on an emotional level. It is the means by which the provider demonstrates to individual prospective clients that the basics (convenience, cost, and quality) are already met and that their service provides the added value needed to benefit the employer and potentially to solve some of their health-related problems.

Special attention should be given to new companies that move into the area. Often, the first provider to contact them will get their business.

Approaches to Occupational Health Sales

Generally speaking, there are three different approaches to occupational health sales.

Approach #1: By Marketing Only

New business can be brought in without engaging in any sales whatsoever by simply executing a strong marketing plan. If the provider can enhance brand awareness, define services (see Chapter 16), and emphasize its competitive advantage(s), new business is likely to follow. In some cases it may even be more effective to design and execute an astute marketing plan than to meet face to face, one by one with prospective clients.

Effective marketing often paves the way for subsequent sales even if the marketing itself does not attract incremental client business. The more familiar the occupational health service and program name is to the potential buyer, the more likely it is that a sales professional representing the service will get in the door and be shown respect.

This approach is most likely to work well for small and medium-sized enterprises. Small enterprises are not sufficient in themselves to generate enough revenue to keep an occupational health service open but if the client base consists of enough medium-sized businesses, small enterprises can piggy-back on the availability of better services in the community than they would have otherwise.

Approach #2: By Just Showing Up

In the words of the great philosopher Woody Allen, "80 percent of success is showing up." Many times an occupational health sales professional is the only person *ever* to visit a company and to talk about their health issues. If so, why would the company want to consider any other option?

The first two approaches work best for medium-sized enterprises. Small enterprises may also be responsive but the cost of accessing them individually is hugely disproportionate to the revenue, making Approach #1 the only viable option for the smallest business sector. Larger companies that use a disproportionate amount of occupational health services are most likely going to make or break an occupational health program. Just one or two contracts with a big employer can anchor the financial viability of the occupational health service, although it is always wise to diversify with smaller clients for stability through the business cycle and to prevent business catastrophe in case a contract ends. Such large companies are unlikely to make a decision based solely on name recognition or a brief drop-in visit. Thus to Approach #3.

Approach #3: The Classic Sales Process

This is where selling really begins. At this level, success is often contingent on either being in the right place at the right time, or *targeting* prospects. Targeting involves directing the sales effort to the potentially high-volume companies that are most likely to need or to use the provider's services.

Although it is difficult to pinpoint projected utilization with precision, it is not difficult to estimate the magnitude of likely utilization. The classic approach for estimating service utilization has changed little during the past 25 years: work-related injuries per year can be estimated by multiplying a company's anticipated injury rate (by NAICS code) and the number of full-time employees (FTEs) at that company. Hence, an industrial classification that yields 6.1 injuries per 100 workers per year projects to an estimated 18.3 injuries per year at a company with 300 employees.

Two other predictors are often used to rank ordering of prospects by their potential value: the distance between the company's headquarters and the clinic(s) location, and the company's history with your service and/or others in the area. Obviously, an occupational health service stands a better chance of securing the business of a company close to its locations than one that is more distant and closer to competitors. A review of the company's history usually involves a subjective analysis of previous relationships, if any, and the degree of loyalty the client may feel to the competitor. Sometimes this is unknowable, but for large companies the relationships might be revealed in the service of officers on charity and hospital boards.

Few occupational health programs are accustomed to supporting a sales function and most seem unaware of what such a position would even require. Some seem to feel that it is demeaning to talk about sales, as if they were not in business.

For community-based providers embedded in hospital or multispecialty group networks, the commitment to sales is out of synch with the corporate culture of having patients come to them because of their reputation and through advertising. Instead, hospitals and groups usually try to market without sales, using Approach #1 by mentioning occupational health in a long list of medical services advertised, an approach which works poorly in reaching employers. Occupational health sales for these organizations, when they do try it, is frequently a landing place for someone within an organization who has nowhere else to go or a fresh-faced newcomer with no sales experience. Total compensation is often low, which means the candidate pool for sales is proportionately inexperienced.

For results, it is essential to hire an experienced sales professional. It is easier for an experienced sales professional to learn about occupational health and to master the fine points of a provider's service product than for a health care professional to learn how to sell. When recruiting, it is important to communicate standards, to ask questions during a preliminary phone interview to screen candidates for the job, to assess a candidate's demeanor and enthusiasm in person, and to hire someone with a genuine ability to connect with people at the workplace.

Occupational health sales professionals tend to be under-compensated, and many either have no or misconceived incentives as part of their compensation plan. The National Association of Occupational Health Professionals (NAOHP) 2010 national survey of provider-based programs shows a median compensation level of US$58,315 for an occupational health sales professional, with considerable variation by geographic region. Such compensation is markedly low compared to many industries and suggests that the position is not structured to attract the best and the brightest.

Setting other goals, establishing quotas and monitoring metrics are not necessarily inadvisable. Measures such as phone calls per week, initial meetings, introductory letters, first sales calls, follow-up calls, and percent of closes per live sales calls may be interesting and might be helpful to diagnose a sales problem and help maintain a sales professional's sense of focus, but they are not an appropriate way to measure sales success. Metrics do not translate to gross revenue. For a community-based occupational health service serving employers, the only number that really matters is gross revenue.

One solution is to simplify the compensation model. A sales professional's role should be to increase their provider's gross revenue. The incentive model should therefore be based on incremental gross revenue, comparing performance to previous year's performance, to seasonally-adjusted norms, or to budgeted expectations.

Sales as a Team Effort

The central issue in occupational health sales, aside from a skilled and ethical account services representative, is provider involvement in sales and marketing as a critical component in building sustainable occupational health relationships. However, sales does not come naturally to many, perhaps most, physicians and occupational health nurses. The time is here, in the contemporary rapidly-changing and competitive economy, for every occupational health professional to learn and embrace the basic principles of marketing. Even the strongest occupational health program cannot sustain itself for long without client education, outreach, the ability to articulate value, and an aggressive marketing effort.

Because physicians and nurses are rarely naturals at making sales, they need to accept being "managed up." In other words, the account services representative, acting as the chief sales executive (although often in a one-person sales shop) has to exert some authority and discipline over the, usually, much more senior professional staff. Providers need to learn to accept this, because sales professionals are as specialized for their world as medical specialists are in theirs. Those worlds overlap in very few places but this is one of them and the sales staff has the more critical skill set and knowledge to get the job done. Box 15.3 is a list of critical factors for managing provider involvement in occupational health sales. It is written from the point of view of the account services representative.

The presence of a senior provider or manager in person can be very impressive in the right situation. Involvement in the sales process by a physician or occupational health nurse, service line director, or senior administrator frequently seals the deal on major contracts with large employers. Their presence at a sales call suggests that the occupational health

Box 15.3 Provider Involvement in Sales: Factors that Determine Success or Failure in Occupational Health Sales

- *Factor #1: Know Your Market.* The appropriate degree of provider commitment is related to the nature of your market. A more industrialized market and/or one with unique workplace exposures suggest the need for a greater on-site provider presence. Likewise, a new start-up occupational health service or one that is not the local market leader should use its providers more often as a vehicle for winning market share because they are playing catch-up. Many smaller markets remain "high touch," person-to-person markets. In many respects, it is more essential to ensure provider visibility in a community like Pocatello, Idaho (where everybody knows everybody else) than in a larger market, such as Seattle.
- *Factor #2: Evaluate Sales Strengths.* The broader effectiveness of the sales team is an important variable in a provider's role in sales and marketing. Programs with a strong sales team or exceptional sales professional often find there is less need to use a provider in a sales role.
- *Factor #3: Consider the Provider's Personality.* Providers, like other professionals, run the gamut of personality types. If a provider is outgoing and an effective communicator, encourage frequent trips to the workplace. Many providers are technically gifted but may be shy or lacking in people skills. In this instance, it may be better to promote their technical expertise but keep their sales and marketing activities to a minimum.
- *Factor #4: Define the Provider's Time Commitment.* Spell out the degree of a provider's involvement in advance. The provider might be expected to participate in two worksite visits every Wednesday afternoon for the first year and one visit per week thereafter. A typical dilemma for many programs with a strong provider is that they want to use the provider more often for sales and marketing activities without simultaneously eroding their clinical availability.
- *Factor #5: Establish Participation Parameters.* Most providers have little or no training in sales and marketing and are likely to know little about handling objections, discerning between features and benefits, or how to close. Providers tend to go too far rather than not far enough in these areas, potentially jeopardizing a virtually completed sale.

   Clearly define the breadth of a licensed health professional's role. Generally, the physician or nurse visits a workplace to learn about work conditions and to offer preliminary recommendations, not to sell. The provider should be prepared to ask questions about current working conditions and long-term plans, and provide ad hoc advice. First and foremost, a health carer is a professional and should play that role, and should recognize his or her own limits on the sales side.
- *Factor #6: Hand-Pick Prospects.* When taking a provider on a sales call, target those employers with high injury incidence rates, hazardous conditions, complex or unusual job functions, and/or a large workforce. Ideally, a targeted sales approach is based on market research and part of the program's overall marketing plan.
- *Factor #7: Plan Ahead.* The program director should call or visit a company to obtain a preliminary sketch of special problems, critical job tasks, and current health and safety practices prior to the provider's visit. The site visit team should

develop a game plan before meeting at the company. Being well prepared for an on-site visit enhances the provider's value in the eyes of the employer.

- *Factor #8: Match the Provider with Senior Management.* Effective long-term relationships between providers and employers invariably involve a commitment from a company's senior managers. A provider's presence at a workplace provides an excellent opportunity to meet senior company management—if only briefly. Such a meeting may go a long way toward establishing or solidifying management's sense of commitment to your program.

- *Factor #9: Plan.* The provider–employer relationship is enhanced if it includes a long-term game plan for ensuring optimal health status. Provider involvement is an excellent opportunity to gauge the quality of the current plan and offer suggestions for developing a more comprehensive one.

- *Factor #10: Offer Further Contact.* The provider should conclude his or her visit with an invitation for the employer prospect to contact the provider. Although many inquiries are made through the program director, clearly stated availability of a provider is a compelling feature to most employers.

- *Factor #11: Follow Up.* A follow-up letter or email from the provider should be sent immediately after the site visit. The letter should summarize key issues and recommendations and project a sense of commitment to the employer.

- *Factor #12: Hire Well.* Many occupational health programs are so eager to have an experienced provider that it minimizes the "personality issue." If a provider's role is limited to seeing patients all day, this may work; if the provider is expected to assume an active public relations role, people skills should be factored into the hiring criteria.

- *Factor #13: Be Available.* The provider should be willing to jump in as needed to answer questions from prospects and help retain existing clients.

- *Factor #14: Take the Lead with Internal Marketing.* The provider credibility issue is no less true within your own organization. Attaining buy-in and understanding from the larger organization's senior management team is a critical issue.

- *Factor #15: Market at the Injured Worker Level.* Whether or not your program operates in an employee choice state, marketing to the individual worker is critical. A provider's "bedside manner" is a subtle yet crucial aspect of a program's image.

- *Factor #16: Make Relationship-Building a Cornerstone of the Marketing Plan.* The sales professional and the provider must not only interact, and build relationships with, decision makers and executives, they must also develop a strong relationship with each employer's workers' compensation representative and the employer's workers' compensation insurer representative/adjuster. It should be possible to pick up the phone to speak to the client's key staff in workers' compensation management and occupational health without going through a designated management representative or asking permission. This takes trust. An in-depth understanding of how workers' compensation operates within the given state is vital to successful work injury management.

- *Factor #17: Be Involved in Designing the Marketing Plan.* The provider should have input into, understand, and embrace the program's broader sales and marketing plan.

program places a high priority on the prospective client, is competent and coordinated, with impeccable teamwork, and that the program has blessing from the top.

On the other hand, it looks desperate for a physician, nurse, or senior manager to be selling prospects, especially on cold calls and especially alone. The client may be forgiven for thinking that the enterprise is failing if their most highly skilled professionals are doing sales instead of medicine. Some managers, especially at smaller firms, may be intimidated by physicians. When to bring in the "big guns" is therefore a judgment call, to be decided after the groundwork is laid, and mostly for major employers.

The value of professional involvement in face-to-face meetings also depends on the interest and "stage presence" of the staff member. If they are eager to help, that will usually show in their demeanor during the sales call. Some people light up a room with their presence, others absorb every photon. The account services representative should be selective when involving senior staff, depending on their interest and personal presence.

When the account services representative (acting as the sales executive) involves a senior staff member in a sales call, he or she should:

- Brief them on the objectives of the call.
- Define everyone's roles and limits at the meeting before they walk in the door.
- Emphasize the need for brevity and clear value statements.
- Conduct a debriefing session following the meeting, for example what went well, what did not go well, and what lessons were learned.

Many occupational health programs have an expectation that a health care professional (physician or senior nurse) will go along on a sales call every week or so. Such provider marketing can be helpful in the right situation and keeps the provider attuned to employers' needs, but is it the best use of a provider's time? Programs rely on providers to participate occasionally in important calls and consider such involvement to be the acceptable depth of their commitment to sales and marketing. But a provider can do so much more without an inordinately large commitment of their time.

An alternative is to minimize a provider's time for sales calls by shifting their time to telephone calls to prospects. Box 15.4 lists ways that the account services representative, acting as the chief sales executive, can maximize provider value in sales by leveraging their time. For example, if a provider calls up to five companies every week the day before the sales professional's initial sales call, it allows the sales professional to "hit the ground running" and is not as problematical as showing up in person. Most calls or voice mail messages take just a few minutes and can be scripted by something such as:

> Hello, this is Dr. David Webb calling from Community Occupational Health. I understand that one of our sales professionals—Donna Rust—is scheduled to meet with you tomorrow at 3:00 p.m. I would like take a few minutes to learn about the health challenges your company is facing before you meet with Donna so she will be better prepared and we can save you considerable time by cutting to the chase.

Calls can be made at times that are convenient for the provider or even after hours. This is because voice mail is often more effective when the recipient is listening to the message without any pressure or expectation that they will have to respond in the moment. At the same time, they are unlikely to hang up on a well-crafted and very brief message by a respected physician that seems to address their needs. As long as a number is given for the manager to

Box 15.4 Provider Involvement in Sales: Methods for the Efficient Use of Providers in Sales

These tips can be given to a new account services representative, as part of their "marching orders":

1. *Set the Stage for a Sales Call.* Imagine how valuable it would be for a sales professional to have their two most important initial sales calls each week preceded by a call from your Medical Director. The provider's time on the phone need not be lengthy; even a voice mail will do. The provider should state something akin to, "As the Medical Director for Work Well, I find it useful to learn a little about the challenges a company faces before they meet with our sales professional…" Just two credibility-building calls a week help position the sales professional for success.
2. *Send Out Email Blasts.* Most occupational health program email blasts directed to employers are sent by the Program Director or sales professional. Why not send a number of such blasts under the name of a program's clinicians? His or her name will add substance to your communication and increase the likelihood that the message will be read.
3. *Leave Scripted Voice Mail Messages.* A periodic voice mail campaign emanating from a provider (e.g. "I am calling to advise you we are expanding our clinic hours as of April 1.") provides considerable value. It takes little time for the provider to make such calls.
4. *Write Letters.* Use multiple modalities (email, voice mail, regular mail) to "stay in the face" of your prospects and clients. Send a letter to all companies on your mailing list once a quarter. One of those four letters should be sent annually from a senior provider.
5. *Appear on your Website.* Create a series of 30-second videos in which your clinicians offer gems about prevention and workplace health practices. Offer a new video clip each month on the home page of your program's website, or, even better, post it on YouTube and link from your website. This will spur interest in revisiting your website and showcase your clinicians. A side benefit is that it will give the staff a morale boost.
6. *Project a Pleasant Demeanor.* Most service websites provide a dry and unimaginative overview of their primary providers. Personalize each provider's biography and use a confident, congenial head shot.
7. *Be Available During Clinic Tours.* Most clinic tours should involve a brief face-to-face encounter with a program's provider. The provider can show a genuine interest in the client/prospect by asking a few simple questions germane to their workplace.
8. *Be a Public Health Advocate.* If a provider is passionate about the public health aspects of their responsibilities, they should speak periodically on related topics at community forums and employer gatherings. If they do not enjoy public speaking, a cogent written advocacy piece can be an effective alternative. Blogs are an excellent means of generating interest but require commitment so that they are of high quality and appear regularly. Letters to the editor of your local newspaper have a good chance of being published, as do more lengthy pieces for in-house and local employer publications. The more your market views you as *the* authority the more your services ride the credibility wave.

9. *Participate in High-Profile Sales Calls.* Coming full circle, in most cases your providers can be helpful participants in targeted sales calls provided he or she:
    – Clearly understands their role going in.
    – Does not dominate the sales call.
    – Demonstrates sincere interest in the company and your program's ability to customize services.
    – Improves their own understanding of the workplace by participating in a walk-through of the workplace at every opportunity.
10. *Obtain Referrals from both Internal and External Sources.* As professionals of stature in the community who are likely to meet their peers in business and local government, the committed provider can do wonders for their program by proactively reaching out to others for referrals and introductions.

call back (they rarely will) or an email address is provided, the brief recorded message will have made its point, with considerable time saved on both sides.

Such referrals may be made through other internal staff or virtually anyone throughout the community. Many people simply find it hard to turn down a physician. The provider can query fellow medical staff members, senior administrators and/or department heads, if they are embedded in a large network. Their central question should be something akin to: "You can really help our program if you can refer us to a contact of yours who may not be a client of ours at the present time. A personal introduction would even be better."

The same approach should work equally well with contacts in the community. Providers may know well-connected people within their neighborhood, fitness clubs, or through various civic activities. A personal and credible introduction easily carries as much weight as 20 cold calls.

Recommended Reading and Resources

Beckwith H (1997) *Selling the Invisible: A Field Guide to Modern Marketing.* New York, Warner Books.
Gitomer J (1999) *Customer Satisfaction is Worthless, Customer Loyalty is Priceless: How to Make Them Love You, Keep You Coming Back, and Tell Everyone They Know.* Austin TX, Bard Press.
Leoni F (2012) *Marketing Healthcare Services to Employers.* Santa Barbara CA, Seahill Press.
Parinello A (1994) *Selling to VITO: The Very Important Top Officer.* Holbrook MA, Adams Media.
Renvoise P, Morin C (2007) *Neuromarketing: Understanding the Buy Buttons in Your Brain.* Nashville TN, Thomas Nelson.

16 Services and Service Lines

Tee L. Guidotti and Craig Karpilow

A successful occupational health service, in the sense of a service provided, is one that is appropriate to the needs of the organization it serves, efficiently managed, and provides benefit in relation to cost. This chapter deals with what occupational health providers do, what these evaluations and interventions are called, how they relate to one another, and how communication can be simplified so that what is needed can be delivered by the provider.

Occupational health is a field with many ambiguities and sources of confusion in language. This has many practical implications for communication, training, and marketing. An occupational health service (providers) provides occupational health services (something needed) and it is unfortunate that the word "service" is the same in English for the provider organization (as in a hospital service) and the word for what it delivers (as in a clinical service).

Unlike other branches of medicine, where a particular procedure or surgical operation has a clear and unambiguous name, the vocabulary for common services in occupational medicine is all over the place. This is because much of the vocabulary is colloquial among workers and managers, and often differs from employer to employer. Terminology should be standardized by the occupational health service provider to prevent confusion and to convey the idea that there is a clear structure for occupational health services. For example, a test is performed at intervals to determine whether a worker is adversely affected by a working condition and that protective measures are effective. The occupational physician is likely to call it by its proper name, a "periodic health surveillance evaluation," the contract physician to call it a "screening exam," the nursing staff to call it a "medical exam," the secretary to call it an "annual physical," and managers to call it a "medical." This is not acceptable. (Most workers are likely to call it a "medical," regardless, because that is the term most often used in the community.)

To prevent confusion and ensure clear communication and accurate marketing, terminology should at least be accurate and consistent within the provider network. Soon, managers throughout the employer's organization will begin to adopt more consistent terminology as they interact with the occupational health service and the objective of the service becomes clear. However, if staff use colloquial rather than professional terms, in a misguided effort to develop rapport with workers in this way, there will be as much confusion and muddle as ever. Worse, careless terminology suggests that there is no professionalism in what is being done.

Essential Occupational Health Services

These essential services should precede others, such as wellness and worksite health promotion programs, which are only appropriate once an employer has taken care of the basics. This chapter shows how these simple services can be developed into product or service lines.

The most basic priority needs in occupational health must be provided reliably, at high quality, at a reasonable cost, and expeditiously. This is basic. These services are:

1   Acute care for illnesses and injuries.
2   Periodic health surveillance (including OSHA mandated surveillance, see Chapter 20).
3   Preplacement, periodic health, and other fitness-for-duty evaluations (see Chapter 22).
4   Prevention-oriented services (see Chapter 30).

For an expanding occupational health service, these services are also building blocks for later development.

Successful and worthwhile occupational health services should be designed to meet the real needs of the employer and the workforce, determined by an objective analysis of the company's health hazards, the characteristics of the workforce, and the workforce's illness and injury experience.

Occupational Health Service Lines

Occupational health service providers exist to deliver leadership, support, and technical services to both the employer and the employee in all areas relating to health and safety in the workplace. They do this by providing specific occupational health services that relate to fitness for duty, occupational risk, and the consequences of personal health issues (primarily as it pertains to capacity to do the specific job) to individual workers and to the workforce as a whole.

The list of specific occupational health services is long (Box 16.1), often confusing to employers, classified in different ways (see Chapters 1 and 6), and difficult to market on the basis of value added. However, these individual services can be organized into rational packages or service lines that are easier to plan, market, and support together. It is much easier, then, for employers to see how packages of services are designed to meet their specific needs.

It is useful to think of occupational health services in three dimensions (individual/ population, occupational/personal, present/future) in the form of a 2 × 2 × 2 "service cube," a graphic for thinking in three dimensions, as schematically represented in Figure 16.1. (This service cube is different from the one used in Chapter 8.) Particular occupational health services relate to either occupational health and to personal health (including the evaluation of employability and future health risk), to either individuals or the workforce as a whole (including evaluating worker health to ensure that protective measures are working correctly), and to either present health status or future health risk.

Figure 16.1 implies that some services are designed for the individual worker, others for the workforce in general, such as periodic health surveillance (which is certainly a service provided to the individual worker but which is not focused on any particular worker and is really intended to ensure that health protection measures actually work). Some services are provided to address health conditions that arise out of work and others address personal health concerns, such as employee assistance programs (because substance abuse is not considered an occupational injury or illness). Figure 16.1 also implies that some services are intended to serve the worker's need today, such as clinical services for injured workers, and others are intended to protect them from future risk or from failure, such as fitness-for-duty evaluations.

Not every one of the eight permutations of these three variables applies to occupational health services. For example, within the role of the occupational health provider, there is

Box 16.1 Occupational Health Services, Organized by Consolidated Service Line

1. *Case Management.* Managing the *present condition* of the *individual worker*
    1.1. Acute care
    1.2. Diagnosis and treatment (more complicated levels of care)
    1.3. Disability management (advisement on rehabilitation planning, how to prevent future disability, and how to overcome limitations imposed by disabling conditions through accommodation)
    1.4. Substance abuse (employee assistance, identification, employee-centered management).
2. *Occupational Health Protection.* Protecting the *workforce* from *future risk*
    2.1. Hazard identification and control
        2.1.1 Proactive role of occupational health in spotting problems
        2.1.2 Workplace risk assessment and management
        2.1.3 Health hazard investigations (as part of team)
        2.1.4 Fatality investigations (as part of team)
    2.2. Periodic health surveillance (performed for the purpose of protection, not fitness for duty)
        2.2.1 Mandated (by Occupational Safety and Health Administration (OSHA) or other occupational health standard, e.g. asbestos, lead, mercury, benzene, silica, cholinesterase-inhibiting pesticides, noise)
        2.2.2 Discretionary (for workforce protection in the absence of a regulatory standard, e.g. welding fumes, pulmonary irritants)
        2.2.3 Monitoring health experience (when the health effects of an exposure are not known and cannot now be anticipated, such as nanomaterials)
        2.2.4 Specific job assignment (e.g. hazardous materials responders, laboratory workers)
    2.3. Personal protection
        2.3.1 Respirator clearance for use and fit testing
        2.3.2 Self-contained breathing apparatus (SCBA) clearance
        2.3.3 Other
    2.4. Occupational psychology
        2.4.1 Stress prevention and management
        2.4.2 Psychosocial hazards
    2.5. Emergency management and disaster planning
        2.5.1 Catastrophic events—support for business continuity
        2.5.2 Disaster planning
        2.5.3 Workforce protection as required during the emergency
    2.6. New facility planning and review (tertiary or executive level of occupational health).
3. *Work Capacity.* Managing employment issues involving the present work capacity of the *individual worker* and preventing *future risk* to self and others
    3.1. Fitness for duty (FFD)
        3.1.1 Preplacement evaluation (time of hire or reassignment)
        3.1.2 Return-to-work evaluation (after absence or injury)
        3.1.3 "For cause" fitness-for-duty evaluation (referral for declining performance)

3.1.4   Substance abuse screening (for fitness for duty and safety-sensitive positions)

3.1.5   Confined space entry certification

3.1.6   Special evaluations

    3.1.6.1   Commercial drivers (based on Department of Transportation standards)

    3.1.6.2   Security and law enforcement officers (LEOs)

    3.1.6.3   Firefighters

    3.1.6.4   Seafarers

    3.1.6.5   Aviation (based on FAA standards)

    3.1.6.6   Diving

    3.1.6.7   Other (e.g. offshore oil and gas workers, remote area assignments)

3.2.   Disability management and impairment assessment

3.2.1   Impairment assessment for disabling conditions not arising due to work, objective to identify accommodation

3.2.2   Impairment assessment for disabling conditions arising due to work (permanent disability).

4.   *Health Risk Management.* Managing *future risk* for the *individual worker's personal health issues*

4.1   Employability and prospective risk (a health care liability function)

4.2   Support for health promotion programs

4.3   Stress management and resilience (life skills)

4.4   Absence evaluation (on referral)

4.5   Substance abuse prevention (intervention for benefit of worker)

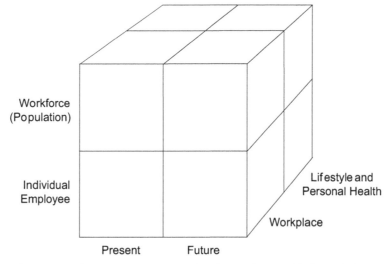

Figure 16.1 Service cube for occupational health, showing services provided to individual workers of the workforce as a whole, managing present or future health issues, which arise out of work or from personal health issues. This service cube is different from the strategic planning cube in Chapter 8 and relates closely to the pyramid of occupational health care in Figure 1.3, in Chapter 1

Table 16.1 Consolidated Service Lines of Occupational Health (simplified)

Service Line	Time frame	Level	Objective
Occupational health protection	Future	Workforce (Population)	Protection from risk
Work capacity	Present	Worker (Individual)	Fit for duty
Health risk management	Future	Worker (Individual)	Health enhancement
Case management	Present	Worker (Individual)	Health care

no provision of care for present personal health conditions for an entire population, for example—that would be the role of an entire health care system! This simplifies things.

From a marketing perspective, these clusters of related services can be organized into "service lines," as shown in Table 16.1, which consolidates the common individual services into broad product or service lines based on the natural placement of occupational health services in the three dimensional scheme. These service lines are the counterpart, for occupational health services, of the clinical service lines developed by hospitals and managed care organizations. In addition to marketing and process efficiency, however, the objective of redefining occupational health services into broad service lines is also to shift the mission of the unit toward a different balance. Making these service lines explicit has the effect of balancing acute medical care for individual workers with preventive occupational health, programming services for the workforce as a whole, and emphsizing future risk, and in so doing expands the scope of what the employer should expect the occupational health provider to achieve for them. The service lines can be used to drive marketing, plan information technology (IT) requirements (automatic selective data call-ups before scheduled clinic visits for a particular purpose), and standardized data fields in the electronic medical record.

There are four important consolidated service lines (Table 16.1):

- Services that *manage* the *present* medical condition of an *individual worker*: Case Management.
- Services that *protect* the *workforce* (population) from *future risk*: Occupational Health Protection.
- Services that evaluate the *present* medical condition of an *individual worker*, and its implications for the present or immediate, not distant, future: Work Capacity
- Services that manage the *future risk* and ability to do the job of one individual worker at a time but only in the context of standards applied to the *entire workforce*: Health Risk Management.

The individual services in Box 16.1 are classified under these headings. Table 16.2 is a simplified version, more explicit in where key services fit within the designated service lines. A major advantage of grouping services into consolidated service lines is that it is now possible to define data requirements for just four service lines rather than every single service (especially all the many fitness for duty and periodic health surveillance programs), so that on each clinic visit, selected and relevant parts of the medical record can be viewed, without searching.

Table 16.2 Summary of Service Lines and their Principal Component Services

Service Line	Clinical	Non-clinical
Occupational health protection	Periodic health surveillance Sentinel events	Proactive risk management Investigations Emergency management
Work capacity	FFD Impairment evaluation	Consultation on workplace accommodation
Health risk management	Wellness services Substance abuse	Support for health promotion Stress management (organizational)
Case management	Clinical case management Disability management	Stress management (individual)

- *Case Management* services, including clinical care, are based on the evaluation and management of individual health care needs in the present, and may involve clinical preventive services to limit disability or to support wellness in an employee who has a chronic condition. Using this term, or calling it "clinical case management," also introduces an important concept, which is that from the beginning of acute injury care to return to work, the case as a whole should be managed, beyond just treatment for the injury. This means, at a minimum, communicating clearly, from the first encounter, when an injured worker is likely to return to work to both the injured worker him or herself and the employer, monitoring progress, and evaluating the injured worker for his or her fitness for duty when recovery appears to allow safe return to work, as early as safely possible. These services require common data elements, including personal health information, at every clinic visit.
- *Occupational Health Protection* services are preventive in nature, oriented toward future risk, and although they may be provided to individuals one at a time, they are primarily for the purpose of protecting the workforce as a whole. Safety and industrial hygiene services exist for "primary prevention": to control or prevent exposure to the hazard in the first place. Clinical occupational health providers have a limited role in the primary prevention of bad outcomes from occupational hazards: they may educate or facilitate use of personal protection or learn about some lapse in practice during a medical interview, but otherwise a medical encounter does not in itself prevent exposure. Rather, the role of the clinical providers in occupational health protection is "secondary prevention" (screening for early signs of disease) in the form of periodic health surveillance. Secondary prevention is a backup to primary prevention, never a first line of defense. Screening for occupational disease, for example chest films to detect asbestosis in rip-out workers, is undertaken without actually expecting to find it, because asbestos-related disease should never be present in a well-managed workplace. If it occurs at all, its appearance represents a failure to control the hazard, with implications for the entire workforce in that job assignment. Periodic health surveillance is therefore primarily a strategy for secondary prevention for workers at risk, not an individualized medical service for individual workers. Occupational health protection services require common data elements, including detailed exposure assessment and workplace descriptions, but not detailed personal health information.

- *Work Capacity* services are based on the evaluation and management of individual work capacity in the present (not in the future, as prognosis is not a valid indicator by which to judge future fitness for duty and is not allowed under the Americans with Disabilities Act). Work capacity evaluation may involve judgments of short-term fitness to return to work, fitness for duty for a particular job assignment, or may involve chronic and permanent medical conditions and separation. However, they all involve matching the employee's capacity with job requirements (in the case of permanent disability evaluation, any job). These services require common data elements, including detailed job descriptions and requirements, but not detailed personal health information.
- *Health Risk Management* services are based on the evaluation and management of an individual employee's health risk in the future, for reasons of health promotion. These services may involve clinical preventive services at all three levels ("tertiary prevention" is the prevention of disability) and support for programs in health promotion. Disability prevention is a major objective in occupational health in order to avoid impairment and loss of personal quality of life, to protect the future employability of the workers, to protect against loss of income, and to preserve productivity. This service line may include dealing with substance abuse (see Chapter 28), as one form of disability prevention. These services require common data elements, including personal health information.

Within these service lines, individual services may be clinical or non-clinical. Most health care providers (such as physicians and nurses) are more accustomed to classifying services as "hands-on clinical" (diagnosis and treatment, done wearing a white coat or a nurse's uniform) or non-clinical "administrative" (programmatic, done wearing business attire). However, this mindset unnecessarily limits the vision and therefore the scope for integration of information and expansion of the occupational health provider, and obscures the common goals of clinical and non-clinical services.

Licensed health care providers have a role in non-clinical services as well as clinical services. Their participation in non-clinical services often requires a team approach and this helps to build rapport with other occupational health and safety professionals.

Communication with Managers and Supervisors

An employer must support its health service with a well-defined policy which addresses the interests of the employees and which is accessible to them. The company's policy is the keystone which supports the entire array of delivery programs and establishes the importance which the company gives to the maintenance of employee health and safety. The company occupational health and safety policy should originate with, or at least be clearly endorsed by, top management. It must be more than a mere statement of good intent. Specific policy statements on environmental hazard control, employee health monitoring, confidentiality of personal health information, rehabilitation post-injury or illness, and informing workers of hazards and of their monitoring results should be included. The policy statement should be accessible to all company employees.

Employees are frequently referred to the occupational health service by their supervisors, who may be concerned about their ability to work, performance problems, or about a health-related problem. Other times, an employee may be referred by the manager, a more senior level of supervision, because there has been a pattern of absence (see Chapter 24), a pattern of injuries or near misses, or some other reason to question the health and fitness of the worker. These situations happen more often in corporate or in-plant occupational health services than in community-based services.

Effective problem solving requires clear, accurate, and complete communication on many levels, including:

- Clarity of requests for assistance or query. (Manager → Provider)
- Information on specific hazards in the workplace. (Manager → Provider)
- Information specific to individual cases for supervisors (specifically, fitness for duty). (Provider → Supervisor)
- Training of managers for their responsibilities (including confidentiality of medical records). (Provider, Employer → Manager)
- Education and training of supervisors, employees, contractors, and suppliers on occupational health. (Provider → Manager)
- Feedback from the occupational health service to the line manager, on health issues affecting workforce. (Provider → Manager)
- Feedback to the worker to ensure that he or she understands the process and where his or her case may be at any given time. (Provider → Worker)
- Feedback on process and satisfaction of service. (Worker, Supervisor, Manager → Provider)

One of the more common ways in which communication breaks down is when managers and supervisors do not know what to ask for. The result may be a referral to the occupational health service that is vague, off-point, or inappropriate. It is more important for managers simply to tell the provider what they need instead of specifying a particular service by name. Eventually, managers must be trained through briefings and exposure (which is why consistent terminology is so important) to provide occupational health with the information it needs to do provide the right service.

Box 16.2 outlines the minimum information the occupational health service will usually need when a case is referred. Generally, for in-house occupational health services the best way to do this is electronically, with a single-window of contact, privacy protection, and a simple, web-based form that prompts the manager or supervisor for the critical information so that it will be available at the time of encounter with the employee. For community-based services, a paper form (requiring explanation and delivery of a supply to employers, and therefore unlikely to be used) or secure website may be required.

Three difficult situations are unfortunately all too common in corporate occupational health services:

- *The Mystery Referral.* This occurs when the employee arrives at the occupational health service with no documentation or referral request. The provider is then forced to ask, "Why are you here?" Not infrequently, the worker does not know or (if it is a performance issue) may be evasive, so the provider must call the supervisor, much valuable time is lost, and nobody is satisfied with the encounter.
- *The Cryptic Referral.* Referral to the occupational health service is arranged by the manager, who has become involved because a situation has escalated out of the control of the supervisor. There is a reason given but it does not sound right. Behind the referral may be a question of deteriorating performance in a previously well-performing employee and often a genuine concern for whether this is a health-related problem. On the other hand, the manager may have in mind firing the worker but does not want to commit too much in writing before a decision is made and so does not

Box 16.2 Checklist of Information Needed When Referring a Case

Provide at least the following information for all cases referred for medical evaluation:
- Reason for the referral.
- Question to be answered (as specific as possible).
- Job description, with clear statement of unusual hazards or requirements.
- Duration of employment:
    - With the employer.
    - In the current job assignment.
- Performance issues with this employee.
- Pre-existing disability, if any, and job accommodation (adaptations made to help a person with a disability to stay on the job).
- Expectations for this employee.
- Whether this is a general problem (i.e. affecting several employees) or specific to this one employee.
- Who to contact for further information.

provide enough information. The referral is uninformative and often useless because key information is lacking.
- *The Dump.* The most difficult common scenario is when a manager, usually in the human resources department, refers a worker for evaluation as an inappropriate disciplinary measure, often as a last step before firing them. This usually happens after a long sequence of threats, reassignments, and attempts to alienate the individual and induce them to leave (constructive dismissal), often to employees who are perceived as difficult, uncooperative, or insubordinate. The unstated objective on the part of human resources is for the occupational health service to find grounds, on the basis of health and fitness, to dismiss the individual. The hidden agenda is that the human resources department either does not believe that it has strong enough documented grounds to fire the individual or it may fear that the employee will lodge a complaint or appeal, resulting in a major legal or administrative battle. So, they would rather have someone else trigger the dismissal action and take the heat for it.

Obviously, it is not for the occupational health service to play a disciplinary role or to get the human resources department off the hook for taking action based on performance. The occupational health service is on firm ground objecting to this practice. The US Equal Employment Opportunity Commission requires referral for medical evaluation to be strictly for the purpose of business necessity, and has stated: "An employer cannot require a medical evaluation solely because an employee's behavior is annoying, inefficient, or otherwise unacceptable" (see Chapter 22). Even so, the pressure from within the employer's organization can be quite intense to play along. The occupational health provider, the worker, and, ultimately, the employer are best served by clarity of communication and complete documentation. Another reason for seeking clarity in referral information is therefore to document exactly what is happening so that the occupational health provider is not vulnerable and unprotected in a situation that could get ugly.

Executive Health Services

Major corporate executives are valuable to their companies. Executive health services are very attractive to medical group practices and hospitals as a way of increasing profitability and catering to an affluent clientele who may in the future choose the institution for various health care needs and for philanthropy. The value added for executive health services compared to evaluation by a private physician at home is convenience of scheduling and efficiency, personalization of care, and prestige. These services are expensive. The costs are justified as a direct employer expense because executive health services are intended to identify and correct health problems in key management personnel at an early stage to avoid expensive disruptions in executive succession, business continuity, or poor judgment.

Executive health services are rarely, if ever, combined with more traditional occupational health services, despite the obvious parallel to evaluations for fitness for duty and periodic health surveillance. However, they are often offered in another department (such as internal medicine) of a hospital network and often involve occupational health practitioners. They can be considered to be high-level wellness programs (see Chapter 30).

In recent years, executive health services have thrived in high prestige settings such as the Mayo Clinic, the University of Pennsylvania, and the Cleveland Clinic. The great advantage of these centers is that the executive will leave satisfied that his or her health has been evaluated by the best physicians available.

The executive health experience features expedited access, by appointment, to diagnostic and imaging services in a logical sequence, following which all results are available for review in a session with an appropriate medical specialist (usually an internist), with sufficient time to initiate treatment for minor problems or investigations for positive findings. This usually takes two days, with time for relaxation or business communication.

There is a long history of establishing clinics in resort settings where major executives can have health evaluations in a week combined with tourism, recreation, and fitness programs. The attraction of a resort atmosphere has led to highly successful executive health operations in places such as The Greenbrier (White Sulphur Springs, West Virginia), and the Mayo Clinic in Scottsdale. This option appears to be less popular than it once was, however, as executives come under more pressure to be available for work around the clock and are constantly traveling for business. Spouses of executives can also participate in the social amenities.

Executive health programs present an excellent opportunity to encourage sound health practices. Participants are likely to be more receptive to health promotion interventions than they might have been at home.

Executive health programs are now almost always based on sound principles of preventive medicine, behavioral medicine, and health promotion. In the past, when the emphasis was more on travel as an executive perquisite, they were often disparaged for relying on obsolete screening protocols and excessive clinical testing. The tests incorporated in the program should be reasonably cost-effective, reliable, and safe, but the screening protocol is usually more intense than for the non-executive subject.

Managing Travel Medical Services

Travel medicine services are mostly provided to the many workers and executives who travel on business to parts of the world with less developed health care systems and with higher risks. Tourists, aside from ecotourists, extreme sports enthusiasts, and adventure seekers, tend to stay in areas that present less risk.

The vast majority of workers who travel are "well" (referred to in this book as "subjects" rather than "patients"), and so it is the responsibility of the provider to help maintain their health while they are working abroad and above all to "*do no harm*" when providing travel medical care, immunizations, chemoprophylaxis, and other preventive measures.

One should allow at least 30 minutes for a consultation appointment in order to exercise best practice in travel medicine.

Travel-Related Services

The health requirements of employees who travel have become much more diverse and complex. Global health issues and the distribution of health risks change constantly. The staff of occupational health services delivering travel medicine care needs to be well informed and up to date with best practice. In addition to anticipating infectious health risks while traveling, such as malaria, travel medicine should feature education on risks the traveler may not have thought of but which can be serious in some parts of the world, such as a high rate of traffic injuries, the need for foot care (because an injured foot interferes with ambulation and complicates everything else), dental emergencies, and rabid dogs.

An occupational health service offering travel medicine should deliver the following basic services:

- Comprehensive travel health "risk assessments" to determine what health advice, immunizations, and prevention/ prophylaxis is needed in the particular case.
- Provision of general travel health advice and education on topics such as: the prevention and treatment of travelers' diarrhea, the prevention of mosquito bites, HIV/AIDS prevention, and blood-borne infection awareness.
- Hepatitis B immunization.
- Prescription, provision, and administration of "routine" travel vaccines including typhoid, hepatitis A, and updates of routine vaccines, that is, tetanus and diphtheria (Td), polio, measles, mumps, and rubella (MMR).
- Prescription and provision of malaria chemoprophylaxis and the use of emergency standby malaria medication, post-exposure prophylaxis, following blood-borne virus exposure.
- Advice for employees with underlying medical conditions or who are traveling during pregnancy.
- Vaccine safety evaluation for individuals with special needs (underlying medical conditions, immune-compromised, experienced previous adverse events following immunization).
- Administration or rapid referral to obtain more unusual travel-related vaccines such as: Japanese B encephalitis, rabies, tick-borne encephalitis, and BCG.
- Evaluation of need for and rapid referral to obtain yellow fever vaccine and indications for the prescription, provision, and administration.
- Provision/vending of travel health-related equipment such as water purification filters, insect repellents, mosquito nets, condoms, sunscreen, etc.
- Evaluation to recognize the likelihood of acquired disease in recent travelers (especially malaria, tuberculosis, HIV/AIDS) and to refer them to specialized centers for diagnosis and treatment.

Travel medicine is a rapidly evolving specialty and as such it is essential that practitioners utilize recognized, reliable, and up-to-date resources. Online travel health websites are now considered essential tools to achieve quality of care in travel medicine. They are listed at the end of this chapter.

Vaccine Inventory

Certain standard vaccines should be kept on hand (see Chapter 11). These include the current year's influenza vaccine; vaccines such as tetanus-diphtheria (Td), polio (IPV), measles, mumps, and rubella (MMR), hepatitis A and B, and possibly, especially if there is a significant primary care component to the practice, pneumococcal vaccine, meningococcal serotype vaccine, and human papilloma virus (HPV).

Which other vaccines should be kept on hand depends on the usual and ordinary itineraries of clients and employees and how frequently they are required. It is not cost-effective to keep most of these vaccines on hand unless there is a regular need for them. Many of them are expensive and likely to expire before use. Some, such as yellow fever and cholera, must be given and stamped by a county health department official or a clinic that has obtained permission to stamp certificates. The more exotic vaccines are available from the various pharmaceutical houses and contact information is readily available through several of the online reference services given at the end of this chapter. For occupational health services that have more than one location in an area, it may be more cost-effective to store infrequently used vaccines in one central location and to have a staff member drive it over to the clinic or have it sent by courier in advance of when it is needed.

Education and prevention

Patient education depends on where the employee is traveling and the baseline medical conditions the employee is "carrying with them." The occupational health care provider should not assume that the worker's or travelling executive's family physician knows or has given appropriate instruction for their conditions regarding upcoming travel to potentially risky areas.

The traveler should be educated on the signs and symptoms of the common health problems of travelers: gastrointestinal infections, animal bites, what to do after traumatic injury, and the top six causes of fever among travelers outside developed areas of the world: malaria, dengue, enteric fever, rickettsioses, acute schistosomiasis, and pneumonia. The use of a mask to avoid infectious diseases on public transportation is as acceptable for foreigners as for locals in certain countries during certain seasons.

In addition to infectious disease, education should cover environmental issues such as sun exposure and the use of SPF 45 or higher sun block, heat stress, humidity, foot care, and significant air pollution.

All travelers should be educated on the risk of thromboembolic disease ("travelers thrombosis"), which is significantly increased during pregnancy. Preventive measures include hydration, frequent movement of the extremities and compression stockings. A history of deep vein thrombosis is quite common, so the provider should be prepared to consider prophylactic injectable anticoagulants and how to manage this.

Emphasize dietary precautions and food contamination, water purification and treatment of traveler's diarrhea, emphasizing prompt and vigorous oral or parenteral hydration, plus the use of Pepto-Bismol®. If persistent, the traveler should know the general indications for use of an antibiotic such as azithromycin, ciprofloxin, etc., especially if the local health care system is unreliable.

Those travelers with chronic medical problems such as hypertension, diabetes, or respiratory disease need to have the signs and symptoms of potential crises reviewed and instructions on when to seek medical care, because they may not have experienced them in the past but may be at high risk while traveling. For women who may be pregnant, education should include obstetrical complications such as bleeding, contractions, rupture of membranes, premature labor, and toxemia if the provider is confident in his or her knowledge. If not, referral back to the woman's obstetrician with a recommendation for this (and suggested references) may be in order.

Substance abuse almost always involves alcohol because drug acquisition and possession is so dangerous in many countries and punishable by the death penalty in some. Expatriate communities, particularly where isolated, often have a very high prevalence of alcoholism. In some settings there is very little diversion after hours and where alcohol is available (including homemade, in countries where it is not legal), individuals without other interests may develop serious drinking problems. If there is a possibility of this, but no current problem can be documented (but which may just be well hidden), confidential referral to an employee assistance program for preventive intervention prior to deployment may be advisable.

Depending on the situation and the experience of the traveler, it is useful to discuss safety issues such as seat belts and fall prevention. Among the most important safety issues for some countries are those related to preventing victimization during a crime: not wearing expensive clothing or jewelry to avoid robbery or kidnapping, dropping to the ground or the floor of the car to avoid bullets in crossfire, being alert to unusual traffic patterns, maintaining "environmental awareness" while walking, and never going to a window to see what has happened after hearing an explosion.

Malaria

Malaria is a critical dimension of travel medicine because it is the most common potentially lethal infectious disease in the world and is endemic in many areas where industrial activity is intense, such as the oil and gas industry. Malaria ceased to be widely endemic in the US or Canada over a century ago, and so very few workers are immune to any strain or type of malaria or resistant to infection and are at risk of full-blown infection which can easily be fatal or cause brain damage in the case of falciparum.

The provider should either be well trained in malaria or know where to refer the worker for immediate assistance. (For hospital and multispecialty groups, this may simply involve arranging in advance for the travel clinic to see such workers on an expedited basis or to have someone from the travel clinic come down to occupational health quickly to deliver the service.) Either the occupational health provider (if this is a frequent need) or the referral partner should then be able to discuss risk/benefit calculation when considering malaria prophylaxis. Regardless of whether chemoprophylaxis is prescribed, the employee should always be counseled on personal protective measures against mosquito bites.

Medical management is beyond the scope of this chapter; however, the principles relate directly to the work issues. The basic risk/benefit calculation for chemoprophylaxis of malaria compares the risk of a serious adverse reaction to the prescribed antimalarial with the risk of contracting falciparum malaria; left untreated, falciparum malaria is a progressive and fatal disease. The true malaria risk facing the employee traveler will in most cases remain unknown and can only be inferred from country-specific information and knowledge of what activities the traveler will engage in. Therefore, the decision to prescribe prophylaxis will be a clinical one, and may vary by practitioner, the experience of similar workers, and national experience. For example, approaches to prophylaxis may vary among the US and UK (which favor chemoprophylaxis), France and Germany (where practitioners often favor "stand-by treatment," as discussed below), and practitioners in the country where the traveler is going (where the perception of traveler's risk may be distorted because of high endemicity within the native population).

Simplistically, the risk of developing malaria should exceed the risk of experiencing a serious adverse drug reaction. However, because chemoprophylaxis is generally prescribed for well or asymptomatic individuals (increasingly including those with stable chronic illness), only a very low risk of serious adverse events from the medication is acceptable. Medication risk obviously varies with the antimalarial prescribed: the lower risk is generally seen with atovaquone-proguanil and doxycycline. Mefloquine is less well tolerated and carries a liability risk because of recent litigation and allegations of side effects.

For the educated employee, there is an alternative approach. Although current recommendations of the World Health Organization (WHO) and the Centers for Disease Control and Prevention (CDC) are that travelers should be prescribed chemoprophylaxis where the risk of falciparum malaria exists, some authorities recommend the use of "stand-by emergency treatment" (SBET). This requires the traveler to be alert to symptoms and to know when to start medication. Because dosages are for treatment rather than prophylaxis, the risk of side effects is proportionately higher.

Strategies currently used to protect travelers against malaria are not 100 percent effective: travelers' compliance with recommendations is problematic. While abroad, the employee may experience significant difficulties in accessing either competent medical care or efficacious medication. (Counterfeit medication circulates in many parts of the malaria-endemic world.) Therefore, travelers who will be in country for more than a few weeks should receive a prescription for treatment doses and take them along for SBET, to self-medicate as a backup to chemoprophylaxis.

Sexual Activity

The topic of sexual activities with the "locals", or with other expatriates, or with imported prostitutes is almost never discussed openly in travel medicine but it is an extremely important part of the risk profile of business travelers. It is unwise to rely on promises of abstinence. There is, of course, a greater risk of contracting HIV/AIDS, gonorrhea, HPV, hepatitis B, and syphilis in areas where the prevalence is high in the local population but an elevated risk also occurs among mobile risk-taking travelers and anywhere there are many sex trade workers serving frequently transient worker populations. Educating traveling workers and executives to the hazards of antibiotic-resistant infections is also valuable. These topics may require tact and possibly storytelling rather than a more direct approach.

If the employee is HIV positive or has other diseases that compromise immunity, they are at higher risk of infection and complications. If the CD4 count is $<200/mm^3$, there may also be interactions with travel medications.

Travelers with HIV-positive status and some other documented diseases (such as Hansen's disease, formerly known as leprosy) may be restricted from obtaining entry visas to some countries.

Recommended Reading and Resources

Most textbooks and references on occupational medicine focus on clinical practice and not provision of services.

American College of Occupational and Environmental Medicine (ACOEM) (2004) *Occupational Medicine Practice Guidelines*. Chicago, ACOEM, 3rd ed., as updated. Purchase includes one-year subscription to online version and regular updates. Available at: http://www.acoem.org/practiceguidelines.aspx. Accessed January 6, 2011.

Guidotti TL (2010) *The Praeger Handbook of Occupational and Environmental Medicine*. Santa Barbara CA, Praeger ABC-Clio. Relevant sections throughout the book; comprehensive.

Guidotti TL (2010) Occupational Medicine. Chapter 6 in Nabel EH, ed. *ACP Medicine*. Hamilton, Ontario (Canada), BC Decker for the American College of Physicians. Discusses overview of clinical services.

LaDou J, ed. (2007) *Current Occupational and Environmental Medicine*. Columbus OH, McGraw Hill, 4th ed. Concise descriptions of many services but incomplete.

Rosenstock L, Cullen MR, Brodkin CA, Redlich CA (2005) *Textbook of Clinical Occupational and Environmental Medicine*. Philadelphia, Elsevier Saunders. Primarily a clinical textbook, with some discussion of individual services.

Smith I (2007) *Occupational Health: A Practical Guide for Managers*. London, Taylor and Francis.

Travel Medicine

Chiodini J and Boyne L (2003) *The Atlas of Travel Medicine and Health*. Hamilton, Ontario, Canada, BC Decker.

Cook G, Zumla A, eds (2003) *Manson's Tropical Diseases*. London, WB Saunders Co. Ltd., 21st ed.

Dawood R, ed. (2002) *Travellers' Health; How to Stay Healthy Abroad*. London, Oxford University Press, 4th ed.

DuPont H, Steffen R, eds (2001) *Textbook of Travel Medicine and Health*, Hamilton, Ontario, Canada, BC Decker Inc, 2nd ed.

Guidotti TL (2010) *The Praeger Handbook of Occupational Health*. Santa Barbara CA, Praeger ABC-Clio. See Chapter 26 on "Global Occupational and Environmental Health."

Jong E (2002) Management of a travel medicine clinic. Chapter 4 in Zuckerman E, ed. *Principles and Practice of Travel Medicine*. New York, John Wiley.

Karpilow C (1991) *International Occupational Medicine*. New York, Van Nostrand Rheinhold. See Chapter 8, 9, and 10, which contain material on the management of travel services in the occupational health setting.

Keystone J, Kozarsky P, Freedman D, et al. (2004) *Travel Medicine*, Phlilladelphia, PA, Mosby.

Lockie C, Walker E, Calvert L, et al. (2000) *Travel Medicine and Migrant Health*. Edinburgh, Churchill Livingstone.

World Health Organization (2005) *International travel and health*. Geneva, WHO. http://whqlibdoc.who.int/publications/2005/9241580364.pdf. Accessed April 16, 2012.

Online Resources

(all websites accessed 10 January 2012)

British Mountaineering Council: www.thebmc.co.uk/.

Fitfortravel: www.fitfortravel.scot.nhs.uk/.

Health Protection Scotland: www.advisorybodies.doh.gov.uk/jcvi/fol_classesofinformation.htm This is the Scottish national surveillance unit, home of the Joint Committee on Vaccination and Immunization.

ISTM TravelMedListserve: http://www.istm.org/webforms/Members/MemberActivities/listserve. aspx.

National Travel Health Network and Centre (NaTHNaC): www.nathnac.org.

Promed: www.promedmail.org.

UK Department of Health: www.dh.gov.uk.

UK Foreign & Commonwealth Office: www.fco.gov.uk.

UK Health Advice for Travellers: www.dh.gov.uk/PolicyAndGuidance/HealthAdviceForTravellers/ fs/en.

UK Health Protection Agency: www.hpa.org.uk (malaria).

UK malaria prevention guidelines: www.malaria-reference.co.uk.

US Centers for Disease Control and Prevention (CDC): www.cdc.gov.

World Health Organization (WHO): www.who.int/en/.

World Health Organization disease outbreak news www.who.int/csr/don/en/.

17 Quality and Performance Indicators

Tee L. Guidotti

At the enterprise level, occupational health and especially safety can be seen as a continuous process of quality improvement. In that sense, occupational health and safety is no different than continual refinements in production or the quality assurance process that has become well known to sophisticated managers around the world and in all industries. The principles outlined in this chapter apply equally to the occupational health experience of employers, the delivery of a specific service, and the overall performance of the occupational health service itself. The difference is in the selection and interpretation of performance indicators. Appendix 1 provides a comprehensive audit instrument that can be used to assess health and safety performance at the enterprise level and provides many of these indicators. However, assessing these indicators is usually not the role of clinicians. Audits are more commonly performed by industrial (occupational) hygienists, health and safety consultants, and managers.

The major emphasis of this chapter is not on how to assess the performance and quality of a clinical service, per se, but on how managers associated with major employers view quality and performance indicators, so that occupational health providers will understand the terminology and concepts when communicating with them.

Clarity of "mission, vision, and values" (MVV), was emphasized by Malcolm Baldrige, a former US Secretary of Commerce and early advocate of quality management, and this concept has become foundational in management theory today. The relevance of quality improvement, and "process engineering" to streamline production while rendering it more reliable, depends on the mission of the enterprise (to make a profit, to produce a necessary good, to deliver a service, to provide a just and equitable public service). Quality improvement also reflects the vision and values of the organization. A commitment to quality represents integrity, just as a commitment to occupational health represents respect and mature acceptance of an employer's responsibilities, suggesting that an employer is reliable and can be trusted. Performance indicators are ways to keep track and to know where improvements should be made. The concept of "continuous quality improvement" has been taken up by industry as a mainstream management philosophy. It applies equally well to running occupational health services.

It may be less obvious but is equally important that occupational health itself is a type of process improvement, because achieving a healthier and more productive workforce supports productivity and reduces costs, just like other process improvements. Communicating occupational health goals and performance in terms of process improvement makes that point to management and expresses the enterprise's occupational health in terms management can understand.

At the same time, the performance of the occupational health service as a department or unit can be measured and tracked using the same system. Managers tend to look at tangible outputs (such as number of injuries), and health care facilities such as specialty group practices tend to look at services provided (a process measure) in evaluating performance. However, neither is appropriate for occupational health services, in which the goal is to prevent something bad from happening and to minimize the need for providing treatment-oriented health care services (which is usually the goal of a health provider) by providing preventive services that may seem unnecessary if bad outcomes are not happening. Because of this conundrum, the performance of occupational health services is very difficult for management to interpret, appreciate, and value. Redefining occupational health as process improvement and measuring progress by using performance indicators that are different from hospitals and clinics expresses occupational health protection in terms management can understand and provides a more accurate picture of what is being done and why.

When performance indicators are introduced for occupational health, it is not unusual for trends in reportable injuries, short-term disability, and absence to go in the wrong direction at first, because the results are more reliable. Improvement in a performance measure that leads to stringent accuracy, always results in injuries being reported that previously would have been concealed, overlooked, or misclassified. This results in a temporary deterioration that can be alarming to management, which was expecting improvement. Ultimately, more accurate reporting unmasks the true situation, which management has usually not appreciated and often does not wish to face.

Inaccurate or poorly monitored performance indicators almost always hide much poorer performance than the indicators show, due to underreporting. Incidents get missed, lost-time injuries are concealed by inappropriate return to work, employees will "forget" about incidents because they do not want to get into trouble, management will discourage reporting cases that would break an apparent (but unreal) exemplary safety record, and teams will keep quiet in order to win awards. For the occupational health service, and especially for safety officers, improvement in the reporting system is therefore a calculated risk. Accuracy, improved data capture, and scrutiny removes many (but not all) ways that incidents and injuries can go unreported or misclassified and data can be manipulated.

The Deming Cycle

The analytical methods of continuous quality improvement, the general approach of enterprise-based risk assessment and management (which underlies control banding and other variations), and the general approach of quality improvement (and many other management techniques) all reduce to the familiar Deming Cycle of "Plan → Do → Study (or "Check") → Act," which is management policy in many organizations already. (Figure 17.1) The Deming cycle underlies the strategy of process engineering and improvement that has been widely accepted in manufacturing and service industries for decades. In this section, the emphasis is on process improvement in the enterprise, but the concepts apply equally well to improving performance of the occupational health service provider's systems and operations.

W. Edwards Deming was a visionary statistician working in the field of quality control who made the transition to leading management thinker by abstracting the concept of continuous quality improvement from the more batch-oriented quality control monitoring protocols of his day, and then applied his insight generally. (Deming himself always referred to the cycle as the Shewhart Cycle, in honor of his mentor, Walter Andrew Shewhart, who devised the theoretical framework of modern statistical quality control.) In the 1950s Deming toured

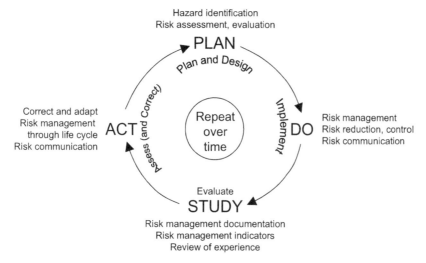

Figure 17.1 The Deming Cycle (ring), the Risk Cycle (outside ring), and Quality Improvement Process (inside ring). The Risk Cycle applies to the management of hazards and risks, at all levels, and so is an important concept in occupational health and safety (see Chapter 21). Most hospitals have adopted some variant of the Quality Improvement Process for general health care

Japan giving lectures on quality control, in order to assist the Japanese in rebuilding their devastated industry. His message was enthusiastically embraced and brilliantly adapted. (In Japan, it became "Plan → Do → Check → Act." Deming himself preferred "Plan → Do → Study → Act.")

The essence of Deming's work was quality improvement and most contemporary quality improvement systems draw heavily on his work and follow the same general cycle. Today, Plan → Do → Study → Act permeates management theory and has been the foundation for other systems, including the Six Sigma process developed by General Electric and widely applied in business, ISO 9000, Total Quality Management, Quality Circles, Kaizen (Continuous Quality Improvement), and Lean Manufacturing (the Toyota method). All of these management systems are commonly used in North America (see Chapter 6). Not surprisingly, given its challenges and the consequences of a defect, the health care sector has been particularly interested in quality improvement systems and has spun many variations of the Deming cycle as applied to health care.

Some systems do not follow Deming's teachings, however. "Business process reengineering" (BPR) features a reinvention of the process, but without reference to the experience with existing processes: it continually starts from square one. Because it is a rethinking rather than a learning system, BPR can be disruptive and can lead to unpleasant discoveries of why production was organized as it was in the first place. "Zero defects," a quality management system popular in the 1960s, was also contrary to Deming's thinking and he considered its goal of perfection to be unachievable and therefore an obstacle to practical management. Zero defects has its counterpart in the goal of "no injuries, no lost time," which in practice can be a perverse incentive to underreporting.

Presenting worksite-level risk assessment as a simple application of "Plan → Do → Study → Act" renders it familiar and demystifies occupational health protection, which seems remote and technical to many managers. Presenting hazard control and enterprise-level risk assessment (see Chapter 21) in the same way turns it from a duty into a management opportunity and a key performance indicator, because performance in occupational health protection is almost certainly among the most sensitive summary indicators of overall management performance. This observation has practical utility because it can be used to advance occupational health in the following ways:

- Enterprise-level risk assessment and management can be readily integrated into enterprise quality improvement and Six Sigma by linking the steps explicitly to the Deming Cycle.
- Worksite-level risk assessment and management, which can appear complicated to the uninitiated, can be easily integrated into the policy of organizations that use the Deming Cycle and progress can be reported in "Deming" terms for rapid management comprehension.
- Corporate policies regarding continuous process improvement can be harmonized with policies on occupational health protection.
- Occupational health protection measures and outcomes can be developed as key performance indicators for the entire organization, since they reflect adherence to the Deming model.
- It has been observed repeatedly that badly-managed companies almost always have the worst occupational health and safety records. Occupational health indicators may therefore be used as performance indicators for the company as a whole, and reflect on management competence.
- The occupational health service can apply these same principles to its own operation and achieve excellence.

Performance Indicators

Performance indicators are measures that can be used to track performance for a business unit. For example, sales are a way of tracking performance of the sales department with respect to quantity, returns following a sale is a way of tracking quality, since they should not be necessary if the product fits the customer's need, service calls are a way of tracking the performance of the product under real-world conditions, and repeat service calls are a way of tracking the performance of the service department.

Performance indicators are universal in industry and familiar to anyone with a passing acquaintance with business. Virtually every business in North America at least tracks quarterly earnings or daily cash receipts. This section looks more narrowly at their use in evaluating the performance of occupational health services.

However, as noted above, standard approaches to performance indicators that might apply in health care (such as number of patients seen, readmission rate, postoperative infection rate, time spent in an office visit) are largely meaningless in providing occupational health, where the objective is to prevent problems, reduce the need for expensive health care, and to get workers back to work early but always safely. Performance indicators for occupational health therefore need to focus on reductions in the frequency of occupational health problems, often based on estimates of cases prevented, quality of service, efficiency, and compliance.

Whatever their type, performance indicators should relate to the core business, not to a peripheral function. Context is everything. The popularity of the food at the lunch counter is of no importance to the enterprise if the food service is operated by a contractor, employees are not dissatisfied, health standards are maintained, and it is there strictly for the convenience of employees. It is of paramount importance if the employer is sponsoring a health promotion and wellness program and has launched a nutritional guidance program.

Performance indicators are essential to manage any business unit, to the extent that in business school there is a saying that "if you can't measure it, you can't manage it" (variously attributed to numerous management gurus and even to a paraphrase of Galileo). Performance indicators drive process improvement and are a way of keeping track of the effectiveness of innovations. They are also important in demonstrating transparency and confidence to stakeholders (such as senior managers, directors, and shareholders). They can be used to track the performance of individual providers, and provide some objective measures for performance reviews, or they can track the performance of teams, departments, or the entire enterprise.

Performance indicators should be easily measured, actionable (should lead to corrective action), interpretable, acceptable to those being evaluated, easily shared, sensitive to poor outcomes, and demonstrate a close correlation to process quality and efficiency. For occupational health, these are difficult specifications, not nearly as readily achieved as in general health care. For this reason, among many others, it is essential that the occupational health service have a deep knowledge and understanding of how every performance indicator works that is applied to its evaluation. Simply applying the same performance indicators to an occupational health service as are used by, say, an urgent care center, or by other parts of a hospital, or by a clinic, will profoundly bias the evaluation. It is a constant battle to educate clinic and hospital administrators to understand this because they value consistency and uniformity, and this is a major reason why it so difficult to manage occupational health services in that environment.

Performance indicators can be categorized in many ways:

- Quantitative indicators, which can be presented as a number and might include indicators of activity (such as number of subjects enrolled in a study or number of patients seen in clinic).
- Practical or operational indicators reflect operations or process efficiency ("cycle time" for completion of a case, waiting times, or percentage of patients who have gone through an intervention or educational program).
- Directional indicators are trends that suggest improvement or warn of decline.
- Actionable indicators are like "idiot lights" on a dashboard—they warn that immediate action should be taken to avert a serious problem (such as failure to have 100 percent of staff complete safety training).
- Financial indicators are used in business performance but are usually not very helpful in tracking progress in occupational or environmental health, except as input as budgeted and return on investment.

Performance indicators are classified as "leading" and "lagging," depending on whether they predict or reflect the final outcome. Leading indicators precede the outcome and usually reflect the process or resources available. Lagging, or "trailing," indicators reflect the outcome and its consequences. In traditional evaluation research methodology, leading indicators are "process measures" because they reflect the level of activity (such as the number of patients seen), the performance of the systems on which performance depends (how many case reviews resulted in finding an error), or the steps in the middle (how many workers were contacted, how many showed up for immunization clinics, how many immunizations were given, how many seroconverted). Lagging indicators are "outcome measures" in traditional evaluation research methodology, because they reflect the final result (how many people got influenza, how many low back pain cases returned to work). Here, business management differs from traditional evaluation research. Traditional evaluation research generally considers process or activity measures to be inferior to outcome measures, except for diagnostic purposes. Business prefers leading indicators because they suggest what the outcome will be and provide a guide for making mid-course corrections to improve performance. They also suggest which aspects of the process are succeeding and which are failing, if they are properly designed.

Lagging health indicators describe outcome and in occupational health are mostly related to the frequency of injury and disease. By then, of course, it is too late to change an outcome that may reflect a lapse or problem that occurred in the past. Lagging indicators in the occupational health arena are summary measures that integrate all the many influences on health (community disease trends, personal risk factors, sports injuries), all the influences on attitudes toward work and compensation (community, family), all the influences on quality of care and outcome (access to care, practitioner competence, compliance), and all the factors that influence management of a case (cooperation on the part of the treating physician, supervisor, injured worker, workers' compensation carrier). The occupational health service controls only a fraction of these parameters and those incompletely. The true measure of success in occupational health services is some metric of what did not happen: health problems that were prevented, lost-time injuries or time off work that did not occur, and workers' compensation costs that were not incurred (see Chapter 18 for examples).

Leading indicators give an indication of process integrity and if the process is linked closely enough with the future outcome they predict eventual performance. Often, however, leading indicators are only loosely correlated with outcome, especially in health care. Leading indicators are informative about the direction that things are going, preferably in sufficient time to make corrections. For example, in a health care setting, one might track the number or proportion of currently smoking patients without smoking-related illness who receive counseling to quit smoking in the course of a visit in order to assess the delivery of preventive services. This would be considered a leading indicator, since an increase is presumed to correlate with an increase in people in that clinic's population eventually quitting tobacco use. If the practitioners in the clinic are not raising the question of smoking with their patients, this deficiency can be corrected. The number of patients who actually do quit would be a lagging indicator.

Performance indicators may be qualitative (often called "traffic lights"), with the assumption that the outcome is either good or bad, or quantitative, with more or less precise measurement. Quantitative measures are easy for financial indicators and inventory. However, the financial and production data that are collected to track the business have no application in occupational health. None of the data collected at great expense by management helps to assess performance in this area.

Measuring the quality of occupational health care quantitatively can be very difficult. Traditional measures of performance in health care, such as volume of clinic visits, are reversed in a prevention-oriented service, in which the whole point is to keep people well and demonstrate their fitness. The clinical procedures performed in occupational health are not technically complicated to perform; it is the application and strategy behind them that is sophisticated. Questionnaires for general health care for services and for outcomes such as quality of care and quality of life usually do not work for occupational health because the instruments available are scaled to a greater level of severity than is useful in occupational care.

Failure to understand this has often led to inappropriate performance indicators being applied to occupational health services. For example, it is perfectly reasonable to evaluate a hospital, emergency room, or clinic on the basis of health service performance indicators: number of patients seen, coding accuracy, referral rate (referrals/provider/day, for example to radiology or physical therapy), utilization of laboratory services, waiting time before patient is seen by a physician. These same indicators are nonsensical when applied to occupational health, because, respectively, occupational health should be judged on success in prevention rather than volume of treatment services, coding is usually not a critical issue in workers' comp cases, most occupational health cases do not require referral, relatively few cases require laboratory tests (other than X-ray imaging), and the time spent before an injured worker is seen by a physician is usually used productively in completing workers' compensation forms, which would have to be dealt with anyway and are critical for documentation.

Likewise, tracking relative value units (RVUs) in order to evaluate productivity and calculate compensation for occupational physicians is illogical in occupational medicine and unfair to providers, because although they describe primary care practice well, they fail to count many common occupational medicine services (such as independent medical evaluations or bundled services such as Commercial Driver Medical Evaluations) and place too much value on procedures. High-value treatments and procedures are rarely required to provide high-quality occupational medical care, where much greater emphasis is needed instead on intensive case management and cognitive services.

For an occupational health service, the relevant performance indicators have more to do with reductions in treatment services over time, increases in non-treatment services, and dollars saved (and income protected) through efficient case management and early and safe return to work. Occupational health practitioners legitimately seek to reduce costs of care and generally stick to proven and relatively conservative management approaches for injured workers, with generally good results and low rates of complications.

Performance indicators that might seem to apply to occupational health also require interpretation, because the context is different than in general health care. Referral rates to physical therapy often appear high in occupational health compared to general medicine, but having the injured worker closely evaluated by frequent visits to a non-physician is much less expensive than having them seen in clinic, and tracks recovery more closely in order to expedite evaluation of fitness to work at the end of rehabilitation. Some widely-published guidelines for expected time to return to work are misleading, because they are based on all patients with the injury, both occupational and community acquired, and fail to take into account the different injury patterns in the workplace (for example, in hand injuries, where carpal tunnel may have very different characteristics when arising from ergonomic factors compared to the disorder arising from the many associated non-occupational risk factors such as diabetes, pregnancy, or obesity), rehabilitation options, incentives and disincentives in workers' compensation, and the distribution of cases (a mean time to return to work for a foot injury may obscure or average out the patterns for different groups: sports injuries in which there is likely to be a lot of soft-tissue strain and trauma in surrounding tissues, and occupational injuries, which are more likely to be simple, except in professional athletes). Another difference is the pre-injury health of the patient. Workers, in general, are likely to be in better condition than the average person in the community and those persons who experience sports injuries are likely as a group to have a higher level of pre-injury conditioning than the average worker but also more likely to have an injury.

Too much is out of the control of the occupational health service to risk a management review that is based on lagging indicators. Occupational health managers should be alert to any attempt to base the service's budget on performance indicators and should avoid business value propositions that attempt to "share the risk" on the basis of cost savings. That does not mean that indicators should not be managed but the flip side of "if it can't be measured, it can't be managed" is that "if it can't be managed tightly, it should not be measured to evaluate the performance of the manager." Occupational health services can certainly strongly influence health in large organizations and can manage the uncertainties around it but they do not control health in the way the chief financial officer controls the flow of money or the chief information officer controls the information technology (IT) system.

Key Performance Indicators

The highest-level performance objectives are called "key performance indicators" (KPIs). KPIs give an overview of functions that are critical to business success. They are benchmarks used in the private sector to determine whether their activities are meeting business objectives that are closely linked and statistically or logically correlated with good outcomes in support of the core mission of the organization. KPIs operationalize the goals by providing numerical targets: they are almost all quantitative. They are derived from data collected within the organization and benchmarked against historical trends, best practices in the industry, or standards that reflect goals. KPIs represent a set of measures that can be used in combination to determine whether the project, product line, or organization is on track to meeting goals or if and where further effort is required to drive the enterprise in the right direction. For that reason, a collection of KPIs that are tracked closely by senior management is called a "dashboard."

KPIs should flow naturally from the business model and reflect important goals of the enterprise, whether it is production or public service. An enterprise has a mission of what it is supposed to achieve, a vision of how it should operate, and goals, short term and long term. The occupational health service operates in support of those goals but also in support of health goals and the protection of workers' rights. In that sense, the occupational health service has a mission that always exists in addition to its role in supporting the mission of the enterprise. This is not a concept that is easy to explain to management at times.

Because data collection is expensive, KPIs should rely to the extent possible on administrative data already collected or relatively easily derived from the enterprise's IT system and the electronic occupational health record. It is customary to say that KPIs should be SMART: Specific, Measurable, Achievable, Realistic, and Time-bound. (The SMART formulation first appeared in 1981 in the writings of management thinker George T. Doran.) In other words, they should be as concrete and quantifiable as possible but based on practical sources, such as existing administrative data, rather than expensive new data collection efforts. Cost is more than an issue of budget, because an excessively costly data system will be unsustainable through the enterprise's business cycle and is unlikely to survive the departure of the manager who champions it. Unfortunately, this all works better for the business as a whole than for the occupational health service.

Special information systems may be necessary to develop the indicators required for tracking occupational health protection and health management. Reliance on KPIs requires a commitment to the collection of data to support them. Little of the enormous data pool collected for management purposes is of much value in evaluating occupational health services. There is also a tendency to base KPIs on data that are available rather than the guidance that is actually needed. This should be resisted.

The occupational health service needs to develop its own relevant KPIs, validate them, and demonstrate their usefulness empirically to management. Blindly accepting the same KPIs that are applied to general medical services is courting disaster, as demonstrated above.

Box 17.1 is a list of candidate KPIs suitable for occupational health services. The list of indicators tracked should be narrowed to those KPIs that provide the most useful information and that do not duplicate each other or closely track together (and therefore can be assumed

Box 17.1 Examples of Key Performance Indicators in Occupational Health

Leading Indicators

1. Number of completed risk assessments for workplace hazard evaluation. (Measures activity, not quality.)
2. Percentage of "health risk assessments" completed, by business unit. (Measures completion, not just activity.)
3. Percentage of completed "health risk assessments" resulting in a recommendation that was implemented. (Measures follow-through directly and quality indirectly.)
4. Percentage of workers at risk that have completed worker education and training programs appropriate to their positions.
5. Percentage *exceeding* a standard response time for medical emergencies, with documentation as to why. (Note that *average* response times are of virtually no interest or usefulness—it is a measure that carries essentially no useful information. What matters is how many responses were inadequate as judged by a standard that reflects medical urgency.)
6. Compliance with clinical care guidelines for work-related injuries. (Assuming that the guidelines are authoritative, such as the American College of Occupational and Environmental Medicine Practice Guidelines, this is a measure of quality of care.)
7. Number of fitness for duty evaluations performed. (Just a measure of activity but has to be known to go further.)
8. Percentage of fitness for duty evaluations with recommendations appended. (This is getting to a measure of quality.)
9. Percentage of workers completing periodic health surveillance evaluations appropriate to their position, over cycle length.
10. Number and description of health impact assessments completed for new projects.
11. Time between diagnosis and reporting of work-related illness.
12. Percent completeness of reporting occupational injury, comparing lowest and highest reporting levels.

Lagging or Trailing Indicators

1. Sentinel event cases detected (indicative of a deeper problem).
2. Frequency of occupational illness (very hard to measure because of latency, underreporting, and appearance of many conditions after retirement).
3. Time since last fatality or serious injury (years).

to measure the same thing). Although it is unlikely that a small number of KPIs will provide an adequate description of comprehensive occupational health performance, the actual number used in practice should be kept to a reasonable limit. Over time, KPIs used for operational purposes, should be evaluated, prioritized, and assessed for cost-effectiveness in data collection. KPIs, once validated, should only be changed after careful consideration and both the old and the newly-revised KPIs should be used together for a while to establish the trend under the new definition.

Recommended Reading and Resources

There are many books on quality improvement in clinical medicine and medical services provision. Virtually none of them focus on occupational health services, which, as noted in this chapter, have unique characteristics.

Deming WE (2000) *Out of the Crisis, Cambridge, MA, MIT Press.* Deming is quoted more often than he is read, in this day and age, but his prose is pithy and provocative. Quote: "Everyone doing his best is not the answer. It is first necessary that people know what to do."

Glass W (1992) The occupational health audit: an organization's barometer. *Management Auditing Journal,* 7(6):13–16.

Guidotti TL, Cowell JWF, Jamieson GG (1989) *Occupational Health Services: A Practical Approach.* Chicago, American Medical Association, Reissued in 2001 by The Blackburn Press, Caldwell NJ, in facsimile edition (http://www.blackburnpress.com/). This is the first edition of the present book. It contains a chapter (Chapter 14, "Program Evaluation") that discusses the performance of occupational health services from an evaluation methodology viewpoint. This chapter was not carried over into the present edition.

Kemp S (2005) *Quality Management De-Mystified.* Columbus OH, McGraw Hill.

McLaughlin CP, Kaluzny AD (2005) *Continuous Quality Improvement in Healthcare.* Jones and Bartlett.

Moser R Jr. (2008) *Effective Management of Health and Safety Programs.* Beverly Farms MA, OEM Press.

Ransom ER, Joshi MS, Nash DB, Ransom SB, eds (2008) *The Healthcare Quality Book: Vision, Strategy, and Tools.* Chicago, Healthcare Administration Press.

18 Benefit and Cost Analysis

Joel Bender and Raymond J. Fabius

Operating expenses and capital costs for providing occupational health services depend upon the size and design of the facility, personnel expenses (both professional and staff), and the services provided. The budget for providing community-based, corporate or plant occupational health services should be based on realistic work plans and established goals developed and administered by an occupational health professional. It should be prepared with the help of the company's financial personnel, and the support of human resource and environmental safety leadership, with final approval given by the senior executives responsible for the services. The scale of the occupational health service also must be taken into account. In general, it is prudent financially, for quality assurance, and for liability protection to use community providers for clinical support services such as radiology, physical therapy, and laboratory tests. For a large operation at an employer's site or as the occupational health service grows in the community, however, there may be a break point at which it makes sense to have these services provided in-house.

This chapter emphasizes on-site services at the employer's venue. However, most considerations apply equally to community-based services and facilities. In particular, community-based providers who master the skill of calculating return on investment and cost/benefit will have a distinct advantage in communicating with employers.

Construction and equipment costs vary from place to place and change with the complexity of services delivered. Most occupational health services occupy existing buildings rather than purpose-built space. Therefore, estimates are not given here for initial capital requirements or reserves. It is important, however, that the facility and equipment chosen be appropriate to the facility's objectives or the company's needs, financial requirements, and the services that the occupational health service will provide (see Chapter 11). Advice from consultants and potential vendor partners in both architecture and occupational health is always prudent before issuing requests for proposals, obtaining competitive bids, initiating construction, and purchasing equipment and materials.

It is increasingly rare for on-site occupational health services to be limited to just the basic services, responding to occupational illness and injury, and providing medical surveillance exams. More often, such locations are engaged in ergonomics, employee assistance, and medical management of both occupational and non-occupational issues. Community-based occupational health services have been slower to branch out (see Chapter 19) but have been successful when they do so thoughtfully and with preparation. New services will add to costs (and presumably to revenues) with specialized staff and equipment, and with increased general staffing to handle the additional responsibilities. Figure 18.1 shows how occupational health services serving larger employers are leveraging their clinical talent and resources to provide

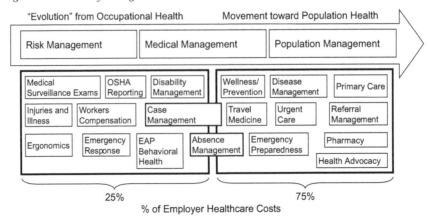

Figure 18.1 Major employers have determined that most of their identifiable health-related costs result from personal and group health issues rather than work-related injuries and illness. Health management is therefore moving from a narrow focus on occupational health to a more comprehensive population health management model

comprehensive medical services and population health for their employees and their dependents. As a consequence of this market trend the calculations of both the costs as well as the benefits of investing in workplace health has become more complicated. Services such as workplace rehabilitation and disability management require additional skilled personnel and equipment.

Direct Operating Expenses

The following expense features and the estimated percent of a total operating budget are fairly typical of occupational health services in industry.

Salaries, Wages, and Benefits

The staff of an occupational health service may include a variety of different professional and administrative personnel. Any or all of them may be employed on a full or part-time, salaried or contract basis. The level of compensation should reflect the qualifications, experience, and level of responsibility. Table 18.1 presents representative levels of compensation for various staff. Contracts for outsourcing services with vendor partners can include the hiring, training, and oversight of some or all workplace health personnel.

This component usually accounts for up to 25–70 percent of the total budget. This figure could approach 90 percent in organizations that do not charge for rent, utilities, and maintenance. An occupational health physician's basic salary range is US$90,000–180,000 per year or US$90–200 per hour. An occupational health nurse's basic salary range is US$40,000–70,000 per year or $25–45 per hour. Full-time employed personnel will also receive a comprehensive benefits package covering such items as disability insurance, life insurance etc. that can be valued at 25–30 percent of their salary. Contract employees generally do not receive a benefit package. If there is a problem determining the physician or nurse's salary or fees, consulting the local medical or nurses' association can be helpful. The salary and contract fees of other administrative and technical personnel vary greatly and will not be listed. Usually, an organization can obtain information regarding salary and contract fees from surveys conducted in the local community.

Table 18.1 Approximate Levels of Compensation of Personnel

Position	Salary Range (US$)	Contract Fee (US$/hour)	Comments
Occupational physician	90,000–180,000	90–200	Fee for service according to medical association-recommended schedule of fees and local availability. Retainer fees may be in addition to hourly rates and vary.
Occupational health nurse (COH)	40,000–70,000	25–45	Adjust for experience and certification.
Nurse administrator	60,000–90,000	45–75	Adjust for complexity of assignment and local availability.

Other: Salaries or fees equivalent to similar positions in other settings:
• radiologists
• psychologists
• physical therapists
• nutritionists/dieticians
• health promotion specialists
• audiologists
• technicians
• clerks
• receptionists
• administrator.

Professional Development Expenses

Funds to pay for tuition, travel, and lodging for coursework and conferences that provide professional development such as continuing education for licensure should be included in the budget. Organizations should also pay for certain professional license fees and memberships in associations. This cost feature will account for 2–5 percent of the operating budget. Major legislative changes, collective bargaining agreements, or citations for failure to comply with regulations may increase this feature substantially for an employer. Attention should be paid to acquiring medical liability coverage, unless a particular service is outsourced and provided by the vendor. Large employers may be able to include this within their umbrella protection package.

Contract Labor—Fee for Service

It is not cost-effective for an occupational health service to provide all professional services in-house and on staff. Contract arrangements can be made with vendors to meet staffing needs for many professional services required, including: radiology, psychology, audiology, nutrition, medical technology, health promotion, and nursing. Certain services required for quality assurance, such as calibration of medical equipment, may be bundled with leases and purchases or provided by a local vendor. Medical surveillance examinations, hearing conservation or educational programs related to regulations or health promotion may be seasonal and if so may require periodic short-term staffing, which could be filled by qualified professionals at a fee for service.

Efficient Use of Labor

All personnel should function at their highest level of training and all personnel should be qualified and trained to do their jobs well, and preferably more than one job for flexibility and efficiency. There are many opportunities for staff to receive appropriate training, through commercial training programs (especially for hearing conservation, pulmonary function testing, and ergonomics), at conferences, and short courses at local educational institutions. Non-clinical services should be delivered by administrative staff. Depending on the size of the population served, defining levels of clinical roles can reduce the costs and need for the most expensive full-time occupational health specialists. Consider hiring nurse assistants, medical technologists, licensed practical nurses, and physician assistants where possible to perform functions at levels commensurate with their training. Reserve clinically intensive diagnosis and treatment for the most highly trained professionals, especially physicians, occupational health nurses, and nurse practitioners and spare their time as much as possible from routine functions.

Facility Expenses

Expenses of rent, light, heat, water, maintenance, and cleaning costs are fixed overhead costs and change little with changes in services, assuming the facility is not modified. They may be included in direct operating expenses for accounting purposes. Periodic repair expenditures are variable costs and can only be estimated until they happen, although they can be projected when calculating the total cost of the facility. Applied to proposals and to formulas for physician reimbursement, however, these costs are usually treated as general overheads and are not readily identifiable. This feature doesn't always appear in a budget. However, it can consume up to 20–30 percent of the operating expenses.

Operating Supplies

Administrative supplies such as files, paper, and postage; medical supplies such as bandages, disinfectants, suture kits, disposable gloves, vaccines and drugs; facility maintenance supplies such as cleaning agents and floor wax, must all be included in the budget. A good inventory control system is required to control costs and ensure sufficient stocks when needed. Competitive bidding is recommended to obtain the best volume discounts from distributors.

Sundry items often too small to have their own expense feature can be included here as well. The extent of primary care and pharmacy services delivered, regulatory requirements, bargained agreements, health promotion, and benefit plan designs for employees will have a significant impact on these expenses. Costs in this feature can range from 10–20 percent of the operating budget.

Information Technology Services

This cost feature generally includes a variety of expenses related to communications and data management such as phone, fax, computer hardware and software, and other technology used in the workplace setting. Capital expenditures for computer hardware and other equipment should be captured under a separate heading in the budget to account for depreciation. Medical records are a large part of this expense category and require close attention. Specialized occupational health software is essential to manage the care delivered, follow periodic health surveillance records, generate necessary reports, comply with Occupational Safety and Health Administration (OSHA) requirements, and determine fitness for duty. Conventional, clinic- or hospital-based electronic health records do not have the flexibility or the depth to do this and attempting to modify existing general-duty software to support occupational health services is usually unsatisfactory. In larger facilities hand-held tablets should be considered to ease the clinician's recording requirements. If there will be on-call responsibilities, the information technology (IT) system should allow for access off-site by authorized clinical personnel.

Depending upon the activities and nature of occupational health services, this expense feature may account for 6–10 percent of the budget. This depends on the desired sophistication of the user, software requirements, regulatory requirements, and extent of integration with medical claims, pharmacy claims, and other data stored in a data warehouse.

Other Features

There may be other expenses, depending upon the size of the organization and the nature of medical services provided at the facility. An important category of expense is access to medical and professional information, as distinct from software. In addition to the IT services mentioned above, the occupational health services will require subscriptions to journals, bundled access to online library resources (including back issues of journals, medical and nursing books, specialized databases), without which professionals cannot function in occupational health. Some these expenses reflect the needs of professional staff to maintain their license and continuing education requirements. These could include memberships and dues for professional staff, training, travel, lodging (for example, at professional meetings), relocation, and professional licensure. Others may involve access to the clinical facilities or medical services in the community. These could include transportation (ambulance services, a clinic van), courier services, and food service (usually on contract).

Indirect Operating Expenses

Many community-based occupational health services apply overhead to the cost of providing occupational services at a clinic facility in order to derive the price (allowing for a margin for profit or to fund future investment). These expenses include charges for administrative, facility, financial, and human resources support. The overhead is then applied as a percentage to the cost of service. For example, if a clinic has a 60 percent overhead rate (not uncommon in hospitals and multispecialty group practices), then the actual cost for a service may be 1.60 times the direct cost of providing the service. Under such an arrangement, physicians (but not nurses, because they do not generate revenue directly), would be expected to return a multiple of their salary in earnings in order to cover overhead expenses and the operating margin: a factor of three is typical. Expenses for executive examinations, special compensation, or even separation allowances can appear in the overhead rates as indirect operating expenses.

In in-house corporate or in-plant services, overhead is more likely to be accounted and calculated as indirect cost in the budget rather than applied as a formula.

Cost/Benefit Review

An occupational health service is engaged by employers for various reasons. The organization may believe that there is a competitive advantage to providing health services that support employee well-being. In other cases, the employer must comply with pertinent laws, regulations, or collective bargaining agreements. The strongest incentive from a business perspective, however, is that in both the short run and the long run, occupational health services of good quality will save money and create a positive return on the investment. In the short term, the assumption is that occupational injuries will lead to early and safe return to work and that workers' compensation costs will be minimized by effective case management. In the long term, the assumption is that occupational injuries will be managed properly to reduce the risk of disability, that occupational diseases will be prevented, and that personal risk factors of workers will be modified to enhance their health, leading to an improved quality of life and morale and to increased productivity. Skeptical employers may demand proof of these statements.

Whatever the motivation, the costs of occupational health services are always more readily apparent than the benefits. Expenses incurred to support occupational health services are relatively easy to capture. Determining the financial benefits is more elusive. However, it is crucial that an organization conduct realistic analyses to determine the financial benefits for occupational health services, whether in a department, within an organization, a clinic, or a private consultant retained on a full or part-time basis.

The components of the cost/benefit analysis will vary according to the size, type and nature of the organization. Although its accuracy will only be as good as the data being collected, trends can be demonstrated using best assumptions and simulation. The newer the occupational health service, the harder it is to measure its financial impact, as it is unlikely to be fully or properly staffed, and its policies and programs will not be fully developed or implemented yet. Nevertheless, the evidence that will be used to measure the impact of the occupational health service (such as wellness, workers' compensation, absence management, and days lost due to accidents or sickness, etc.) should be chosen early and recorded as soon as possible. For example, if the occupational service is dedicated to reducing occupational injury and illness then it should be tracked monthly and efforts to convert improvements to cost reduction should be pursued and agreed with management. If the purpose is to reduce disability days away from work then this should also be recorded and reductions should translate into productivity gains and dollars saved.

Costs

The budget for the occupational health service should be prepared and administered under the direction of the most senior person in the occupational health service, with the help of the organization's financial advisors.

Separation between implementation expenses versus ongoing fixed and variable costs should be a focus of the budgetary process. There are two components of operating costs. Fixed costs are incurred regardless of the volume of work and include heat, light, essential equipment, basic support staff, and the IT system. Variable costs are proportional to the volume of work and the services that are provided and include supplies, specialized personnel, additional staff required to handle increasing numbers of patients, special-purpose equipment, and computers.

The capital budget will be most significant when the occupational health service is first constructed and at times of major renovations. Since these costs are fixed and will vary greatly according to the size and location of the occupational health facility, they will not be discussed here.

The operating budget lists the funding needed to run the occupational health service on a day-to-day basis. The budget contains many expense features but the largest will be compensation and benefits for staff. If the occupational health service is a department within an organization, such as an employer or a military unit, its operating expenses will be consolidated into a total operating budget. Overhead items such as rent and utilities may not be specifically identified.

If the occupational health service provider is external to the employer, the employer might only budget for a bundled service that represents the aggregate occupational health cost. In this situation, the occupational health service will need to provide an operating budget (often in the form of a bid or a proposal), which usually will need to be detailed for purposes of accountability. The following discussion will not cover all circumstances but will emphasize expense features commonly encountered in the preparation of a typical budget for an occupational health service.

Benefits

It is difficult to quantify reductions of human suffering or unrealistic to put a value on the absence of fines or court action. Clearly, however, these have presumptive value, may escalate the costs of judgments against the employer, and should be mentioned in any cost/benefit analysis. There are certain identifiable direct and indirect savings that can be calculated or estimated. When workers become ill or are injured at the workplace they will require medical care. The first cost/benefit of a workplace health center is to supply these services and remove the need to pay community providers for this service. Studies have demonstrated that early assessment and treatment markedly reduces the need for disability claims. Most large employers offer disability health insurance for their employees for non-occupational conditions.

Calculating Cost / Benefit

Table 18.2 shows several years of direct savings for workers' compensation (WC) and health disability insurance (HDI) costs. All the amounts shown are examples.

Another element of the analysis estimates the cost savings that result from the reduction in health-related absences. This can be best impacted through early assessment of workplace injuries and illness as well as programs such as modified work. The total cost of an absence includes wages and benefits for the absent employee, wages paid to a replacement, overtime costs, costs for extra supervision and co-workers' time, cost of training a replacement, and administrative costs. Some studies have shown these costs can total ten times the wage of the absent employee.

Table 18.2 Direct Savings Projected from Occupational Health Services (Example)

Assume base year costs: Workers' compensation (WC) = US$1,000
                          Health disability insurance (HDI) = US$1,000

Year	Workers' Compensation Costs	Savings Related to Base Year	HDI Costs	Savings Related to Base Year	Total Savings
1	800,000	200,000	900,000	100,000	300,000
2	750,000	250,000	700,000	300,000	550,000
3	700,000	300,000	650,000	350,000	650,000
4	600,000	400,000	600,000	400,000	800,000

Compensation insurance for conditions occurring on the job is an important expense of doing business. In some companies these premiums and associated costs represent a significant and even crippling expense. A well-run occupational health service can have a profound effect by reducing these costs. Measures such as timely intervention for work-related accidents, health surveillance programs, fitness-to-work programs, and health promotion can have an effect on reducing health-related absenteeism and employee turnover while increasing productivity and performance.

To calculate the reduction in health insurance costs, a base year should be chosen for comparison purposes. This year should be from a time prior to when the employee's occupational health policies and programs were fully operative. Clearly, then, if these costs go down over time compared to the base year, the occupational health service can justifiably take some or all of the credit for the reduction. When doing this analysis, one must keep comparing back to the base year, year after year, because the cost reductions may occur slowly, from time to time, or may be large at the beginning and then taper off as a minimum cost level is reached. In effect what is being shown is not only what has happened because of the actions of the occupational health service, but also what might happen again if the service or program is removed. Sometimes this analysis can only show how costs have been kept at a certain level. In this situation additional information from the insurance company will be necessary to learn what the costs might have become if the employer's performance had not been enhanced by workplace occupational health services.

The following example, a hypothetical appliance manufacturer, shows how to estimate these costs.

Assume that the average hourly rate, including benefits, is US$18 per hour for general employees. An eight-hour day's compensation cost is US$144, and if one assumes a very conservative factor of threefold (four or five is more common) for the related (indirect) costs, the cost of a one-day absence, direct and indirect $(1 + 3 = 4)$ is 4×144 or US$576.

Now one assumes that the occupational health service records show that acute care and return-to-work interventions by the service have resulted in 100 employees returning to work on average five days earlier than they would have otherwise, thus the estimated cost savings is as follows:

100 employees $\times$ 5 $\times$ 576 = US$288,000

In other words, the employer avoided 500 days of absence costing US$576 per day because of effective health interventions. If the company also has a health promotion program that includes fitness and smoking cessation programs, further cost savings can be estimated in the same way. Many studies have shown that regular exercisers lose less time than less active workers. If, say, 100 employees now exercise regularly because of a fitness program, saving an average three days per year, the following productivity savings can be estimated:

$100 \times 3 \times 576$ = US$172,800

Smokers are said to be absent about an average of three days per year more than non-smokers, so if 20 workers stopped smoking, additional productivity savings can be estimated:

$20 \times 3 \times 576$ = US$34,560

Furthermore, if the occupational health service has looked after a few executives whose salaries are twice that of the general worker (or US$1152 per day in absence costs) and assuming that there are ten executives who lost five days fewer and who now exercise regularly (three days) and who have stopped smoking (three days), one can make the following estimate of productivity savings:

$$10 \times 11 \times 1152 = US\$126,720$$

Using rather straightforward assumptions, therefore, this example of an occupational health service, by helping only 110 participants in total, prevented the company from losing $622,080 in health-related absences! In year four of the occupational health services, using the numbers from the health insurance savings table (US$800,000), the total estimated savings directly due to the health interventions would be US$1,422,080. This adds up to a convincing argument indeed for management.

This example is very conservative in its assumptions, and therefore all the more persuasive. In a real situation these numbers are likely to be much higher. The estimated cost savings would therefore be even more impressive to a client employer.

Return on Investment

To extend the cost/benefit analysis into a return-on-investment (ROI) proposition, one may assume that in the example the occupational health services costs US$350,000 to operate. Such a service would probably have a full-time occupational health physician, three to four occupational health nurses, and several clerical support staff. An operation of this size certainly could serve an employee population of three to four thousand. The original conservative cost savings estimate was US$1,422,080. If one divides this by the cost of the service, the calculation results in a 300 percent return or an ROI of 3:1.

In publicly-traded companies, one can bring the cost/benefit analysis directly to the bottom line by showing the impact on earnings per share. To do this, one first subtracts the costs from the estimated cost savings to get the net benefit (i.e. 1,422,080 less 350,000 = US$1,072,080.)

If one assumes that the company has 20,000,000 common shares outstanding, the earnings per share contribution is:

$$1,072,080 \div 20,000,000 = 5.4 \text{ cents per share}$$

This 5.4 cent benefit therefore contributes to the earnings of the company distributed to or retained by each shareholder in the year that the benefit accrues. However, shares are priced by their longer-term market value, typically in multiples of their earnings in any given year. Assuming that this hypothetical company is trading at a price per earnings multiple of 10:1, benefit per share price contribution is 54 cents. This contribution provides 54 cents of value per share × 20,000,000 common shares or over US$10 million of additional market value, independent of the share value at any given time. Such numbers make a real impression on senior management.

The target audience for these figures is usually, roughly in reverse order of skepticism, the chief financial officer (CFO), the chief operating officer (COO), and the chief executive officer (CEO), the executives which in colloquial business vocabulary are collectively called "the C-suite." The legal counsel for an employer may also be very interested because these measures not only provide an impressive return on the investment but reduce the employer's liability. The COO and individual product line managers may also be heavily influenced by another line or argument, based on equivalent productivity and sales.

Another method for speaking effectively to the C-suite is to convert the savings into the estimated units of goods that would otherwise have to be manufactured and sold to achieve an equivalent amount of income. Using the same example above, one may assume that this large appliance manufacturer makes US$100 per dishwasher in profit. Therefore, to achieve the same revenue required to save or gain US$1,072,080, the organization would need to produce and sell an additional 10,720 dishwashers. If one production line can produce 200 dishwashers in a day and it takes 90 days to sell them on average, it would take that line 50 workdays to build the number of units necessary and the sales force would need to sell them all over the following 90 days in order to reap an equivalent benefit for the company.

A third way to look at the benefit is to calculate the "present value" of a health event or disability that is projected to occur in the future that is prevented by occupational health management in the present. Calculation of this figure depends on many assumptions, chief among them the "discount rate," which is often taken to be the rate of a bond or other instrument of equivalent value which would represent an alternative investment of the money during the same period. For example, the present value of an event costing US$200,000 in ten years is approximately US$101,670 at a discount rate of 7 percent (representing the nominal yield of an equivalent investment). That figure can support the argument that in order to cover the future cost (fund the liability) of an injury of that magnitude in the future, the employer would have to divert almost half that amount to nonproductive uses in the here and now. It is much cheaper to prevent the problem in the first place. The present value argument is particularly useful for CFOs, corporate counsel, and risk management officers because it brings the cost of the future home to the present and counters the natural tendency to consider costs in the future as speculative and "not real."

This example has already shown a remarkable return by focusing only on two areas, reduced medical costs and reduced health-related absence costs. An effective occupational health service ought to be able to demonstrate that it can produce substantial additional economic benefits in reducing the indirect costs of injury- and illness-related absence (for example, retraining, substitute labor, and lost efficiency) and reduce worker's compensation costs. Preventive services through health promotion, ergonomics, and facilitated personal prevention such as vaccinations have also been shown to reduce medical costs and absence. Maintaining OSHA compliance prevents fines from being levied and the corporate brand from being tarnished.

For global companies, an investment in travel medicine and ensuring safe business journeys can provide particularly high returns. Preventing a single air ambulance evaluation from a remote location can pay for a corporate travel medicine program many times over. Organizing an emergency response team to prevent a death from a single heart attack episode at the workplace can be priceless for morale, life saving, and hugely significant to a company's bottom line. This is why automated external defibrillator devices (AEDs) have become so popular.

A similar analysis can be made on the basis of productivity, using measures of absence (from work) and presenteeism (health-related low efficiency while at work). Absence can easily be counted, as it is reflected in attendance. Presenteeism must be measured, usually by a standardized questionnaire. It is prudent in conducting a cost/benefit and ROI analysis to avoid basing it too narrowly on reducing absence. This is because absence rates depend on company policies with respect to leave and the demographics of the workforce. When employers try to reduce absence too vigorously, they risk having people come to work who should be staying home, both for the health risk of other workers (for example, with upper respiratory infections) and for their own productivity. Absence rates and presenteeism rates are to some degree reciprocal, because if people come into work feeling poorly (for example, with migraines or bad allergies), absence may be reduced but presenteeism may soar, with an equally bad effect on productivity (possibly worse if the quality of work is critical). That is why effective wellness programs target the root cause of employees' health problems (through prevention) or effective management of the problems (case management of chronic disease) rather than absence.

19 Primary Care-Level Clinical Services

David G. Lukcso

There are many models for providing occupational health care to multiple employers within the private sector. The most common are:

- occupational medicine in primary care practice
- individual or partnership consultation practice in occupational medicine
- multispecialty group practice
- hospital-based clinics
- managed care or health maintenance organizations, such as Kaiser-Permanente
- occupational medicine centers, defined here as high-volume, free-standing centers specializing in the delivery of occupational health services.

This chapter will emphasize the occupational medicine center (OMC). These are the new generation of occupational health services that grew out of the "industrial medicine clinics" of the past. The other models are discussed in previous chapters (see Chapter 1).

The old model of industrial medicine clinics was often criticized for having had an excessive emphasis on profits with little regard for the quality of care provided and little to no commitment to preventive services. They were often staffed by physicians with marginal qualifications. There were, however, a number of exceptions, including the Detroit Industrial Clinic, PC (1920) in Southfield, Michigan, and the Occupational Medical Clinic, Ltd. (1961) of Phoenix, Arizona. These high-quality clinics provided the model for what later became a success story in health care.

During the 1980s and 1990s, OMCs began to proliferate as many well-qualified occupational and enviromental medicine (OEM) physicians left corporate medical departments and entered practice in the community. Other physicians entered occupational medicine practice in mid-career, because of the new opportunities. The result was a substantial upgrading in the profile of physicians practicing occupational medicine in the community. Additionally, the proliferation of OMCs made quality occupational medicine services easily accessible to small businesses that were previously available only to major employers, thereby benefiting both employers and their employees.

The OMCs, as free-standing facilities that provide services to many employers in a well-defined geographical area, have been an attractive model for entrepreneurial physicians interested in providing direct health care services in settings with low overhead. The maturation of the industrial clinic into the OMC has brought about improvements in the quality of medical services provided while advances in technology have greatly improved information management. There has been significant consolidation in this sector in recent years and it has been dominated by several providers on a national scale including US HealthWorks Medical Group and Concentra Inc.

The OMC focuses on cost-effective management of minor workplace injuries and periodic health evaluations. The successful business model consists of providing high-volume basic occupational health services that all employers are required to provide, in a streamlined and highly efficient process to control overhead costs. The patients are generally drawn from local employers and the employees of national employers with whom they have contracts or informal arrangements. The basic marketing strategy includes offering mandated services such as Department of Transportation (DOT) commercial driver exams, Occupational Safety and Health Administration (OSHA) compliance exams (asbestos, respirator, cadmium, lead, hearing conservation, etc.) and drug and alcohol testing at very competitive prices. Some OMCs will offer the alcohol and drug testing just above cost or as a loss leader, then entice the employer to direct (depending on the workers' compensation regulations in each state) injured employees to the OMC for the treatment of work-related injuries. Revenues are generated from direct payments from the employer for the mandated services and workers' compensation fees (often the majority of revenues).

The major business advantages of the OMC are the streamlined and highly efficient process with which services are delivered, followed by efficient and effective management of the associated paperwork. Employers are naturally anxious to minimize the time an employee spends out of the workplace; the OMC must meet this critical demand in order to retain the client. The OMC must provide high-quality medical care to employees; two critical elements in efficient process and time management are staffing and information management systems.

Staffing

In general, OMCs rely on a medical staff supervised by a chief of staff or medical director and an administrative staff supervised by a full-time administrator. The medical staff consists of the medical director (an occupational medicine physician) and in large clinics includes primary care practitioners and physician extenders, both nurse practitioners and physician assistants. Many large OMC groups also provide specialty care in the same or separate offices. The advantage of such an arrangement is that the OMC retains control of the treatment of the injured worker through recovery as well as the financial reimbursement of the specialty care.

In order to maximize the profitability of the OMC, the structure of the center must provide sufficient support to the physicians and medical staff such that the majority of their time is spent in performing revenue-generating services that only they can perform, with little time spent on routine or low-yield activities. One effective staffing model includes one nurse in support of several physicians. The nurse coordinates the flow of patients into and out of the examination rooms and maintains maximum efficiency by ensuring that medical assistant support staff performs support services such as ensuring that paperwork is complete prior to the physician evaluating the employee, setting up supplies in treatment rooms, applying bandages, applying splints, and performing gait training for injured employees needing crutches or a cane. To ensure that medical support staff performs to the expected high standards, it is imperative that the medical chief of staff participate in their selection and training (see Chapter 14).

Responsibility for administrative functions is often vested in a full-time administrator who establishes systems for financial oversight and billing, supply, and support personnel. Support personnel are involved in both the front office aspects, interacting with the injured worker and visitors, as well as the back office component, handling paperwork and interacting with workers' compensation. The support staff carries significant responsibility for the success or failure of smooth and efficient processes in a high-volume center (see Chapter 12).

The front office staff must be very efficient in their work and have a pleasant demeanor, as they generate the first impression of the OMC for everyone entering. A friendly acknowledgement of an individual's arrival and quick determination of the reason for the visit will create the impression of the high quality of services provided. Efficient processing of patients into the system requires skill in the information management system and knowledge of the services provided within the OMC. The front office staff must also have good phone etiquette and the ability to respond to common requests from callers without constant supervision. One common request is document duplication; record handling is best performed by an administrative staff fully conversant with OSHA and Health Insurance Portability and Accountability Act (HIPAA) disclosure guidelines (see Chapter 13).

Efficient running of an OMC requires a number of well trained and polite medical assistants. High-volume OMCs perform a large number of drug and alcohol testing services including both collections and on-site testing. Both employees and employers expect drug and alcohol testing to be very quick, with little wait time. Therefore the physical plant must have several designated collection areas that provide privacy for paperwork along with a separate toilet facility (see Chapter 27). The OMC must employ an adequate number of trained collectors to move donors through the process in a timely manner and qualified staff must be cross-trained to do this as needed.

Attention to customer service is vital to the success of the OMC as repeat visits from individuals who receive any service at the center is essential to the growth and success of the business.

Information Management/Electronic Medical Records

Information management is of vital importance to every provider of occupational medicine services. In order for the OMC to maintain the high-volume flow of patients through the center as well as manage the flow of information appropriately, the OMC must have a sophisticated information management system. The information management software may be developed specifically for the OMC or may be a customized version of one of the many commercially available software packages. Some software designed for hospitals and multispecialty groups have occupational health modules but experience with these has usually been disappointing.

The system must be versatile, allowing information to be viewed from a patient-centered point of view, including demographics and service utilization history, and from an employer-centered point of view, including contact, billing, and protocols, and an integrated billing and invoicing package, and features that allow group data to be analyzed for surveillance testing and other variables. Additional information integration is available with electronic transmission of information from laboratories; this is especially useful for OMC practices that perform Medical Review Officer (MRO) services in-house (see Chapter 27).

An appropriate information management system allows for the delivery of a significant amount of information in a timely fashion without the consuming manpower hours. For example, an employer may be notified electronically via fax or email when an employee arrived, the time the employee was released, and the services that the employee received while at the OMC, captured while these services are being performed. The utilization data are entered into the system during admission and discharge, and will be electronically transmitted to the employer following predefined employer protocols that maintain confidentiality of medical information; many employers find the information useful for tracking employee time as well as for reconciliation with invoices.

Many information management systems allow the employee to enter demographic information, and complete history forms and questionnaires electronically. Some systems allow the employee to enter this information before arrival at the OMC using internet-based access. Other systems allow the employee to enter the information into the system himself or herself through keyboard terminals in the waiting room or by using a tablet over a wireless network within the center. Such advances have created even greater efficiencies in support staff by shifting some of the time-consuming data collection to the employees themselves. Once the information is in the system, it must be checked and confirmed by the front office staff for accuracy as the information will be propagated to multiple documents and forms. (Some of these systems have been piloted by information technology companies in their occupational health services in Silicon Valley.)

The move to electronic medical records (EMRs) over the last decade has increased physician efficiency and sped up document management processes. The EMR also greatly speeds up the billing process. These systems allow for the immediate delivery of invoices and so speeds up collections. They rapidly convey documentation to the workers' compensation carrier for processing and keep a record that it has been sent. The use of electronic forms for many of the mandated periodic health evaluations such as DOT commercial driver exams, and OSHA mandated surveillance exams such as asbestos and compliance with respirator clearances, has proven to be very effective and reduces errors, and the software packages allow both trends over time for the individual worker and groups to be monitored.

Patient demographic data and medical history are automatically entered into all of the necessary forms for each examination. The medical assistant support staff enters the data they gather, such as height, weight, blood pressure, heart rate, visual acuity, and urine dipstick results. The physician has the opportunity to review the history and data online prior to his or her examination of the employee. Once the face-to-face interview questions are answered and the physical examination is completed, the physician then enters the results into the system. More advanced systems have integrated voice recognition software so the physician can dictate into a microphone with immediate transcription. The electronic document may be printed for signature or be signed electronically. Another significant advantage of the EMR is that of storage and retrieval. Storage of paper charts and documents is both cumbersome and subject to misfiling and loss. While the employer is required by 29 CFR 1901.1020 to maintain the results of periodic health evaluations for at least the duration of employment plus thirty years, many OMCs provide an electronic data archiving service for some of their clients. The storage of paper archives is both labor intensive (requiring packing, labeling, and cataloging of documents for later retrieval) and expensive. The electronic format allows for storage of significant amounts of information with minimal physical space for storage, as well as much easier document retrieval.

EMRs for injury care have also increased physician efficiency, although some issues have arisen. There are many different systems, some of which are based on an underlying branching system allowing the occupational health professional to select preset statements which lead to further branching statements. Most systems allow for customization of statements, therefore statements that are used repeatedly such as treatment protocols for common injuries can be very beneficial and increase efficiencies. For example, most physicians use the same medications for the treatment of back pain, and the statement may include the use of a nonsteroidal anti-inflammatory drug (NSAID) with warnings about taking after food, the risk of gastric upset and bleeding, and the use of a muscle relaxer, with advice to avoid driving or the use of dangerous machinery due to the risk of sedation. The EMR systems allow for extensive statements to be printed out with a single click or tap, eliminating the need for actually typing extended statements. The major weakness in the branching statement systems is in the history of the injury or illness. While treatment protocols can be uniform, every injury (even with the same diagnosis) occurs in a different manner that must be documented in workers' compensation cases, because the mechanism of injury is often extremely important to the insurance carrier in the adjudication of the matter. In third-party liability cases it may be important to the court if the matter is ultimately contested and litigated. Unfortunately, the predefined history options of many of these programs are weak and inflexible. They do not provide sufficient information to allow true understanding of the mechanism of injury. In order to provide high-quality history, the physician therefore needs to type in text, some of which is redundant and potentially a dangerous source of confusion and contradiction later because the unsatisfactory menu system cannot be overridden. Such systems eliminate the inherent weakness in the predefined branching statement systems; however, the physician still needs to review for accuracy.

Another problem with some menu-driven EMR systems is that the terminology they use is obsolete (e.g. "health screening" instead of "periodic health surveillance") or even against the law (e.g. "pre-employment" instead of "preplacement") but cannot be changed because the system is inflexible. This is a particular problem with software that was originally designed for hospitals. The cost of reprogramming such software is often prohibitive if it is a customized or network system.

Operations

The primary advantages to injured workers and employers is rapid access to the OMC, focused care, one-stop provision of all essential services, early return to work, and correct and timely reporting. It is well known that delay to treatment is one factor in delayed recovery.

Workers' compensation fees represent the largest part of total revenues for most OMCs, therefore the processes and procedures should be continually reviewed to ensure the delivery of the highest quality of medical care while maintaining maximum efficiency (see Chapter 17).

A detailed discussion of medical quality assurance is outside the scope of this text; however, no medical center can or should exist for long if the medical care provided is substandard.

Medical Supervision

In large multi-provider OMCs, the medical staff is supervised by the chief of staff or medical director. As such, the medical care provided within the OMC is ultimately the responsibility of the medical director. The medical director is often a board-certified occupational medicine specialist or has similar relevant qualifications, and is usually the most senior physician in the OMC. The medical director is available as a resource to the other physicians, occupational health nurses, nurse practitioners, and physician assistants. The medical director must have a process for oversight and review of the care provided within the OMC, which may include chart reviews and direct observation of procedures and skills. In an effort to maintain proficiency and in advancing the skills of the medical providers, the medical director should monitor continuing medical education programs and direct staff to appropriate training.

Expediting Services

Most high-volume OMCs are walk-in facilities, for which injured employees do not need appointments.

For employers, time is money, therefore all employers are anxious to minimize the time an employee spends away from the workplace. Many employers simply assume that the quality of care will be adequate and rate the quality of the OMC above all on the timeliness of the delivery of services and the time that employees are out of the workplace, especially for periodic health evaluations, and drug and alcohol testing.

In single-physician operations employee processing usually follows a "first in, first evaluated" methodology. Unfortunately, individuals presenting for a routine periodic health evaluation may be required to wait for a substantial time if they arrive after an injured worker who requires a significant amount of physician time, if the worker is not triaged out of the center and referred to an emergency room. In larger, multi-provider OMCs, one effective method of minimizing employee time in the OMC and away from work is to develop a fast track for basic periodic health evaluations. One of the medical providers can be dedicated to performing these basic examinations while the other medical providers continue to see patients in a "first in" basis. By using a fast track methodology, employees who present for routine period health evaluations can be moved through the system fairly quickly, to the satisfaction of both the employee and employer.

Additionally, the OMC should either have radiographic capabilities within the center (preferred) or should have an agreement for expediting radiography of injured employees referred to a nearby radiology center. Because a majority of work-related injuries are musculoskeletal, immediate access to radiographic capabilities is a significant advantage. In addition, inclusion of radiology provides another revenue-generating service which can improve the OMCs profitability.

Inclusion of laboratory capabilities within the OMC is most often not a cost-effective component. While many periodic health evaluations require laboratory results, performing these tests requires expensive equipment, laboratory certification and quality assurance measures, and highly-trained personnel. Most tests are not time sensitive from a treatment perspective. Therefore, most OMCs have business arrangements with certified laboratory facilities. Often the laboratory will have the capability of transmitting results electronically to a dedicated printer within the OMC facility, so that all results are available for review within 24 hours. If an injured employee presents to the OMC with an injury which requires immediate laboratory evaluation, it is prudent for the physician to arrange for transport of the injured employee to an emergency department. Injuries requiring immediate laboratory evaluation are very likely to be serious, so that the employee is better served in a facility capable of providing more comprehensive services.

Triage and Specialty Referral

Triage of patients is an important aspect of a high-volume OMC to allow for quality of care while maintaining patient flow. Injured employees presenting for evaluation are triaged, to facilitate immediate evaluation of employees with critical injuries, bleeding, eye injuries, chemical exposures, etc. Each OMC facility should have at least two treatment rooms outfitted for minor surgical procedures and at least one equipped with a slit lamp and supplies for the evaluation of eye injuries.

Some injured employees may require the level of care only provided in an emergency department and should be transported to the nearest one via ambulance. Other injured employees may require the services of a specialist. These employees should be referred to the appropriate specialist as soon as possible. Many large OMC groups include specialist services. The advantages of having in-house specialists include the ability for the primary medical provider to contact the specialist for a quick consult prior to referral as well as having the ability to obtain a timely or same day appointment with the specialist.

While workers' compensation matters provide the greatest percent of revenue for the OMC, the free-standing center has capability limitations. Additionally the business model, based on a high-volume of care, requires maximization of physician efficiencies. These considerations require that complicated cases be triaged to other service providers for appropriate care. The OMC must stabilize the injured employee and then arrange for transportation as necessary.

Dispensing

Most OMCs are set up to dispense common medications (analgesics, steroids, muscle relaxers, antibiotics, and eye drops) and basic orthopedic braces and supplies.

The OEM physician or occupational health nurse can promote compliance by providing medications directly to the injured employee and advising them of the benefits of medication compliance. Non-compliance with treatment protocols delays recovery. The medical literature suggests that approximately 30 percent of patients do not even fill prescriptions that they are given and only about 50 percent of patients complete their prescriptions as prescribed. On each follow-up visit, the OEM physician or occupational health nurse must inquire about medication compliance and any potential side effects.

Physical Therapy

OMCs often offer physical therapy on site, usually under contract. Physical therapy utilization tends to be intensive for two reasons: the goal is to return the worker to the job as quickly as recovery can be attained and frequent visits to a physical therapist are useful in monitoring progress. When the worker is sufficiently improved, the physical therapist can alert the physician at once, without the delay between doctor's appointments that would otherwise result. Because fees for physical therapy are much less than for medical services, this is more cost-effective and efficient for the insurer, whose primary concern is to return the claimant to work as soon as possible in a condition that will not lead to re-injury or further decline in health.

The Future

The first edition of *Occupational Health Services* noted that providers of occupational health services were "coming under pressure from such competitors as urgent care centers. The absence of even a nominal claim to special expertise in occupational health care on the part of most urgent care centers is disturbing." Now, some 20 years since the first edition, with progress in injury prevention and workplace safety, and the resultant decrease in injury rates among private industry employers, many of the national providers of occupational health services have begun providing urgent care services. This integration should be monitored as the process develops to determine whether it will compromise the gains made over the last few decades in the specialized delivery of occupational medicine services.

At the same time, the introduction of "on-site medical clinics" at major employer locations and in retail space (see Chapter 1) has created a new opportunity for blending primary care for employees at those locations with occupational health services, with obvious advantages for convenience and efficient time utilization. As in the case of urgent care centers, the effectiveness of this combination needs to be evaluated as experience accumulates.

Recommended Reading and Resources

American College of Occupational and Environmental Medicine (ACOEM) (2004) *Occupational Medicine Practice Guidelines.* Chicago, ACOEM, 3rd ed., as updated. Purchase includes one-year subscription to online version and regular updates. Available at: http://www.acoem.org/practiceguidelines. aspx. Accessed January 6, 2011.

Bureau of Labor Statistics, US Department of Labor, Workplace Injuries and Illnesses – 2010. http://www.bls.gov/news.release/archives/osh_10202011.pdf. Accessed April 16, 2012.

Guidotti TL (2010) *The Praeger Handbook of Occupational and Environmental Medicine.* Santa Barbara CA, Praeger/ABC-Clio.

Guidotti TL, Kuetzing BH (1985) Competition and despecialization: an analytical study of occupational health services in San Diego, 1974–1984. *Am J Ind Med*, 8: 155–165.

Moser R Jr. (2008) *Effective Management of Health and Safety Programs: A Practical Guide.* Beverly Farms MA, OEM Press, 3rd ed.

20 Periodic Health Surveillance and Monitoring

Tee L. Guidotti

When the risk of a particular disease outcome is known to be increased in a particular industry, the main strategy to determine the group experience with that outcome is called "surveillance." When a particular outcome is not the focus of attention and the overall health experience of the individual or group is to be observed, the strategy is termed "monitoring." The terminology overlaps with health promotion and disease prevention in general medicine and can be confusing. "Health monitoring" and "periodic health evaluation," for example, are terms commonly used for monitoring programs intended for individual health care rather than exposed or high-risk groups of workers. They are not discussed here. This chapter emphasizes periodic health surveillance for workers exposed to known hazards. Workforce protection is the assumption on which mandated surveillance is based, as in standards of the Occupational Safety and Health Administration (OSHA) for noise, asbestos, lead, and other hazards (see Chapter 4).

Periodic health surveillance is not like disease screening programs. The purpose of a disease screening program is primarily to find treatable cases and to prevent progression of a disease in the individual, and secondarily to monitor how prevalent the disease is in the local population. The purpose of periodic health surveillance is primarily to find out whether hazard controls are working effectively and, if not, who is most at risk and why, so that controls can be tightened to protect the entire workforce at risk. It is secondarily (because the overriding objective is to prevent, not detect disease), but no less importantly for the individual worker, intended to identify new cases. This should be done at the earliest possible stage, when removal from exposure, and early intervention or treatment will make a difference. The findings from surveillance must therefore be analyzed, tracked over time, and used for correcting the problem by controlling the hazard (see Chapter 21). If this does not happen, then the surveillance program is a failure, even if it detects many cases that can be cured.

Health care providers often do not think about surveillance correctly: they assume that they are looking for an individual who has a disease and, if they find one, their work is done because that person can then undergo treatment or be protected from further exposure. The error is that the mental model providers use for screening workers for disease is based on the historical model of tuberculosis. Surveillance is different. The real reason they are doing it is to confirm that there are no positive results, ever, as long as the hazard is present and fallible control technology is in place. Follow-up, including tracking results and mapping where the positive results are coming from, is critical, even more important than intervening on an individual basis, as important as that is. The whole point of doing the screening is missed completely if surveillance does not lead to fixing the problem.

Surveillance programs are conducted secondarily for the protection of the individual worker; it is conducted primarily for protection of the entire workforce, including the individual worker. The individual worker who tests positive must be individually protected and for that person the surveillance program has made a contribution to his or her health. However, for every person who tests positive there are usually others who are also at risk but for whom the disorder or preclinical change has not yet appeared. The positive test in that person has additional significance for the workforce as a whole. Of course there will be occasional positive results in the real world, because occupational health protection is rarely as good as it could be. When they occur, prompt treatment or evaluation of the individual worker is necessary but follow-up with the employer to control the root cause is essential and whether the employer acts on the information appropriately may depend on the working relationship between the occupational health service and the employer.

That is why it is a mistake to refer to periodic health surveillance casually as "screening programs" without qualification. Screening is a strategy, not a service. The term "screening" is also commonly applied to fitness-for-duty evaluations, which have a wholly different purpose (see Chapter 22). The point is *why* the screening is being performed.

Periodic Health Surveillance

Surveillance is a strategy to determine a group experience with a particular disease outcome, while monitoring (which has other meanings as well) tracks the overall health experience of the individual or group. Employers in high-risk industries provide surveillance programs at company expense for workers in hazardous conditions, usually because it is required ("mandated") by occupational health regulations such as OSHA standards. Surveillance is applied when the diseases in question are known to be associated with a particular industry, such as asbestos-associated lung disorders. Surveillance is usually restricted to certain high-risk groups and is required by law to be provided at the employer's expense to workers exposed to specific hazards covered by OSHA or other regulations, such as asbestos, noise, or lead.

In the past, individual workers were periodically screened for signs of disease or early changes associated with exposure to work-related hazards as a substitute for controlling their exposure. The only way to protect the health of the individual worker in the absence of effective controls was by finding signs of disease early, when it is more easily treated. Unfortunately, the screening tests of the day were also primitive, so that lead, benzene, and other hazards had to produce clinical disease before their effects were detectable and showed positive in a periodic health surveillance. This may have been the original reason to perform periodic health surveillance in the past, when occupational hazards were uncontrolled and workers were at high risk, but it is not acceptable today.

Today, the primary reason for periodic health surveillance is as a backstop to determine whether the means of hazard control are working effectively to protect all workers at risk of occupational disease. Positive results should be very rare because hazards are better controlled. That we still see them tells us that the means of controlling the hazard in that workplace has failed and the means of control must be improved.

This means that an occupational health service needs to have the capacity to track trends in a group of workers and in individual workers, to see if there are changes in blood lead levels, in threshold shifts in the audiometric evaluation, and so forth, over time and in specific workplaces in the enterprise. Following individuals on an individual basis is not enough. Surveillance in the past was worker (individual) protection; today and in the future, it is workforce (population) protection.

Principles of Screening

The design of monitoring and surveillance programs is advancing rapidly. Screening tests for early detection of abnormalities related to exposure are selected on the basis of sensitivity, specificity, and the prevalence of the abnormality in a complicated relationship. Physicians involved in these programs must understand their rationale and legal framework to make sense of the results. Because the field of study is advancing so rapidly, certain terms have not yet become standardized. In reading other sources, one should determine exactly how an author is using such words as monitoring, surveillance, and screening.

The selection of a screening test is based on three variables: the "sensitivity" and "specificity" of the test, and the "prevalence" of the disease in the community. Sensitivity refers to the proportion of diseased persons in the population who are identified by the test. (For example, the percentage of people in the community who have tuberculosis and are detected by the QuatiFERON-TB ® gold test. For an occupational example, the percentage of workers in a beryllium-exposed workforce who actually have beryllium disease who test positive on the lymphocyte beryllium proliferation test, LBePT, assay for beryllium sensitivity.) The higher the sensitivity of the test, the more effectively it will identify the diseased individuals. The specificity of a test refers to the proportion of non-diseased individuals in the population who will have a negative result, in other words how reliably the test rules out disease in people who do not have it. The higher the specificity of a test, the more reliably it will exclude non-diseased individuals. Put another way, an insensitive but specific test may yield many false-negative results, whereas a sensitive but nonspecific test may give many false-positives. The ideal is a combination of high sensitivity and high specificity. The diagnostic efficiency of a test is called its predictive value and depends heavily on the prevalence, or frequency, of the condition in the population at the time of screening. Textbooks of clinical epidemiology and, increasingly, general medicine usually have chapters that provide more detail on the calculation of test performance when applied to a population with a certain prevalence of disease.

Test performance degenerates rapidly the lower the prevalence of the disorder in the population. Many clinical tests perform well for diagnosis in patients because the clinical features that caused them to be referred for the test indicate that they have a high probability of having the disease. These same tests may perform so poorly when applied for screening purposes on workers and the general population (who have a much lower probability of having the condition) that they are counterproductive and contraindicated for screening. One example is serological testing for anti-nuclear antibody (ANA) and other tests for lupus, which because of their high sensitivity but low specificity are first-line diagnostic tests in the clinic but useless for population surveys.

A test with low sensitivity but high specificity, such as a posterolateral (PA) chest film for the detection of asbestosis, will detect most but not all of diseased individuals, but a positive result will be a reliable indication that disease is present in an individual. However, a negative test result will not reliably rule out the disease, and in the case of workers with asbestosis many of those with negative chest films will be found to have low-grade disease on high-resolution computed tomography (CT) scan. A test with high sensitivity and low specificity will correctly identify most true cases but will also yield false-positive results for many individuals who do not, in fact, have the disease. For example, in years past, many employers insisted on low back screening X-rays in order to evaluate the risk for future low back pain. In addition to being an unacceptable test because of the radiation dose to bone marrow involved, the test was highly sensitive in identifying anatomic abnormalities, most of which are silent, but completely useless in identifying workers with current low back pain, let alone predicting the risk of low back pain in the future. Low back screening X-rays are now considered unethical.

The declining prevalence of many conditions in the community and therefore among the workforce, such as tuberculosis, has rendered useless many tests, such as the baseline chest film, that were traditionally used in "pre-employment" evaluations, before they became preplacement evaluations (see Chapter 23). If a disease is rare in the population, the false-positive results of a sensitive but nonspecific test will usually outnumber the true positives, requiring additional diagnostic tests to confirm the result. These diagnostic tests are usually more invasive and much more expensive and may have their own unfavorable test characteristics. Tests should never be ordered unless the physician has a clear idea of what to do with the results.

For reasons of cost, legal defense, and reliability, occupational health surveillance programs tend to be simple, to utilize a few well-established tests, and to be rigid in their testing requirements. For example, the surveillance program mandated by OSHA for workers exposed to high noise levels relies on an annual audiogram covering prescribed frequencies and performed by certified personnel with specified training, using equipment with prescribed specifications. The surveillance program for lead uses blood lead levels. Both tests have been around for years, are known to be reliable, and can be easily interpreted. There are many more sensitive tests available but their reliability and predictive value is questionable and they are not so readily interpreted. When errors arise from test performance problems and from the premature use of experimental methods, "state-of-the-art" testing can be very dangerous for employers because they may lead to discrimination and to bad decisions on preplacement and work assignments. This creates risk for workers and liability for employers. (Because of the imminent use of modern genetic testing, the Genetic Information Nondiscrimination Act of 2008 was passed, which makes it illegal in the US for preplacement evaluations to include any kind of genetic information, including family history.) There was a long history of invalid and experimental testing in the early and mid-twentieth century in Europe and the US, which led to workers being denied jobs. This led to the many strictures in codes of ethics against using unconventional and unvalidated tests. This is reflected in many of the provisions in the international code of ethics for occupational health (see Chapter 5).

Surveillance Programs

When a specific health outcome is known or suspected, the task of observing a population's health experience is much simplified. Surveillance programs are targeted to specific high-risk or high-exposure groups as defined by workplace assignment, known exposure history, and environmental monitoring data.

Two dozen standards promulgated by OSHA require specific surveillance procedures for workers exposed to certain hazards (Table 20.1). When a surveillance procedure is required by regulation, it is termed "mandated surveillance" (discussed below). The National Institute for Occupational Safety and Health (NIOSH) has issued voluntary surveillance recommendations applying to a larger number of exposures. Most large employers have a broader program of periodic health surveillance than is required by OSHA standards, including more chemical exposures depending on the process and exposure opportunity. These health surveillance evaluations may be part of the employment contract between the employer and the worker, and therefore are required.

Surveillance programs are applied in many ways. The primary function is to ensure adequate workplace protection by identifying cases of occupational disease that occur

Table 20.1 OSHA-Mandated Surveillance

Hazard	Frequency	Body Systems Emphasized	Special Test	OSHA Standard (CFR)
Acrylonitrile	Preplacement + annual, emerg/exp, term	Respiratory, GI, thyroid, skin, neurological (Ca risk)	CXR, stool guiaic	1910.1045(n); 1926.1145; 1915.1045
Arsenic, inorganic	Preplacement + annual, emerg/exp, term	Respiratory, skin, nose (Ca risk)	CXR	1910.1018(n); 1926.1118; 1915.1018
Asbestos (General Industry)	Preplacement + annual, term	Respiratory, cardiovascular, GI (Ca risk)	CXR, PFTs	1910.1001(l)
Asbestos (Construction and Shipyards)	Preplacement + annual	Respiratory, GI (Ca risk)	CXR, PFTs	1926.1101(m); 1915.1001
Benzene	Preplacement + annual, emerg	Hematopoietic (Ca risk)	Urine biomonitoring	1910.1028(i); 1926.1128; 1915.1028
Bloodborne pathogens	Post-exposure only	Infection risk	Serology	1910.1030(f)
1,3-Butadiene	Preplacement + annual, emerg, term	Skin, immunol, hepatic (Ca risk)	CBC	1910.1051(k); 1926.1151
Cadmium	Preplacement + annual, emerg, term	Respiratory, cardiovascular, renal, prostate (Ca risk)	CXR, urinary biomonitoring, CXR, PFTs	1910.1027(l); 1926.1127; 1915.1027; 1928.1027
Carcinogens (Suspected)	Preplacement + annual, emerg/exp	(Ca risk)	Variable	1910.1003–1016(g); 1926.1103; 1915.1003–1016
Chromium VI (Hexavalent)	Preplacement + annual, emerg, term	Respiratory; skin (Ca risk)		1910.1026(k); 1926.1126(i); 1915.1026(i)
Coke oven emissions	Preplacement + annual, term	Respiratory, skin (Ca risk)	CXR, PFTs	1910.1029(j)
Compressed air environments	Preplacement + annual	(Not specified)		1926.803(b)
Cotton dust	Preplacement + periodic (annual)	Respiratory	PFTs	1910.1043(h)
1,2-Dibromo-3-chloropropane (DBCP)	Preplacement + annual, emerg/exp	Repro, GU	Sperm count, hormone levels	1910.1044(m); 1926.1144; 1915.1044

Substance	Frequency/type of exam	Target organs/systems	Tests	CFR regulation
Ethylene oxide	Preplacement + annual, emerg/exp, term	Respiratory, skin, neurological, repro, heme, ocular (Ca risk)		1910.1047(i); 1926.1147
Formaldehyde	Preplacement + annual, emerg/exp	Respiratory, skin, ocular (Ca risk)	PFTs, if respiratory protection	1910.1048(l); 1926.1148; 1915.1048
Hazardous chemicals in laboratories	Preplacement +periodic when required by other standards, emerg/exp	Neurological, cardiovascular, skin, oral, GI, renal, (variable) (Ca risk)		1910.1025(j); 1926.62
HAZWOPER (hazardous waste operators and emergency response)	Preplacement + annual, emerg/exp, term	(Variable) (Ca risk)		1910.1048(l); 1926.1148; 1915.1048
Lead	Preplacement + annual, emerg/exp, term	Neurological, heme, renal, cardiovascular, repro, GI, oral	Blood lead, hematologic testing, ZPP, renal function	1910.1025(j); 1926.62
Methylene chloride	Preplacement + annual, emerg/exp, term	Respiratory, cardiovascular, skin, neurological, hepat, (Ca risk)		1910.1052(j); 1926.1152
Methylenedianiline	Preplacement + annual, emerg/exp	Hepat, skin (Ca risk)	LFTs	1910.1050(m)
Noise	Baseline + annual	hearing	Audiometry	1910.95(g); 1926.52
Respiratory protection	Screening questionnaire with follow-up, annual in certain circumstances	Respiratory; facial characteristics that pertain to fit of mask	Fit testing for respirators; CXR and PFTs may be required	1910.134(e); 1926.103
Vinyl chloride	Preplacement + annual, emerg/exp	Respiratory, hepat, skin, renal, spleen, (Ca risk)	LFTs	1910.1017(k); 1926.1117

Key: Ca = cancer; CBC = complete blood count; CFR = Code of Federal Regulations; CXR = chest X-ray; emerg/exp = evaluation following an emergency or exposure event; GI = gastrointestinal; GU = genitourinary; heme = hematology; hepat = hepatology; immunol = immunology; LFTs = liver function tests; PFT = pulmonary function test; repro = reproduction; term = termination; ZPP = zinc protoporphyrin test.

despite proper industrial hygiene measures. A surveillance program that identifies no disease outcome despite suitable screening procedures suggests adequate control of the exposure in question and should be judged a success. If previous cases have been observed and the control measures that have been instituted have not been extensive, however, suspicion should be raised either that new cases are being missed because the surveillance program itself is inadequate or that insufficient time has elapsed for new cases to appear.

A secondary function of surveillance, as noted, is to identify new cases as early as possible to prevent the progression of disease in the individual. Surveillance programs have sometimes been proposed as alternatives to workplace exposure controls. This is an unacceptable compromise because the mere detection of a disease is not a substitute for its prevention.

Surveillance programs may be conducted in-plant, or by an outside medical facility or physician under agreement with the employer. The tests to be conducted and the frequency of screening must be clearly specified, and the referral process for individuals found to have a disorder, as well as the employer's response to these individuals, must be spelled out in advance.

An important complement to any surveillance program is environmental monitoring, which involves periodic or continuous measurements of the potential exposures in the workplace. In toxicological terms, this provides information on the potential exposure received by an individual or group of employees, while medical monitoring or surveillance indicates the potential response. If an association exists or is suspected between a given exposure and a disease outcome, the data from environmental monitoring and either medical monitoring or surveillance can be used to construct an exposure–response relationship. The demonstration of a strong exposure–response relationship is powerful evidence in support of a suspected association.

Monitoring the environmental levels of hazards is one of the most important functions of an occupational health service, more important even than periodic health surveillance, but surveillance backs it up to ensure that hazard control is working. It can be completely preventive in the sense that, in circumstances where dangerous levels are found, it may be possible to take corrective action before harm comes to the employee. Environmental monitoring data from industrial hygiene surveys should be made available to the worker's physician, if possible, and must be disclosed to the worker. The worker's physician will normally need help interpreting exposure data, as this lies far outside the scope of practice of most practitioners.

Mandated Surveillance

Surveillance that is required by law or regulation is called "mandated surveillance" and is mandatory for both employers and employees, who cannot opt out (except for religious reasons, which is very rare). The occupational health professionals who perform surveillance should always read the original standard, or an authoritative summary from OSHA or the competent authority in their state or country (the occupational health regulatory agency) before conducting these evaluations. They are not difficult or complicated but the regulation must be followed closely to avoid legal liability and potential lapses in worker protection.

Table 20.1 compares the mandated surveillance requirements of OSHA standards, all of which are published in the Code of Federal Regulations (CFR), where abundant documentation is to be found. Most of these standards rely heavily on the physical examination and symptom interview, clinical methods that tend to be imprecise and insensitive for the purpose of surveillance. Several rely on special tests, most often pulmonary function studies, making it essential for an occupational health service with high volume to have the capacity to perform at least spirometry and audiometry. The timing of the evaluations depends on whether a preplacement or baseline evaluation is needed to benchmark the worker's health status, whether there are acute effects that require post-exposure or emergency evaluation, and whether an exit evaluation is required when an employee leaves the job (termination). It can readily be seen that some of the tests are obsolete (ZPP for lead exposure, for example, which is never performed in practice) and others are highly insensitive (pulmonary function tests for asbestos related disease, for example). Oddly, there are different, although similar, standards for General Industry and for Construction and Shipyards for both lead and asbestos. The differences mostly have to do with whether a preplacement or termination evaluation is required but there are also differences of substance. For example, the medical removal provision for lead workers in construction is slightly different from general industry. These inconsistencies and idiosyncrasies reflect the history of the legislation and the scientific understanding that preceded the promulgation of the standard, often by some years (see Chapter 4). For political reasons, it has been difficult or impossible for OSHA to change more than a handful of standards or to adopt new ones, which has led to the adoption of more generic standards such as those for "hazardous waste operators and emergency response" (HAZWOPER) and otherwise unregulated or unidentified carcinogens.

There is a very high risk that mandated periodic health surveillance evaluations will be taken for granted, especially when positive findings are infrequent. It becomes too easy, once they are routine, to forget their importance for the workforce, for the individual worker, and for liability of the employer. Reports often go unread and patterns unrecognized because those conducting the examinations do not bother to track year-to-year changes for individuals or to review results in a way that patterns are visible for work areas. Audiometric evaluations for noise-induced hearing loss have a particularly unfortunate record for missed abnormalities, missed opportunities for correcting problems, misinterpreted findings, overlooked reports, and bad outcomes resulting in preventable hearing loss. A famous court case involving an unreported abnormality on chest film played a pivotal role in defining the scope of responsibility in occupational health practice (see Chapter 3).

Biological Monitoring

Biological monitoring and toxicological monitoring are conducted primarily to assess the level of exposure that a worker has experienced. They are surveillance tests in the sense that they are surveillance for recent exposure, rather than health outcome. Occupational health practitioners use them for diagnosis and validation of the exposure history. Industrial hygienists use them to assess the levels and distribution of exposures in the exposed workforce.

Biological monitoring includes techniques to determine the magnitude of an effect the exposure is having on the body without direct measurement of the toxic substance. Measuring plasma or red cell cholinesterase levels after low-level exposure to organophosphate insecticides is an example. (Although common practice, it really is not necessary to do both and plasma cholinesterase is much less expensive.) Toxicological monitoring includes tests to determine, by direct measurement, the levels of a toxic substance or its residues in tissue body fluids or excreta. Testing for blood lead levels is a common example of toxicological screening. Some practitioners refer to surveillance using clinical findings, such as a physical examination, or chest films and other imaging techniques as biological monitoring. Imaging and clinical examination were not part of the original definition of biological monitoring but fell under the general rubric of "medical monitoring." The distinction is breaking down, however, and the term "medical monitoring" is falling out of use.

With both biological monitoring and toxicological screening, the intent is to detect potentially toxic exposures before their effects become manifest. Often, however, disease due to hazardous exposure cannot be detected during the subclinical phase. Some diseases, because of their natural history and biologic characteristics, are already in an advanced stage by the time detection is possible, and a targeted intervention to change the outcome is fruitless in all but a handful of cases. These tests do not benefit the individual worker much more than regular periodic health evaluation by their personal physician. Unfortunately, that has been the case in screening for lung cancer with sputum cytology and monitoring by chest film and computed tomography (CT), although advanced methods of imaging (spiral CT scanning) seem to be approaching a breakthrough.

Biological monitoring, strictly speaking, involves testing exposed employees to determine the uptake or the health effect of a hazard. The particular test used must directly reflect the hazardous substance, its passage in the body, the chemical change it may undergo, its effect on body tissue, its route of excretion or its place of storage in the body. "Shotgun" screening or testing for multiple unrelated variables is usually wasteful and the results usually present more questions than answers, because of low predictive value.

Example: Trace Element Analysis

Trace element analysis is a good example of a common "shotgun" test and one that presents a special problem of interpretation when a physician orders a complete panel. (This is actually more efficient for toxicological evaluation because the technology for trace element analysis can determine levels for 15 as easily as for 1.) The problem comes when a clinician orders a panel without knowing why or what to do with the findings and expects to interpret them as if they were conventional laboratory tests. Often patients will request this and have expectations or beliefs for what the test will show, based on a lay understanding or reading online.

Trace elements are metals and semimetals (such as arsenic and selenium) that are present in very low concentrations in body fluids (therefore excluding iron, magnesium, and calcium). Some of them, such as cobalt, copper, vanadium, and selenium, are nutritional requirements (although at such low levels that deficiencies are very rare). Others, particularly the more toxic metals (lead, mercury, cadmium, arsenic, and manganese) are not, to the best of contemporary scientific knowledge (there is recent evidence that extremely low amounts of arsenic and manganese may actually be required metabolically). When laboratories screen for trace elements, the reports that they return are almost always interpreted as if the trace element had a "normal range" predicated on a statistically normal distribution, which these elements do not. Metabolically-required elements, such as calcium, iron, and electrolytes, are kept under strict homeostatic control and so have a normal range. Trace elements are not and their distribution is highly variable, depending entirely on exposure. Their concentration in body fluids is not normally distributed in the population, the way electrolytes are. A determination of "elevated" levels in body fluids, even as high as double the mean seen in the population or more, is usually meaningless in these reports toxicologically. It simply reflects exposure to the metal at work (for example cadmium, which is intrinsically toxic, may be elevated in welders but at low levels), supplemental intake (zinc being especially common), an unusual diet (many foods are rich in selenium, particularly nuts, but also crustaceans, certain fish, braunschweiger, and waffles), cigarette smoking (specifically cadmium), or simply recent ingestion of a food rich in the element (commonly, elevated arsenic levels after consumption of shellfish, although the arsenic is in an organic form that is virtually nontoxic). These exaggerated reports cause considerable unjustified concern among workers, the physicians and nurses who care for them, and employers. A welder with a "very high" molybdenum level is simply not a medical concern.

Elevations in the more toxic metals (listed above) should be compared against thresholds for toxicity, not the distribution of values in a reference population. Some trace elements have complicated kinetics and so biomonitoring for them can be misleading. Manganese exposure, specifically, is not reliably reflected in body fluids and so testing for it is not useful. This problem with trace elements is compounded further when the medium is hair analysis, which is an unreliable matrix for biomonitoring in the first place. Hair should never be the basis for a biomonitoring program and the findings of spot hair analysis should always be viewed skeptically and in most cases ignored.

Voluntary Monitoring

Whether biological monitoring should be mandatory or voluntary on the part of workers has been controversial, especially among advocates for workers' rights. Historically, sensitivities have been particularly strong in Germany and Canada. This fact alone is justification for using a high degree of judgment in selecting surveillance tests. A requirement for employees to undergo testing may be made a condition of employment, but must be accompanied by adequate worksite hazard monitoring and control, and by employee health hazard information and education. Monitoring is not a substitute for controlling hazards.

Mandatory monitoring, either under a regulation or under an employment contract, has the advantage of ensuring that all workers at risk are regularly screened. Whenever abnormal results occur, appropriate action can be taken at the earliest possible time to protect the workforce and the individual worker. It also means that the occupational health service is able to collect sufficient health data with respect to the hazard to have a complete and unbiased record of the effectiveness of their preventive program.

With a voluntary monitoring system, a significant number of exposed workers may never be monitored if a large proportion opts out. It may then become impossible to draw valid conclusions about the condition of the subpopulation of workers who are at risk. Do acceptable levels found in volunteered samples indicate that all workers at risk are remaining healthy? Did the workers who agreed to be monitored do so because they are the conscientious and safe workers, whereas those who declined are more slipshod in their approach to personal health? Are workers in the latter group afraid to reveal what could be significant absorption of the hazardous substance? Are they possibly just taking a stand on a personal belief that their health is their own business? It may be impossible to know for certain.

On the other hand, making monitoring voluntary may avoid labor unrest caused by worker's concerns that the employer is unilaterally imposing its will on employees. Clashes over these issues in the 1960s and 1970s led to the formulation of guidelines such as those presented in the next section.

One situation clearly favors voluntary monitoring and that is when a new product or chemical exposure is introduced and there is no relevant experience with its effects. This is the current situation with respect to nanomaterials, for which there are no exposure standards as yet. There is no reliable toxicological guidance at present. Close monitoring of the health experience of workers exposed to these materials is a means of detecting early, unknown health problems and to gain experience for the eventual setting of protective standards.

New or Purpose-Designed Programs

It is estimated that 85,000 chemicals are in common use around the world, 2500 in "high production" (as defined by the US Toxic Substances Control Act), and that 2000 more are being introduced into commerce every year, 7 per day, according to the California Environmental Protection Agency. Sometimes a familiar chemical that is not regulated or is not known to be a hazard may be used in a form or setting that raises the possibility of health effects. With the advent of nanotechnology, this is becoming a common issue because each new nanomaterial may have unique, often quantum-level characteristics that are different from the same chemical in bulk quantities. (NIOSH has recommended two different exposure limits for titanium dioxide, for example: one for fine particles and one for ultrafine nanoparticles.) Some of these new, newly formulated, and emerging chemicals and nanostructures are likely to become occupational hazards and so employers who use them in processes or produce them are faced with a need to design and conduct new purpose-designed monitoring or (for hazards with known outcomes) surveillance programs for emerging or poorly understood hazards.

Monitoring programs for exposed workers are usually limited to situations in which the outcome is unknown, and are used most often in presumably high-risk working populations when the exposure is new, for example in workers exposed to nanomaterials, where the technology is too recent to fully understand its health risks, or for community residents exposed to perfluorooctanate (PFOA), for which the toxicology is not well known. When the experience of a group of workers is followed over time, patterns of illness may appear which suggest either unusual characteristics of that working population or exposures requiring control.

An answer to the question whether or not to monitor (in the absence of a regulatory requirement to do so), may be difficult to find, particularly one which will be acceptable to both the employer and his workforce. Naturally, local circumstances come into play, but there are recognized criteria that should always be considered when deciding whether or not a particular biological monitoring program should be implemented.

The following are suggested criteria for deciding whether to start or to discontinue a biological monitoring procedure:

1   The information obtained must be of demonstrable importance to the health or safety at work of the employee being tested.
2   The test should not be a substitute for eliminating or controlling the hazard.
3   The test results should be applied for the purpose of improving the health and safety situation at the worksite and maintaining or improving the health of the individual tested.
4   If the test is to determine absorption or intake of a substance, it should be specific for that substance.
5   If the test is to determine an effect, it should detect early signs of exposure.
6   The employee's baseline level for the substance, before exposure in the workplace, should be known in order to permit later interpretation.
7   The test must be acceptable to the employee; a test that is painful beyond drawing blood or very uncomfortable or inconvenient must be clearly justified and agreed upon by the workers subjected to it.
8   The advantages of using the method should be greater than the advantages of using alternative measures to identify cases of excessive exposure.
9   Each employee should be informed of individual and group test results and their meaning and implications for health.

Even when mandated by law or contract, a new surveillance program should have the approval and understanding of all workers involved, through their union or through direct worker education programs in the case of a nonunionized work force. The education program should explicitly state the purpose of the surveillance, the measures being taken to control workplace exposure, the measures that employees can take to minimize personal exposure or to reduce the risk of the outcome in question, and the right of an employee to withdraw from a voluntary program.

A surveillance program must be built around the best available testing procedure that is in established use at the time the program is started. A test that is very controversial or is difficult to interpret will lead to considerable confusion and may delay prompt action. Thus, the most widely applied OSHA-mandated surveillance procedures utilize relatively simple and straightforward tests: the lead standard is based on determination of the blood lead level, the noise standard on audiometric screening, and the asbestos standard primarily on the chest film and spirometric testing.

A surveillance program may incorporate an experimental test, but when a new screening test is validated and introduced as a replacement for an older test of less reliability, both tests should be performed for a period of several years so that the findings can be compared and trends will not be obscured by the transition.

The frequency of testing in a surveillance program depends on convenience and the biological characteristics of the disease. Most surveillance procedures are repeated annually, since one year is a convenient interval and the actual elapsed time is somewhat arbitrary. The OSHA noise standard, for example, requires annual audiometric screening for workers exposed to 85 decibels (dBA) or more of noise. This is the "action level" at which monitoring is triggered as a mandatory requirement; the OSHA permissible exposure level is 90 dB. However, most observers believe this is too high. (At this level of noise exposure, some workers may be expected to develop noise-induced hearing loss.) There is nothing inherent in noise-induced hearing loss that makes annual testing optimal, but testing less often may lead to undetected progression of hearing loss between tests and to inadvertent omission of tests. Testing more often than every year would incur an additional cost and is unlikely to identify a significantly higher proportion of new cases.

Before adopting a test, it is critical to know in advance what the results will mean and how to interpret them. This is just as important for an occupational health service providing periodic health surveillance or monitoring as it is for a clinician ordering an unusual lab test.

A second challenge is to know, again in advance, exactly how to communicate the results to workers, as one must. A number like 200 seems large: it is bigger than 20 and much bigger than 2. However, if that number is 200 µg/L, which are typical units for trace elements, it is one-hundredth of 20 mg/L and one tenth of 2 mg/L, which is the concentration range more familiar for conventional laboratory tests, because the units are different by a factor of 1000. (A typical magnitude for detection limits and variation in laboratory technology might be 200 nm/L.) To make risk communication even more difficult, most laboratories outside the US express their findings in mol/L, not mg/L, so someone without a technical background who goes online for answers is almost certain to be confused. Some laboratories inside the US report mg/dL (= mg/100 ml) rather than mg/L. (The OSHA lead standard is written in deciliters, which has perpetuated this convention in the US.)

For example, a plasma vanadium concentration of 0.10 µg/dl looks much worse when it is expressed as 1000 ng/L and if the subject is told that it is at the "upper limit of normal," when in fact this level is ordinary (the word normal should not be used) for an unexposed person, relatively low for a welder, or someone working on boilers, or around fly ash (typical sources of exposure to vanadium), and far below any toxic threshold for vanadium or levels that might be expected for the significant number of people who take vanadium supplements (unnecessarily, because nutritional vanadium deficiency is almost impossible because the element is required in such minute amounts).

Deciding whether or not to start a monitoring program is one problem; closing down an existing program is quite another. Occasionally, biological monitoring that has been carried on for some time—possibly for many years—may be found not to be cost-effective. Analysis of the results obtained over the time the program has been in operation may reveal that few or no positive results have been obtained because the level of potential exposure, even under worst-case scenarios, does not justify the program. (This is different than demonstrating the effectiveness of control technology where the potential for exposure still exists.) If workers are no longer at risk because the process has changed, then the cost in time and dollars is not justified. For example, benzene exposure used to be common and widespread but now is confined to a few exposure opportunities, mostly in the petrochemical sector. Even in the petrochemical industry industry-wide surveillance is not warranted.

Recommended Reading and Resources

California Environmental Protection Agency. Emerging chemicals of concern. Available at: http://www.dtsc.ca.gov/assessingrisk/emergingcontaminants.cfm. Accessed July 1, 2011.

Gochfield M (1992) Medical surveillance and screening in the workplace: complementary strategies. *Environ Res*, 59(1): 67–80.

Guidotti TL (2010) *The Praeger Handbook of Occupational and Environmental Medicine*. Santa Barbara CA, Praeger ABC-Clio. See Chapter 5 on "Monitoring, Surveillance, and Screening."

Hoffman H, Phillips S (2012) *Clinical Practice of Biological Monitoring*. Beverly Farms MA, OEM Press.

Mitchell FL (2007) *Instant Medical Surveillance: The Evaluation of Chemical and Biological Dangers*. Beverly Farms MA, OEM Press, 2nd ed.

Nasterlack M (2011) Role of medical surveillance in risk management. *J Occup Environ Med*, 53 (Suppl.): S18–S21. Case study of nanomaterials; this distinguished German author uses "surveillance" in sense that "monitoring" is used in this chapter.

Occupational Safety and Health Administration. Medical screening and surveillance. Available at: http://www.osha.gov/SLTC/medicalsurveillance/index.html. Accessed December 22, 2011.

21 Hazard Evaluation and Management

Tee L. Guidotti

Most of the chapters in this book tell the occupational health care professional how to do things. This chapter tells the occupational health care professional why certain things are done, in order to cement the health care professional more firmly in the occupational team and position him or her to add value to occupational health services.

Identification and evaluation of hazards in order to assess and manage risk in the workplace is the foundation of occupational health and safety. This is primarily the domain of industrial hygienists and safety professionals, whose responsibility is to manage hazards. When occupational injuries and illnesses occur, they are the result of a failure in prevention. Every incident and case, some more than others, reveals flaws in occupational health protection, many of them behavioral. Likewise, every case that goes to workers' compensation or, tragically, to fatality investigation, has a story behind it that must be documented accurately and thoroughly. Therefore, an understanding of hazards, risks, and controls in the workplace is key knowledge that distinguishes the committed occupational health professional from the dilettante. It also allows the health professional to speak easily with other members of the occupational health team (such as industrial hygienists, who normally take the lead on hazard-related issues) with workers (whether they are patients or undergoing screening tests), and with employers.

Occupational health providers also need a working knowledge of exposure assessment for patient care to understand what they are dealing with, to understand proposed standards, to relate exposure to outcome in assessing causation and assessing risk, and to interpret the literature. Physicians and nurses in occupational and environmental medicine (OEM) are frequently called upon to interpret the hazard presented by a given exposure to a chemical or to correlate a clinical diagnosis with a history of exposure in either an individual patient or a group of workers. Sometimes occupational health care providers learn about lapses or hazards from their worker-patients during interviews or even casual conversation. At a tertiary or policy-making level (see Chapter 1), occupational and environmental physicians may be called upon to weigh evidence for setting exposure standards in the workplace or environment based on data that cannot be interpreted without an understanding of exposure assessment.

Unfortunately, accurate measurements of exposure associated with a particular patient or case are almost never available to the occupational and environmental physician in clinical practice. Physicians, in the course of their medical work, no longer perform exposure assessments themselves, although they commonly did decades ago. In fact, the profession of industrial (or occupational) hygiene arose out of occupational medicine practice, when the American Industrial Hygiene Association was founded by non-physician members of the

American Association of Industrial Physicians and Surgeons (now the American College of Occupational and Environmental Medicine) in 1939.

The approach to hazard and risk assessment outlined in this chapter is consistent with how hygienists approach exposure assessment in their mission of "anticipation, recognition, evaluation, and control" of chemical, mechanical (and ergonomic), physical, and biological hazards, and also applies in a general way to psychogenic hazard. In recent years a simplified approach to hazard and risk assessment has become available through the work of British and European regulatory agencies and standards-setting bodies, called "control banding". This approach is a robust method for evaluating hazards that was simplified for most relatively straightforward workplace risks, obviating the need for expensive and scarce professional evaluation for routine management. The approach lends itself well to most situations that might be encountered by occupational health professionals. However, it does not match the professional standard of a trained industrial hygienist or safety professional, who remain indispensable for more difficult problems. Familiarity with the approach is not only practically useful for dealing with minor problems but intellectually useful as a template for thinking about risk assessment.

The assessment of risk depends on knowing the level of exposure in the workplace, how frequently the worker is exposed, and the risk associated with that level of exposure. Practical hazard identification and risk assessment in the workplace depends on identification of the hazard, how much is present in the workplace, the opportunity that a worker may have to encounter the hazard, controls that are already in place, availability of personal protection, and many additional factors, such as level of training and awareness, that are not usually considered. Exposure information is used to determine acceptable levels of exposure in setting standards, assessing causation when workers become ill, and to establish risk through studies.

Hazard and risk assessment can be undertaken on many levels. Worksite hazard and risk assessment focuses on the specific workstation, usually involves an inventory of hazards to identify the most problematical, and is usually conducted by a supervisor or a safety officer. Workplace assessment might evaluate the hazards present and the risks they bring to a building or area, and is usually conducted by a hygienist or safety officer. Enterprise-level risk assessment examines the distribution of hazards and the risks associated with them across the entire organization and is usually conducted by hygienists and loss prevention officers.

Definitions

A "hazard" is something that has the capacity to cause harm, whether it is a chemical or a condition in the workplace. A risk is the probability of something bad happening, such as an injury or health effect. A consequence is the result, the occurrence of that bad outcome. A hazard, or threat, causes a risk of injury or disease when a person is exposed to it. (If a person is not exposed to it, or if there is no hazard present in the workplace, then there can be no risk from it.) Box 21.1 lists the five general categories of hazard found in the workplace and traditionally identified by occupational health professionals. This classification of hazard, although widely taught, is too limiting and will be expanded upon later in this chapter. It is important to know, however, because this or a similarly conventional formulation is used universally in the literature of occupational health and safety.

"Risk assessment," in the context of occupational health and safety, is a general approach to evaluating the probability and consequence of the effects of known hazards. "Risk management" is what is done about these risks once you identify or estimate them. The

Box 21.1 Traditional Categories of Workplace Hazards

- Chemical.
- Physical (associated with illness).
- Mechanical (associated with injury).
- Biological.
- Psychological.

terms have somewhat different meanings in other contexts, such as regulatory policy and standards setting, and in loss prevention and liability management. In this chapter, the terms "risk assessment" and "risk management" are used only as they are used in occupational health and safety, except where specifically noted, not as they are used in environmental health and public policy. The level of risk assessment occupational health professionals are most concerned with is workplace-level risk assessment, which brings occupational health protection down to the worksite and the specific work environment. Workplace-level risk assessment and management is primarily intended to empower managers to take control of and to mitigate occupational hazards in the workplaces and business units under their responsibility. Enterprise-level risk assessment is the assessment of risk on the scale of a company or operating division.

A "health hazard evaluation" (HHE) is an investigation with the objective of recognizing a potential or actual health problem in the workplace. (The term comes from the inspections of that name conducted by the National Institute for Occupational Safety and Health.) An HHE is usually conducted by a "walk-through" inspection of the workplace and an interview with managers, production supervisors, and workers in the specific workplace in question. An HHE is conducted as a team, usually led by an industrial hygienist and involving other occupational health professionals, such as a physician or occupational health nurse as needed. The outsourcing of occupational health from in-house to a community-based program has led to a decline in the involvement of health care professionals in multidisciplinary HHEs.

Hazards

The categories of hazard identified in Box 21.1 represent a traditional and very general way of looking at hazards. ("Physical" sometimes includes "Mechanical," but experience suggests that it is more helpful to consider mechanical hazards related to traumatic injury separately from other physical exposures, although both involve uncontrolled release of forms of energy.) It is too limiting to accommodate modern ideas of hazard, exposure, consequence (or outcome), and risk. In practice, hazards are more complicated.

Box 21.2 is an unconventional and longer taxonomy of risk but one that is likely to be more useful in practice. Although slightly longer, the major headings in this list, once memorized, constitute a useful checklist to keep in mind while taking a history, walking around a workplace, designing a periodic health surveillance system or a preplacement evaluation, or mentally noting the problems likely to arise in a particular contract or request for services.

Ergonomic hazards, matching the workplace to the worker's capabilities, are predominantly but by no means exclusively mechanical in nature. "Geography" represents a different way of looking at hazard, one becoming recognized more broadly in the oil and gas industry, particularly. It is helpful in conducting a risk assessment to consider location as a category of

Box 21.2 Expanded Classification of Hazard

1. Chemical
    1.1. That cause toxicity
    1.2. That cause allergy
    1.3. That release energy.
2. Physical (Forms of energy)
    2.1. Ergonomic
    2.2. Electromagnetic
    2.3. Radiation
    2.4. Heat, cold
    2.5. Noise and vibration.
3. Mechanical (safety hazards for injury).
4. Biological agents
    4.1. That cause infection
    4.2. That cause allergy
    4.3. That produce toxic chemicals.
5. Psychological Stress
    5.1. Work organization
    5.2. Interpersonal stressors.
6. Geography (clusters of hazard that attach to location and geography rather than a work process, such as malaria, traffic accidents).

hazard in itself, because so many individual hazards (such as infectious risk, traffic hazards, and pollution) cluster together in the real world and are associated with location rather than specific job duties. Geography also carries its own occupational risk. Offshore location in the oil and gas industry, for example, carries with it a cluster of issues related to safety (fire, explosion, cold water emersion), access (helicopter evacuation), and weather conditions.

The probability of consequences resulting from these hazards defines the risks that are being prevented. In other words, hydrogen sulfide is a *hazard*; *exposure* to hydrogen sulfide has the potential *consequence* of causing a knockdown, which may be lethal. This does not occur in every case but occurs with a certain probability, given the circumstances. This probability is the *risk* that is being prevented or controlled. Risk assessment, at the workplace or enterprise level, is discussed in the next section in more detail.

The outcomes of an exposure are what happen as a result of the consequences of exposure to the hazard. Table 21.1 shows how experienced experts in occupational health and safety tend to view the outcomes of exposure to hazards. Note that it is subtly different from simply labeling disorders as acute and chronic, and that cancer, in particular, is not in its usual place as a "chronic disease." The types of injury and illness that result from exposure to these hazards fall into one of three general categories:

*   *Acute.* Acute disorders happen right away. Managers and health care providers usually know what they are dealing with and the impact is obvious. Examples include traumatic injuries, most asthma attacks, immediate poisonings, and temporary threshold shift (TTS) in hearing due to noise exposure.

Table 21.1 Categories of Consequence for Health Outcomes in Occupational Health

Category	Acute	Chronic	"Stochastic"
Chemical	Acute toxicity Chemical incident	Chronic toxicity	Cancer Allergy
Physical	Acute effects (e.g. TTS*)	Delayed and chronic effects (e.g. PTS*)	Cancer
Mechanical and ergonomic	Trauma	Repetitive strain	Fatality
Biological	Infection	Infection	Infection Allergy
Psychogenic	Workplace violence	Stress-related illness Depression	Decompensation of mental illness
Location	Any of above	Any of above	Any of above

*Temporary threshold shift (TTS) and permanent threshold shift (PTS) in audiogram.

- *Chronic.* Chronic disorders develop over time and last for a long time, often the rest of the person's life. They are hard to count accurately and to attribute to any one cause but together preventable chronic disorders add up to a huge burden on society and the company. Examples include heart disease, lung disease, arthritis, and permanent threshold shift (PTS) due to noise.
- *Stochastic.* Stochastic disorders (stochastic means related to chance) look random. Some people get it and others do not. The frequency of the outcome increases with the exposure level but not the severity. (This is because an infection, a cancer, or sensitization, once started, follows its own pathway.)

In this schema, acute and chronic disease are "deterministic," meaning that for a given level of hazard, the outcome for an individual is certain, taking different levels of susceptibility and manifestation of symptoms into account. A fall from 8 feet causes four times the damage in terms of energy released than a fall from 4 feet. (Basic physics: energy release is the square of velocity.) Exposure to carbon monoxide at a blood level of 20 percent causes headache in everybody and usually visual symptoms. The mechanisms work inexorably.

Stochastic disorders are characterized by probability on a group basis and uncertainty on an individual basis. Increasing exposure increases the risk of a stochastic disorder on a group level, and increases the risk for all the individuals in the group, but for the levels of exposure commonly encountered in the workplace no one can tell in advance which worker will get the disease and who will not. In other words, if a group of workers is exposed to the exact same level of a cancer-causing chemical, called a carcinogen, they will not all get cancer. Who among them will get cancer will be unpredictable. But they will all have a higher risk than members of another group that is not exposed at all to the carcinogen or that is exposed at a lower level. Likewise, many people may be exposed to an antigen, but only a few will become sensitized to that antigen. Similarly, exposure to an infectious agent usually does not infect everyone in a group of people (even in the case of influenza pandemics) but the attack rate is higher the higher the level of exposure. Fatalities, being rare events in occupational health (relatively speaking) and usually the result of more than one factor going wrong, are treated as stochastic in this schema.

Consequence is what happens when the adverse outcome occurs. At this stage, it is no longer a risk but an actualized event. Consequences can be evaluated on the basis of how many people were or would be affected, the severity of illness or injury that did or might result, or the magnitude of loss that did or might occur. Consequence assessment is the key to prioritizing risks for management.

In this chapter, a simple, straightforward approach to risk assessment and management in the workplace is laid out that will enable the health professional untrained in occupational health to understand the process, engage in the role of responsible team member, and speak in the terminology commonly used.

Risk Assessment

"Risk assessment," as the term is used in occupational health and safety (but not environmental health or public policy), is a systematic search for hazards that can result in significant consequences and assignment of a priority for control and mitigation, which is called "risk management."

Some risks are complicated and involve multiple ways in which things can go wrong. For example, an upset in a refinery is much more complicated than a welding accident. These complicated risk profiles can be modeled using well-established, now-conventional methods from engineering. "Fault tree" analysis is an evaluation based on a flow charts showing how an adverse event (such as a fire, or a blowout, or a spill) could happen. Fault trees work backwards to determine what failure could cause the event and then what factors could cause the failure and so forth, until a clear picture emerges of what would have to go wrong to result in a serious event. In many cases, more than one failure is required for an adverse outcome. "HAZOP" (hazard and operability) analysis is used to predict what could go wrong when a part or a process fails. They emphasize consequences and are particularly useful for complicated situations where there may be unanticipated consequences. These advanced methods are not required for most risk assessment activities in the workplace. Health professionals are almost never involved directly but are often called upon to respond to the results when the time comes to do emergency planning (see Chapter 31) and should know that these methods exist.

Fault tree and HAZOP analysis are in the domain of engineers, assisted by safety professionals, and hygienists, and are far beyond the scope of this book. For most purposes, simple methods such as checklists, grids, Excel spreadsheets, and physical inspection are enough. Occupational health and safety professionals can do many of the simpler analyses themselves, or can help walk management through it. Most important of all, understanding how it is done leads the occupational health service to be more responsive, proactive, and helpful to employers, and demonstrates engagement and relevance to employees.

The first step is a walk-through and inspection to compile an inventory of hazards in the location. This has usually already been done in the case of large employers.

After the hazard has been identified, it has to be evaluated. In occupational health and safety, this is done by determining how serious a risk it poses to employees, contractors, or other people who are likely to be exposed. Three pieces of information are most important:

- *Exposure opportunity.* How likely is it that people will come into contact with the hazard (most often by inhaling it) at levels that could be harmful? This level will be called "over-exposure" for simplicity, because exposure at low levels is not of concern here.
- *Quantity.* How much is used or is present in the workplace? Quantification may be by mass (micrograms, pounds, kilograms, tons, tonnes) or volume (milliliters, liters, gallons, barrels, tanks) and does not have to be exact.

- *Level of hazard*. How dangerous is the hazard? A crude indication of relative hazard is to go by the applicable occupational exposure standard, to consult standard references or to refer to the manufacturer's information on the material safety data sheet (MSDS) or some other reliable data source. It is almost never necessary to go back to the toxicological literature (in which case a consultant toxicologist is advisable) unless the hazard is new to industry and there is little information available in standard references.

In practice, the level of hazard is usually determined by reference to the appropriate occupational exposure standard that applies to the hazard. Recognizing that such standards were not designed for this purpose, they are based, particularly the newer ones, on scientific data. Because the OSHA PEL (permissible exposure limit, see Chapter 4) is known not to be protective for many workplace hazards, it is usually better to use the American Conference of Governmental Industrial Hygienists (ACGIH) Threshold Limit Value (TLV®) or the National Institute for Occupational Safety and Health (NIOSH) Recommended Exposure Limit. (Canadian occupational exposure limits (OELs) are usually closer to TLVs®.) It is also important to keep in mind that for many outcomes, such as noise-induced hearing loss and allergy, some workers may still experience effects at current OELs.

Given the information above, the next step is to answer the following two questions:

- How severe will the consequences be if an (over)exposure occurs?
- How likely is it that an incident resulting in (over)exposure will happen?

With the information from worksite risk assessment, risks in the workplace can then be classified and prioritized in two dimensions, frequency and magnitude of consequence, as in Table 21.2.

Frequency or probability information can be drawn from historical data or HAZOP analysis, which is usually more sophisticated than truly needed for basic risk assessment. However, in practice, probability is usually a relatively informal estimate based on realistic projections of what might happen in a worst-case scenario. Assumptions inevitably have to be made.

The most important dimension of risk prioritization is how serious the consequences of an incident involving the hazard might be. Consequences may range from catastrophic to trivial in each of many categories, ranging from human life (which trumps all other concerns) to environmental impact to asset damage to lost revenue to reputational damage to interference with relationships in the community and among vendors and customers. A more sophisticated and comprehensive tool for estimating how severe the consequences of

Table 21.2 Prioritization of Risks for Management

Probability of Occurring	Magnitude of Consequence →		
	Low	*Medium*	*High*
High	Medium Priority	High Priority	Highest Priority*
Medium	Low Priority	Medium Priority	High Priority
Low	No Priority	Medium–Low Priority	Medium–High Priority

* indicates a risk that should not exist in the workplace, that should have been controlled already.

an event might be is given in Table 21.3. It is an example of a more detailed consequence analysis, taken from the oil and gas industry. For most purposes, however, such sophistication is not necessary and would not be expected from health professionals, since risk assessment is not normally their responsibility.

In general, whoever is doing the assessment, usually the supervisor, manager, or hygienist, should give greater weight to the potential severity of the consequences of an incident involving a hazard than to the likelihood of an incident occurring. The probability of an incident is more difficult to predict than the consequences and rare events do happen. It is not a good idea to assume that if a catastrophic event has not happened in the recent past it will not happen in the near future. Hazards that have the potential to cause serious harm must be attended to even if the likelihood of an event is low.

Hazards that are unlikely to occur and that result in little risk of harm if they do occur are not important and are given no or low priority. Hazards resulting in risks that do not result in significant loss are not a priority, especially if they happen rarely, but should be managed as part of regular operations because they often interfere with efficiency and morale. For example, asbestos lagging (insulation) can be left in place as long as it is intact and not disintegrating, in order to prevent inadvertent release of fibers. Asbestos should only be removed when it is possible to seal off the area and use proper protective measures. This is usually best done during a plant overhaul or renovation, when the area would be disrupted anyway.

Risk Management

Risk management in the workplace is mostly a problem of hazard control. This is a very general approach. The solutions to the control of hazards tend to be technical and depend on changes in the workplace. The technical details will be different for each problem. Control or management of occupational hazards is usually the responsibility of the supervisor or manager, with the assistance of an industrial hygienist or safety professional. Occupational health professionals are seldom involved except in qualifying workers for use of respiratory protection (respirator fit testing). Even so, it is useful to know the vocabulary in order to be able to take a history and to discuss management measures with the hygiene and safety staff.

The basic options available for control of hazards are as follows, in declining order of effectiveness as a general solution:

- *Elimination and substitution.* Removing the hazard from the workplace entirely and replacing it with something safer is the ideal solution.
- *Containment and isolation.* Moving the potentially hazardous process away from the worker, behind a barrier, or inside a sealed chamber.
- *Engineering controls.* Engineering controls are mechanical or electronic devices, such as guards on machinery or interlock systems, that protect the worker by creating a safer environment and interface with the hazard. They are generally highly effective, in part because they do not depend on the worker changing behavior.
- *Ventilation.* Actually a subset of engineering controls, ventilation is a highly effective form of protection for airborne hazards when properly installed and airflow is balanced. This is a specialization of industrial hygienists.
- *Personal protection.* The use of personal protective devices, such as respirators, impermeable gloves, aprons, footwear, eye protection, hardhats, and hearing protection, depend on worker training, cooperation, and motivation. For this reason, they are considered much

Table 21.3 A hypothetical consequence analysis for upstream oil and gas production

	People	Environment	Building	Equipment	Wastage	Production	Revenue	Reputation	Relationships
Fire									
Explosion									
Blowout									
Spill									
Gas release									
Structural failure									
Cable snapping									
Theft									
Etc.									

For each column, rate the worst case for risks by the following scale (10 for catastrophic risks, 1 to 5 for all other, using illustrations below for selected categories):

10 = fatality, total loss of significant assets, shutdown in production
5 = disabling injury, major property loss, prolonged interruption in production
4 = serious injury, significant property loss, interruption in production
3 = injury, reparable damage, one-day interruption in production
2 = minor injury, minor damage, brief interruption
1 = any injury, damage, interruption to production
0 = no impact whatever

This grid does not imply that the outcomes are comparable across rows by the same measures of lost value. Injury to people and environment weigh much more heavily than material loss, revenue loss, and social consequences. There is no generally agreed-upon scale or valuation to compare outcomes of different types less reliable than the previous methods, although they may be very effective when used properly. They are indispensable in situations where the work environment cannot be controlled or in emergency situations.

- *Administrative measures.* Rotating workers through hazardous areas to ensure that no worker receives an overdose, or relying on shift scheduling and other management measures to protect workers is useful as a backup to prevent overexposure but it not considered reliable because there are too many ways for it to fail.

- *Behavioral measures.* Training, behavior-based safety, and incentives are generally considered the least reliable and effective approach to managing hazards when used alone. However, behavioral methods can be very useful in reinforcing and motivating compliance with more effective modes of protection, such as proper use of personal protection and housekeeping, and in discouraging behavior that undermines safety (such as removing machine guards because they are in the way). Behavioral methods work best when there are environmental changes that support safety (such as engineering controls) and cues to remind workers. Posters and signs have very limited value.

- *Housekeeping.* Housekeeping in the shop and on the factory floor can be very effective for protection against dust, chemical hazards, and certain types of injury (such as slips, trips, and falls), but this is highly variable, difficult to evaluate, and depends on the hazard. Preventing dust accumulation, cleaning up spills promptly, and picking up loose objects certainly helps to maintain a safer work environment. Alone, housekeeping probably ranks above administrative controls but its practice and standards usually mirror management engagement and attention to safety and so its effect is intertwined with these. A workplace that follows good safety procedures is usually also good in standards of housekeeping as well. A workplace that is deficient in housekeeping also sends a signal to workers that management tolerates sloppy conditions and is lax in other ways.

Recently a new approach has gained ground that makes it possible for managers to handle most occupational health issues without expensive technical assistance. "Control banding" is a simplified way of addressing hazards in the workplace, making it feasible for supervisors and managers to deal with straightforward problems on a small scale without expensive professional help. The control-banding approach is a simplified approach to the recognition and categorization of hazards that points to a "menu" of control measures.

In practice, control banding follows a procedure much like that described above for workplace risk assessment.

Control banding is primarily geared for middle to small enterprises, not large corporations. However, the approach is useful in resolving simple problems in workplaces of any size. It is also a useful way of thinking about the control of hazards, helping managers to see the need for proactive measures to mitigate risk, to set priorities, and to know when to call in the experts.

Business View

In addition to the technical view of risk management presented above, there is also a broader business view of the problem that senior managers and loss prevention specialists work from (Figure 21.1). In this view, risk is treated as an unwanted commodity, not unlike waste. The objective is to avoid it, minimize it, or get rid of it, and to fund liability for whatever residual risk is left. Understanding this point of view makes it easier to speak to employers.

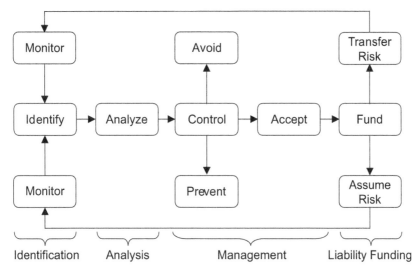

Figure 21.1 Business view of risk management. Financial management of residual risks is a corporate function and never a substitute for control

The first step, in this conceptualization, is to identify significant risks after reviewing all the activities of the business unit, together with its assets (buildings, equipment, management system), and people who may be affected (employees, contractors, visitors). The essential questions are: what can go wrong, what is the worst that would happen if something did go wrong, and who would be affected?

An analysis may then be undertaken to match the likely risks and their consequences with the most likely targets to determine the upper range of plausible losses: life or health, property, production, revenue, reputation. This information is required to prioritize the risks, as before. Here the key questions are: what is the worst that can go wrong and how bad could it be? As before, this can be done qualitatively if the problem is simple or quantitatively if the issues are highly technical.

Once the major risks have been managed to the extent that they can be, there is still likely to be some risk left, some possibility of something bad happening. This is called the "residual risk" because it is what is left over after the control measures are put into place. The residual risk is managed as a financial liability. Risk management on the level of the company also includes managing financial aspects of the residual risk, most commonly through insurance.

The business model treats residual risk as an unwanted byproduct of production, with a (negative) market value (i.e. a price for getting rid of it). If it can be avoided altogether (as by substitution or isolation) or prevented, then no further management is needed. If not, it should be controlled down to a minimum risk level. The residual risk which is unavoidable is a liability that is carried into the future. To the extent possible, this liability is quantified, using "actuarial" (insurance-based) methods, and projected future losses can be funded or insured. The financial management of residual risk may involve transferring the risk to another party (as by taking out commercial insurance), sharing the risk (through deductibles and indemnifying loss on a partial basis), or assuming the risk (either managing it by self-insurance or accepting exposure with an unfunded liability).

The business approach is not fundamentally different from the technical approach to risk management. However, it applies financial measures to manage the residual risk. In large companies, this level of risk management is handled at a corporate level. This does not mean that a high residual risk is acceptable. Financial risk management is not a substitute for technical risk management which controls or reduces the hazard. It is only a practical approach for minimizing future losses and reducing the impact of a risk that cannot be reduced further.

Recommended Reading and Resources

Guidotti TL (2010) *The Praeger Handbook of Occupational and Environmental Medicine*. Santa Barbara CA, Praeger ABC-Clio. See Chapter 14 on "Hazard Control."

Hathaway GJ, Proctor NH (2004) *Proctor and Hughes' Chemical Hazards in the Workplace*. Hoboken NJ, Wiley-Interscience, 5th ed.

Hopwood D, Thompson S (2006) *Workplace Safety: A Guide for Small and Midsized Companies*. Hoboken NJ, John Wiley & Sons.

US National Institute of Occupational Safety and Health. Qualitative Risk Characterization and Management of Occupational Hazards: Control Banding (CB). Literature Review and Critical Analysis. Cincinnati OH, DHHS (NIOSH) Publication No. 2009-152, 2009.

22 Fitness for Duty

David G. Lukcso

Fitness-for-duty (FFD) evaluations are objective assessments of the health of applicants and employees in relation to specific jobs. They are an essential and common occupational health service, usually performed many times a day in an active primary-level service. The primary purpose of FFD evaluations is to provide an objective opinion, in which the employee is fairly evaluated for his or her ability to safely perform the essential tasks of a position, while ensuring that the individual will be able to perform the job as required by the employer without posing a safety concern for themselves or others. FFD evaluations therefore have three very explicit objectives:

1   To ensure that candidates or current employees can perform the tasks of the specific job for which they are applying or currently hold.
2   To assess whether they may be a hazard to themselves or others.
3   To identify any gap between requirements and abilities and identify accommodations that may eliminate the discrepancy.

The FFD evaluation also has a secondary benefit to the employer, because it objectively document's the applicant's health status at a specific point in time, at the beginning of employment or an assignment, providing a benchmark against which future health claims may be compared.

The FFD evaluation is performed by qualified occupational health professionals. Occupational health nurses often conduct the screening tests in preplacement evaluations, with the physician reviewing the results and conducting the physical examination. Highly sensitive evaluations from a legal or management standpoint, such as performance-related FFD evaluations (conducted when the employee's performance has deteriorated to determine if he or she is fit to continue in the job), may require considerable time and effort by an occupational physician. Whatever the procedure, however, it is critical that these evaluations not become a boring routine, dismissed as something to be gotten through quickly, or result in just "going through the motions." When health issues are missed or gotten wrong in FFD evaluations, there can be serious consequences and liability. To do them correctly and without missing important findings requires close attention, motivation, and an understanding of their purpose. This is why they should be done whenever possible by the occupational health service and generally not by primary care providers, who often minimize the implications of health conditions in their patients for work capacity, or by clinical specialists, for whom they are usually of little interest. These evaluations have a significant impact on applicants, employees and employers and must be performed with the same level of commitment and care as other medical services.

FFD evaluations must be conducted in compliance with the Rehabilitation Act of 1973, or the Americans with Disability Act (ADA; see Chapter 23) and in a manner consistent with law and professional codes of ethics (see Chapters 3 and 5.) Therefore, these evaluations must be applied universally and identically to all employees or applicants for any given position for which they are required and must be specific to the job requirements of the position in question.

The Genetic Information Nondiscrimination Act of 2008 (GINA) took effect on November 21, 2009. GINA prohibits the use of genetic information in making employment decisions and restricts employers from requesting genetic information. The family medical history is included in the definition of genetic information, therefore the occupational health professional must not request the family history of the applicant in a FFD evaluation.

The contents and findings of the evaluation must be kept completely confidential. Confidential medical information should never be disclosed to non-medical persons without the applicant's or employee's written approval, except as required by law (and, rarely, in clear cases of imminent harm). The FFD opinion is communicated to the employer, without disclosing any medical information, using medical terminology, or providing diagnosis. The employer only receives the final determination, which is expressed as fit, unfit, or fit subject to specific accommodations (specified):

- *Fit for duty* indicates that the applicant or employee is capable of performing the essential tasks of the position, but implies nothing more. It does not suggest or imply that the employee does or does not have any medical conditions, nor does it imply any indication about the likelihood of future work-related injuries or illness.
- *Unfit* indicates that the employee or applicant is not capable of safely performing the essential tasks of the position, even if provided reasonable accommodation. Any employee who is considered unfit must be fully informed of the medical findings. It is often beneficial to speak directly with the employer or the human resources department when an employee or applicant has been determined to be unfit for duty, to ensure that no accommodation is possible.
- *Fit subject to accommodation* indicates that the employee or applicant is capable of safely performing the essential tasks of the position if provided with a specific accommodation(s). The restriction may be qualified as temporary, when the impairment is expected to resolve, or may be qualified as permanent for individuals with an impairment that is not expected to improve (see Chapter 23, "Equal Access", including ADA). Accommodations may be workplace modifications, changes in work organization, reduced hours, or assistive devices.

Specific FFD Evaluations

Prior to conducting any FFD evaluation, the occupational health professional must have a job description that specifically delineates the essential tasks of the job against which to assess the abilities of the candidate. By assessing an individual's capabilities against the demands of specific tasks, the occupational health professional can provide a more objective and defensible assessment regarding FFD and can recommend reasonable accommodation for those applicants who have a disability but will be able to perform the essential tasks with some modification.

Box 22.1 lists the reasons for performing a FFD evaluation. Most FFD evaluations are based only on employer policy and follow procedures similar to preplacement, return to work,

Box 22.1 Reasons for Performing a FFD Evaluation

- Safety-sensitive positions (e.g. US Department of Transportation, weapon-carrying law enforcement officers, etc.).
- Periodic FFD evaluations are required by statute or company policy based on nature of position and risks to general public.
- When an employee has been offered a full- or part-time job subject to passing a relevant medical evaluation (preplacement).
- When an employee transfers to a position where the working conditions are significantly different (job transfer).
- When an employee is returning to work after a serious illness or injury and that person's ability to perform the original job is not known (return to work).
- When an employee has returned to work at a modified job and is still undergoing therapy, rehabilitation, or both.
- When the employee or employer identifies health reasons as the possible cause of failing job performance (performance-initiated review).

and performance related. However, many safety-sensitive positions have legal requirements and prescribed protocols for periodic FFD evaluations.

Safety-Sensitive Positions

Positions that include tasks, the mis-performance of which could place the general public at increased risk, are called "safety-sensitive" and normally are subject to periodic FFD evaluations. These evaluations are designed to protect both the individual worker and the public from harm.

There are many safety-sensitive jobs that require FFD evaluations as a legal mandate. Most of these are covered in the US by agencies of the US Department of Transportation (DOT), which requires drug testing as part of the evaluation. The more common of these are described in detail in the next section. Other safety-sensitive FFD evaluations may not be required by statute, (e.g. law enforcement officers and firefighters) but are based on minimizing risk to the general public as well as to the employee.

The content of the evaluations and the criteria against which the applicant or employee is evaluated vary considerably. For example, both US Federal Aviation Administration (FAA) and Transport Canada criteria for airline pilots are quite rigid and cover multiple body systems whereas the Federal Railroad Administration criteria for railroad engineers are less so, with only vision, hearing, and medication standards. Employees of the various agencies of the US DOT undergo periodic FFD evaluations with criteria codified by statute. Other safety-sensitive positions such as weapon-carrying law enforcement officers and firefighters undergo periodic FFD using various occupation-specific guidelines. An important example is the National Fire Protection Association (NFPA) Standard for Professional Qualification of Firefighters (NFPA 1001).

The most common safety-sensitive FFD evaluations performed by occupational health services are evaluations for commercial drivers (trucks and buses), followed by railroad engineers and merchant marine. It is recommended that health care providers receive training in performing these exams before attempting them (see Box 22.2 for DOT agencies with

Box 22.2 US Federal Agencies with Medical Standards for Civilian Employees

Federal Aviation Administration (FAA)
14 CFR Part 67
http://ecfr.gpoaccess.gov/cgi/t/text/text-idx?c=ecfr&tpl=/ecfrbrowse/Title14/14cfr67_main_02.tpl

Federal Motor Carrier Safety Administration (FMCSA)
49 CFR Part 391.41
http://ecfr.gpoaccess.gov/cgi/t/text/text-idx?c=ecfr&sid=dc032b301d49de31def7ff84722ceefd&rgn=div8&view=text&node=49:5.1.1.2.34.5.11.1&idno=49

Federal Rail Administration (FRA)
49 CFR Part 240.121
http://ecfr.gpoaccess.gov/cgi/t/text/text-idx?c=ecfr&sid=dc032b301d49de31def7ff84722ceefd&rgn=div8&view=text&node=49:4.1.1.1.34.2.125.12&idno=49

United States Coast Guard (USCG) for Merchant Marines
(NVIC) No. 04-08. *Physical Evaluation Guidelines for Merchant Mariner's Documents and Licenses.*
http://www.uscg.mil/nmc/medical/NVIC/NVIC_4_08_with_enclosures.pdf

medical standards). These evaluations are a serious responsibility. Failure to perform these evaluations correctly may create a liability for the health care provider and, more important, an unsafe situation for the public by allowing a safety-sensitive worker to operate unchecked.

The Federal Motor Carrier Safety Administration (FMSCA) covers drivers of commercial motor vehicles weighing 26,001 pounds or more, carrying 16 or more passengers including the driver, or transporting hazardous materials. The FMCSA requires medical certification at least every two years and has criteria for a number of conditions aimed at ensuring the driver maintains the ability to safely control the vehicle. For example, the driver must have visual acuity of at least 20/40 in each eye individually and binocularly and be able to distinguish red, green and amber, the colors of a traffic signal. Conditions with a significant risk for loss of consciousness and therefore loss of control of the vehicle are considered absolutely disqualifying, such as the diagnosis of epilepsy requiring treatment. Other significant conditions such as insulin-dependent diabetes mellitus, vision in only one eye, or loss of part of a limb may be certified if a waiver is obtained. Conditions that could affect safety but are under control, such as hypertension, diabetes, and cardiovascular disease, require FFD evaluations and certification on a yearly basis.

Similar provisions apply in Canada but without mandatory periodic drug testing. The competent authority for drivers is the Canadian Council of Motor Transport. Medical practitioners are required to report disabling conditions in drivers, including alcohol abuse (see Chapter 27) and poor vision, to the provincial licensing authority, which result in suspension of the license. There are also guidelines for non-commercial drivers developed by the Canadian Medical Association that are extensively used.

The Federal Aviation Administration (FAA) promulgates rules covering three classes of pilots: first class are passenger airline pilots, second class are commercial pilots, and third class are private pilots. The criteria for pilots vary by class, for example first and second class pilots must have visual acuity of 20/20 or better in each eye while the criteria for third class pilots allow for visual acuity of 20/40 or better in each eye. Physicians performing these evaluations must be certified by the FAA as Aviation Medical Examiners. Occupational and environmental (OEM) physicians interested in becoming an Aviation Medical Examiner must contact the FAA and request to be considered for training and certification. The FAA selects candidates based upon the location demands for aeromedical certification services. Canadian and international standards are similar.

Other positions covered by DOT regulations include railroad engineers (Federal Railroad Administration, FRA), and pipeline operators (Pipeline and Hazardous Materials Safety Administration, PHMSA). Mariners' medical certification is mandated by the US Coast Guard (USCG), which is now a part of the Department of Homeland Security.

Many other safety-sensitive FFD evaluations, such as those for weapon-carrying law enforcement officers, are performed against criteria based on guidelines, not regulations. Most police and firefighting functions are uniform or at least similar across most law enforcement agencies or fire services. However, each public safety agency should perform a job task analysis of the actual duties of its officers, as this guides FFD evaluations, identifies special or unusual requirements, and provides insight for administrative actions such as disability evaluation. Each agency, with the assistance of their occupational health provider, will determine the medical standards against which to evaluate their applicants and employees. For example, the American College of Occupational and Environmental Medicine (ACOEM) has produced a detailed *Guidance for the Medical Evaluation of Law Enforcement Officers*. Another example is NFPA 1582 standards for firefighters.

Private employers may use similar guidelines for their safety-sensitive personnel. Many of these have been developed by industry-sponsored associations. Offshore oil workers are subject to particularly rigorous medical standards that are broadly consistent across companies and have been developed by organizations such as the Canadian Association of Petroleum Producers and recently codified for international use by the Energy Institute (London).

Preplacement and Job Transfer Evaluations

Preplacement (sometimes "pre-placement") evaluations are conducted to determine the ability of an applicant to perform the essential tasks of the position for which they are being considered. When an employee moves from one position to another with job tasks that are different, most employers would benefit from performing what is essentially a new preplacement FFD evaluation, just as if the position were being filled with a non-employee applicant.

Promulgation of the ADA changed the nature of medical screening related to employment; it prohibits medical inquiry until after an offer of employment, it prohibits the employer from asking an applicant about the existence, nature, or severity of a disability, and it requires the medical evaluation to be tailored to the job and not to the applicant. Preplacement evaluations are often called "post-hire, contingent evaluations" because under the ADA they are performed after the decision has already been made to hire the individual based on their occupational characteristics but contingent on passing the FFD evaluation. The formulation of preplacement evaluations replaced the traditional "pre-employment" evaluation, in which candidates for a job were medically screened as part of the selection process, a system that discriminated against disabled applicants who could perform the job. Pre-employment evaluations effectively made the occupational health professional responsible for hiring decisions. Hiring should always be a management decision, not a medical one. Preplacement evaluations occur only after the employer has made an offer of employment (see Chapter 23).

Return to Work Evaluations

Not all employers conduct routine return-to-work (RTW) evaluations, although many require evaluation of returning workers when there is an unusual duration of absence or following a severe illness or injury. The goal of the RTW exam is to ensure that the employee has regained the ability to safely perform the essential functions of the position. Either premature or unduly delayed RTW may cause both employee and employer difficulties. Premature RTW raises the risk of reinjury and poor outcomes for employees, with concomitant expense for the employer and sometimes a risk to other workers. Unduly delayed RTW causes unnecessary costs to the employer, impedes reintegration of the worker into the work environment, and, if prolonged, may result in deconditioning and a less fit employee. A rigorous and timely evaluation can reduce over-all lost time and risk for the employee, and can improve productivity and reduce expenses for the employer.

Performance-Related Evaluations

Performance-related FFD evaluations are medical evaluations performed in response to observations of poor or deteriorating performance. If the supervisor, human resources department, or personnel officer has "a reasonable belief, based on objective evidence, that an employee is unable to perform an essential function or will pose a direct threat because of a medical condition" the Equal Employment Opportunity Commission (EEOC) has determined that the ADA permits an employer to request that medical information be provided to the occupational health service or to order a medical evaluation, but this evaluation must be strictly job related and consistent with business necessity.

Employers should have clear policies regarding performance review procedures, appropriate inquiry regarding performance, and when performance FFD evaluations can be suggested or requested. If they do not, they are placing themselves at risk for violation of legal protection under ADA and antidiscrimination laws (equal-employment opportunity, EEO, in the US; human rights in Canada).

The reason that a performance-related FFD evaluation is requested must be absolutely clear to the physician (physicians normally conduct these evaluations), the employee, and the employer, but often they are not (see Chapter 16). They usually involve employees who are facing disciplinary action or dismissal for cause as a result of failing job performance. If a valid health reason is found to be the cause of the failing performance, then no discipline or dismissal for cause should follow, and a reasonable plan for accommodation and management may be worked out. Separation may still be necessary if the employee cannot do the job, but the process is then less fraught and the employee is often eligible for separation benefits. If, however, no valid health reason is found for the performance problem, then discipline or dismissal for cause will proceed. These evaluations are the most sensitive of FFD evaluations and can easily run awry of the Rehabilitation Act or ADA, therefore great care must be taken.

Supervisors who notice a change in an employee's performance or attendance should discuss the performance or attendance issue with the employee and follow the employer's disciplinary policy. If in response the employee states that a medical condition is the cause of the performance or attendance issue, the employer may request that the employee undergo a FFD evaluation. These performance-related FFD evaluations are confined to the reported medical condition and its affect on job performance and safety. The performance-related FFD may result in a referral to employee assistance programs (EAP) (see Chapter 28). When appropriate, this allows for possible interventions and rehabilitation. A FFD evaluation is normally also performed when an employee resumes his or her normal duties after having been off work while being treated under the auspices of an EAP.

Unfortunately performance-related FFD evaluations are commonly abused by employers (see Chapter 16). As noted, the EEOC interprets the ADA as allowing an employer to request medical information (through the occupational health service) or to order a medical evaluation related to job performance. However, the EEOC is strict about business necessity and does not tolerate frivolous intrusion into an employee's medical information for the purpose of solving personnel problems. The EEOC has stated, "An employer cannot require a medical evaluation solely because an employee's behavior is annoying, inefficient, or otherwise unacceptable." Many performance-related FFD evaluations are requested by supervisors and human resource departments who have not been documenting performance issues and want to find a medical excuse to terminate a poorly performing employee. This situation most commonly arises when the supervisor is trying to avoid initiating a messy disciplinary action, when the grounds for dismissal are shaky, or when the real reason for dissatisfaction is a personality conflict or office politics. The occupational health service must resist the pressure to "find something, anything." The occupational health professional should not be used as an enforcer or terminator; the occupational health service is not there to do the work of supervisors or the human resources department. The occupational health professional should not participate in biased evaluations; doing so discredits oneself and undermines trust and confidence in the occupational health service.

Job Descriptions

An accurate determination of the individual's capability to perform the essential functions of the position requires a detailed description of the job conditions and requirements. Therefore prior to the performance of a FFD evaluation, the occupational health professional must be provided with and review an adequate job description which specifically delineates the essential tasks that make up the job. The occupational health professional then evaluates fitness for duty based upon a medical evaluation matched against the documented work requirements.

Performing these evaluations requires a clear understanding by the occupational health professional of the working conditions and activities of the specific job. Ideally, this comes in the form of detailed "health standards" formulated by a detailed "job analysis" based on documentation of ergonomic and physical requirements specific to the job. Such health standards are becoming more readily available for municipal government positions through the continuing work of MedTox, a firm that pioneered the derivation of health standards from detailed job analyses in the 1970s based on work in San Bernardino County, California. Likewise, the ACOEM and NFPA guidelines referred to above are based on job analyses. However, for most jobs, especially in the private sector, no such guidelines are available and detailed job analyses are either unavailable or not current.

More often, there is a more or less detailed job description formulated primarily for human resources and recruitment purposes. The occupational health provider must then infer the physical requirements of a job from the job description. An adequate job description includes a detailed description of job tasks, environmental conditions of work (outside, in a refrigerated room, etc.), hours of shift, all identified safety and health hazards, psychosocial demands of the job, and any special requirements of the position. The more familiar the occupational health provider is with common jobs in the economy, the more likely it is that the FFD process will be conducted accurately.

If the process of developing specific health standards is based on a clear understanding of actual working conditions, and the clinical opinion is in turn based on a medical evaluation that is relevant to those health standards, a proper FFD opinion can be made. Such an opinion is more likely to be viewed as fair and valid not only by the employee and the employer but also by concerned observers, such as union representatives, EEOC, proponents of human rights, legislators and other health professionals. Finally, the occupational health professional will be able to act ethically by protecting the patient's right to confidentiality of medical information, because only the outcome of the process will be revealed—the FFD assessment of fit, unfit, or fit with accommodation.

It is therefore in everyone's interest for the employer to conduct a formal job analysis whenever possible. General statements such as "must be able to lift 50 pounds" are not especially helpful. A more specific description of the task; "employee lifts 50 pound box from floor level to conveyor belt 36 inches above floor level 10 to 12 times per hour for entire 8 hour shift," will greatly assist the occupational health professional in making the final determination of an applicant's capabilities.

Recommended Reading and Resources

American College of Occupational and Environmental Medicine (ACOEM), *ACOEM Guidance for the Medical Evaluation of Law Enforcement Officers*. Available at: http://www.acoem.org/LEOGuidelines.aspx. Accessed December, 10 2011.

Demeter, SL, Andersson GBJ (2003) *Disability Evaluation*. 2nd ed. St. Louis MO, Mosby.

Equal Employment Opportunity Commission. *The Americans with Disabilities Act: A Primer for Small Business*. Available at: http://www.eeoc.gov/facts/adahandbook.html#medical. Accessed April 17, 2012.

Equal Employment Opportunity Commission. *The Americans with Disabilities Act: Applying Performance and Conduct Standards to Employees with Disabilities*. Available at: http://www.eeoc.gov/facts/performance-conduct.html. Accessed April 17, 2012.

Guidotti TL (2010) *The Praeger Handbook of Occupational and Environmental Medicine*. Santa Barbara CA, Praeger/ABC-Clio. See Chapter 18 on "Capacity for Work."

Hartenbaum N, Hegman K, Wood E (2010) *The DOT Medical Examination: A Guide to Commercial Driver's Medical Certification*. Beverly Farms MA, OEM Press, 5th ed.

MedTox. *Medical Guidelines*. Available at: http://www.med-tox.com/medstand.html. Accessed December 10, 2011.

National Fire Protection Association (NFPA) *NFPA 1582: Standard on Comprehensive Occupational Medical Program for Fire Departments*, 2007 ed.

Palmer KT, Cox RAF, Brown I (2007) *Fitness for Work: The Medical Aspects*. London and New York, Oxford University Press, 4th ed.

Rondinelli RD, ed. (2010) *Guides to the Evaluation of Permanent Impairment*. Chicago IL, American Medical Association, 6th ed.

Talmadge JB, Melhorn JM (2007) *A Physician's Guide to Return to Work*. Chicago IL, American Medical Association, 6th ed.

23 Equal Access

David G. Lukcso and M. Suzanne Arnold

Employers, employees, and even governments, all have roles to play in assisting people with disabilities to find appropriate jobs and to keep working. Employment should be seen as an important outcome of the treatment of illness and injury. The present need for accommodation in cases of physical or psychological disability is imperative and is anchored in legislation to ensure that this group of workers, already at risk, is not disproportionately disadvantaged.

People with disabilities have normally been included in society, not excluded, since history has been recorded. In earlier days, workers with disabilities retired into their families for care and support, contributed to the common good by assuming appropriate chores (baking, farming) and continued to be held in high esteem within their communities. The current era, post-industrialization, has often resulted in jobs and workplaces being unyielding to change, requiring the disabled worker to adapt to the workplace, change jobs, or leave work altogether, risking financial security and social role.. This usually meant changing to a lower-paying job and sometimes one that was out of sight, sheltered, and marginal to society.

The modern concept of disability provides the underpinning for the integration of disabled individuals into all aspects of society including the workplace. Critical to this evolution is to understand that the basic terms, "disability" and "impairment," although often used interchangeably, are distinct in meaning. Impairment is a medical concept identifying a change in one's health status resulting from illness or injury, a deviation from the norm of human body function. Disability, on the other hand, is a non-medical, vocational issue. The same impairment can result in different degrees of disability, depending on the specific work situation. For example, the partial amputation of the leg of a professional track star will leave that individual totally disabled for that occupation, but that same amputation will have less effect on an office worker. The impairment is the same but the work is different; and so therefore the disability is different. A worker's disability arises out of the interaction between the worker's impairment and the external requirements of the job— the degree of disability is the gap between what the worker can do and what the worker needs (or wants) to do.

Understanding the difference between impairment and disability is essential for occupational health professionals, company human resources personnel, risk managers, and disability management professionals. As the responsibility and accountability increases for returning impaired employees back to work, disability managers are now attempting to modify work or work environments for accommodative purposes in order to allow workers to return to work, thereby reducing and managing the level of disability.

The pivotal legislation for disability rights in the US is the Americans with Disabilities Act. The most common application of its provisions is in fitness-for-duty evaluations, which are discussed in detail in Chapter 22.

Legislation

Disability rights are rooted in American, Canadian, and British law and society. In 1973, as part of its enlarging emphasis on individual civil rights, the US Congress passed the Rehabilitation Act. This was followed by the Americans with Disabilities Act (ADA) in 1990 which changed the landscape at the time with respect to perceptions of disability and work capacity. Rulings from the US Supreme Court between 1990 and 2008 narrowed the definition of "disability" and increased the degree of impairment required for an individual to be covered under the ADA. In 2008 Congress passed the Americans with Disabilities Act Amendments Act (ADAAA) in which it clarified the intent of the ADA and expanded the definition of disability. The implementation of the ADA and ADAAA has been a pervasive influence in shaping what is perceived to be appropriate with respect to work requirements and individual capacity. Canada's long-standing antidiscrimination provisions are included in the Charter of Human Rights and Freedoms (which overrides other legislation), the Canadian Human Rights Act of 1997 (which applies to federally regulated enterprises), and the provincial human rights codes (which apply to everything else).

The Rehabilitation Act

Occupational health care providers who provide occupational medical services to agencies of the US Federal government, or employers who received Federal funding need to be knowledgeable about the Rehabilitation Act of 1973, which prohibits discrimination on the basis of disability by Federal agencies (section 501), Federal contractors (section 503), and recipients of Federal financial assistance (section 504), in programs receiving Federal financial assistance, in Federal employment and in Federal contracts.

The Americans with Disabilities Act

The ADA is a cornerstone of employment and occupational health legislation in the US (see Chapter 3) and is particularly important in fitness-for-duty evaluations (see Chapter 22).

Title I of the ADA, passed by the US Congress in 1990, prohibits private employers, state and local governments, employment agencies, and labor unions with 15 or more employees from discriminating against qualified individuals with disabilities in job application procedures, the hiring, advancement, or discharge of employees, employee compensation, job training and other terms, conditions, and privileges of employment. An individual is deemed to be a qualified individual covered under the Act if the individual, with or without accommodation, can perform the essential functions of the employment position for which he or she is being considered. Under the ADA, employers are required to make a "reasonable accommodation" to the "known disability" of a qualified applicant or employee if it would not impose an "undue hardship" on the operation of the employer's business.

An individual is considered to have a disability if he or she:

1   has a physical or mental impairment that substantially limits one or more major life activities

2   has a record of such an impairment
3   is regarded as having such impairment.

Based on the second and third level of the analysis, a person may be considered disabled even if no impairment actually exists. A person need only have a past history of impairment, or to be currently regarded by themselves and others as having an impairment if, as a result, that person experiences difficulty securing, retaining, or advancing in employment. For example, an applicant for an unarmed security position revealed that he was a recovering alcoholic. He informed the employer that he had been sober for over five years and continued to participate in Alcoholics Anonymous. The employer determined, based on the fear of relapse of his alcoholism, that the applicant did not meet the requirements of the position due to the public safety aspect of the position. Therefore he was considered to have a disability based on the criteria outlined in the ADA. The employer was then required to provide accommodation for the applicant's disability, which in this case was nothing more than providing the applicant the opportunity to perform the job.

Employees or applicants who have successfully completed a supervised drug or alcohol rehabilitation program, are currently participating in a supervised drug or alcohol rehabilitation program (see Chapter 28), and are no longer engaging in such use are considered to be individuals with a disability but not if they are currently using drugs or abusing alcohol. The ADA definition of disability does not include current drug and alcohol abuse; the ADA specifically excludes coverage of "any employee or applicant who is currently engaging in the illegal use of drugs." Additionally, the ADA allows employers to hold employees who engage in illegal use of drugs or who is a current alcoholic to the same qualification standards for employment or job performance and behavior as it holds other employees, regardless of whether the unsatisfactory performance or behavior is related to the drug use or alcoholism of the employee.

"Reasonable accommodation" means the changes and modifications that can be made in the structure of a job or in the manner in which a job is performed. Such accommodation may include modification of workplace facilities, modified work schedules, assistive devices, reassignments to vacant positions, or restructuring the job itself, and often can be done with little or no cost to the employer. Employers have access to assistance with developing and providing accommodation through the Job Accommodation Network (JAN) a service provided by the US Department of Labor's Office of Disability Employment Policy (ODEP).

"Undue hardship" is defined as actions requiring significant difficulty or expense to the employer. A number of factors are considered in this consideration, including the nature and cost of the accommodation, the overall financial resources of the employer, the number of persons employed at the facility, as well as several other factors. The determination of undue hardship is the responsibility of the employer, and outside the responsibility of the occupational health care provider.

The Americans with Disabilities Act Amendments Act (ADAAA)

The basic three-part definition of a disability has remained the same as originally contained in the ADA; however, the definition of "major life activities" and "substantially limits" have changed.

In the 2008 amendment Congress greatly expanded the definition of "major life activities" to include "the operation of a major bodily function, including but not limited to, functions of the immune system, normal cell growth, digestive, bowel, bladder, neurological, brain, respiratory, circulatory, endocrine, and reproductive functions."

Additionally, Congress significantly loosened the definition of "substantially limits" such that "an impairment that is episodic or in remission is a disability if it would substantially limit a major life activity when active" (as may occur in cases of mental health problems), and the determination of whether an impairment substantially limits a major life activity must be established without consideration for factors which positively impact the identified impairment, such as medication, medical supplies, equipment, or appliances.

Congress, by enacting the ADAAA, fulfilled its purpose. The revised definition of "disability," the change in the definition of "substantially limits" and the inclusion of "operations of major bodily function" in the description of major life activities ensures that most individuals who need it will meet the expanded definition of "disability." The question of whether an individual's impairment is a disability under the ADAAA does not require extensive analysis.

The Role of the Occupational Health Care Provider

The occupational health care provider has a general responsibility to ensure that the health and safety of the employee is protected and maintained. To do this effectively, the health care provider should have direct knowledge of the work environment in which the individual being assessed must function. The occupational health care provider must exercise independent medical judgment in conducting employment-related health assessments, regardless of the nature of the health care provider's relationship to the employer requesting the assessment. Additionally, the occupational health care provider must have a strong understanding of the ADA, the ADAAA, and the Rehabilitation Act, as every almost every evaluation of an applicant or employee in the US except for medical diagnosis and treatment is subject to these Acts.

In order to facilitate appropriate accommodation of disabled employees, the occupational health care provider should:

* keep current with evolving legislation and government policies
* develop and communicate a company policy on accommodation
* know the jobs and job requirements at the worksite
* conduct, or coordinate, a pre-placement assessment of the disabled worker, relevant to a specific job demands analysis
* know the various types of accommodation that are available and appropriate
* develop a team approach to accommodation.

Accommodation

The purpose of accommodation within an organization is to achieve equality in the workplace. It requires that the conditions of disadvantage in employment experienced by persons with disabilities be corrected to apply the principle that employment equity means more than treating persons in the same way; it also requires special measures and the accommodation of differences.

There are a number of resources which detail specific strategies to support workers returning to the job after an absence due to disability factors. A review and assessment of several options will allow the occupational health professional to consider the limitations of the worker, and the constraints of the workplace, and to choose strategies which will work in the best interests of all stakeholders and will provide a successful reintegration for the employee.

Box 23.1 lists various accommodations that can be considered in a given case.

A particularly valuable resource is JAN (http://askjan.org/, phone 800 526-7234), a free consultation service of the US Department of Labor. JAN is the leading authoritative source of expert and confidential guidance on workplace accommodations and disability employment issues. Working toward practical solutions that benefit both employer and employee, JAN helps people with disabilities enhance their employability, and shows employers how to capitalize on the value and talent that people with disabilities add to the workplace.

Box 23.1 Examples of Accommodations

Workplace Assistive Devices

- An assistive device, such as large screen for the vision impaired, an amplification system for the hearing impaired, or ergonomic tools that are easier to grasp and use (particularly scissors).
- Communications devices, such as Text Telephone (TTY) and Braille devices.
- Companion animals, specifically guide dogs for the blind, which would be considered an accommodation rather than a modification of a policy against pets at work because guide dogs are not pets.

Workplace Facilities Modifications

- Removing barriers to access to the workplace, such as providing reserved parking spaces for the disabled or use of a different entry point.
- Ensuring that there are no barriers to washrooms.
- Changing workspace configuration such as placing files in lower drawers for easier access to persons in wheelchairs.

Job Restructuring

- Rebalancing job assignments so that the person with the disability does those parts within their his or her capacity and other workers do the rest.
- Restructuring work organization so that medical and rehabilitation appointments can be kept without disruption, responsive leave policies, and modified work hours, if needed.
- Dedicated assistant or assistance with certain tasks: a sign-language interpreter for a worker who is deaf, a page-turner for someone who cannot use their hands, a travel assistant for required business trips, speech recognition and dictation software for a worker who cannot physically write, or computer reader for a worker who is blind.
- Adjustment of examinations and evaluations, as a worker with a cognitive impairment may require more time to finish a test (but a timed test might be acceptable for pre-placement screening if it addresses a specific work requirement, for example the need to read and act on messages rapidly, and it is given to all applicants).
- "Reassignment to a vacant position" is an accommodation mentioned in ADA that would apply to current employees.

Implementation of Accommodation Strategies

When considering an accommodation strategy for a disabled worker, the employer is generally not required to create a new position within the workplace in order to fulfill the organization's duty to accommodate. A job description which involves the employee doing some of the tasks of their original job, plus other unrelated duties, is not generally considered true accommodation. The ideal job position is one in which the disabled worker can perform all the essential demands of the position, with accommodation as needed. There is also no obligation to replace an employee in his or her current job in order to accommodate a disabled worker.

Many people view a disability in terms of a physical limitation (wheelchair), and, therefore, accommodations are often considered in physical terms (ramp). More and more frequently, workplaces are faced with the need to accommodate employees with mental illness or psychological problems. Workplaces, cultures, and jobs vary greatly, as do people with psychological issues. Workers with mental health challenges also have a wide range of talents, abilities and coping mechanisms, thereby supporting the need for case-by-case assessment. Furthermore, questions about applicability of the accommodation, effectiveness, individual preference, cost, and impact on the workplace must also be considered.

Steps in the Accommodation Process

The occupational health professionals within the workplace are well qualified to implement accommodation strategies for a disabled worker. The critical steps in the accommodation process are outlined as follows:

1   *Perform, or coordinate, a pre-placement health assessment of the disabled worker.* A health assessment/medical evaluation may only be performed after a job offer has been given to the employee (hence "pre-placement," not "pre-employment"). All medical information is confidential. No medical information may be gathered from the individual before a job offer has been received.
2   *Consider the employee's original job, and potential alternate jobs, and conduct a thorough physical and psychological job demands analysis of each position.* This can be done with the collaboration of department and line supervisors, as well as human resources personnel. Job demands data should include all essential job tasks, as well as physical and psychological requirements. Some common job functions and workplace activities may be limited by psychological disorders. Research indicates three major areas of functional limitations which can impact work performance: problems in social interactions and group functioning; difficulties concentrating long enough to complete required tasks; and challenges in coping with day-to-day stress.
3   *Involve all stakeholders in the process.* Stakeholders include: the disabled worker, the occupational health care professionals (occupational medical physician, occupational health nurse, and other occupational health professionals), the human resources department, and the department and line supervisors. The objective of gaining commitment from all stakeholders (worker, supervisor, disability case manager, and physician) for the accommodation and return-to-work process is to find solutions that exceed simple strategies of modified tasks and reduced workload. Accommodations that are sustainable are those that consider the triggers and stressors that negatively impact the returning worker. Each employee who is entering or reintegrating into the workplace with a disability will need to find solutions that address their particular situation.

4   *Decide what accommodation is needed.* Simple accommodations may include such things as ergonomic desks and chairs, telephone headsets, and specific parking spaces. More extensive accommodation could involve the design of wider corridors, ramps with handrails and appropriate grading, and accessible washrooms. Modifications for workers with mental health problems could include: flexible scheduling, job-sharing, more frequent work breaks, private work space to decrease distractions, and time away from work for required treatment, such as short-term leave for hospitalization and professional appointments. The issue of leave for hospitalizations may result in some challenges— differentiating between absences as a reasonable accommodation and absences as a performance issue may present a problem in certain workplaces, particularly amongst fellow workers who share the additional workload.

5   *Set job expectations.* The accommodation process for disabled workers must balance the responsibilities of the employer to accommodate the worker, with the worker's responsibility to perform and to be a contributing member of the workforce. The occupational health professional must take into account an understanding of the workplace environment, and consideration of the worker's motivation and current capabilities. Full commitment to the accommodation process must come from the employee. When the worker is fully engaged in the development of a work plan that allows him/her to accomplish the essential elements of the job, everyone benefits.

6   *Monitor the workplace accommodation opportunities.* The occupational health professional, with the collaboration of the supervisor, should monitor the disabled employee's progress to evaluate the effectiveness of the accommodation strategies and to make additional modifications to the job, as needed. Through this evaluation process the occupational health professional and the line supervisor can also assist the worker to adapt to the modified job.

The occupational health care provider also has the responsibility to inform the employer whether or not the individual has a health condition that represents a direct threat to the health or safety of others in the workplace or a disability that places the individual at high risk of suffering serious, adverse health consequences as a result of performing the functions of the job or exposure to the environment associated with the job. In identifying an individual as being a direct threat to others or at high risk of serious health consequences, *all* of the following should apply:

- the nature of the risk
- the severity of the risk
- the probability of the risk
- the scope of the risk.

The dual advocacy of the occupational health care provider—ensuring the health and safety of applicants and employees, while controlling risk for the employer/client—can be accomplished along with meeting society's goal of assuring equality of opportunity and economic self-sufficiency to people with disabilities. It requires a strong understanding of the ADAAA and Rehabilitation Act supported by the occupational health care provider's specialized knowledge of the workplace. Following the principles outlined in this chapter allows the occupational health care provider to enhance the process of recruiting and retaining qualified employees, and to assist individuals with disabilities achieve their personal goals and function effectively within society.

Outsourcing Disability Management Services

Accommodation and disability management services in the workplace can be provided by the occupational health department, in-house, or through a contracted external service provider. Each format has its advantages and limitations, which need to be considered and analyzed, based on individual organizational needs. Whatever arrangement is chosen, the sponsoring company must be actively involved in overseeing the accommodation/disability management program. Organizations can contract out services, but remain liable and accountable for the provision of those services. This means that organizations must plan strategically.

Among the reasons organizations may choose to look for an external provider for accommodation/disability management services, the following are commonly cited:

- Lack of specific expertise within the organization.
- Insufficient number of services required resulting from too few injured or disabled workers, making external contracting cost-effective.
- Expertise required to successfully achieve a cultural change within the workplace.
- Remote or geographically complex service requirements.
- Company goal of procuring leading-edge knowledge and skills in the evolving field of disability management.

Assessing and determining the qualifications for disability management practitioners is currently rather challenging. Disability management professionals come from a variety of backgrounds including but not limited to: nursing, occupational therapy, social work, and kinesiology. Many others do not have any "health professional" qualifications. Historically, knowledge and skills in accommodation strategies and disability management were learned on the job. There has been a movement in recent years to develop ongoing specialty education and credentials for disability managers. Currently there are more than 35,000 Certified Rehabilitation Counselors (CRC) in the US, and a significant, though fewer, number of Canadian Certified Rehabilitation Counselors (CCRC) in Canada. However, there are no standards of practice currently accepted universally within the practice arena for disability management professionals.

The occupational health department or the human resources department usually assumes responsibility for the process of assessment of organizational needs and evaluation of potential external service providers for accommodation and disability management.

The following steps are recommended in the search for the most appropriate external service provider:

- *Develop a disability management plan, to include the implementation of accommodation strategies for disabled workers.* An assessment of current needs, based on the analysis of site-specific illness, injury, and return-to-work data is imperative. An evaluation of the current process of accommodation should highlight gaps and identify areas where the need for improvement is most critical. The development of a framework on which to build the external service will enhance the chances of success.
- *Establish the service criteria.* The organization must be able to list the specific services required, describe the level of service quality anticipated, determine the professional qualifications and expertise required, and clarify communication links between the service provider and the organization.

- *Clarify performance measures.* Typical evaluation data would include:
  - −service response time
  - −service provision turn-around time
  - −satisfaction (surveys) of workers and business units
  - −compliance with legislation, regulations and policies
  - −short and long-term disability durations
  - −the percentage of disability cases that include modified work and accommodation strategies
  - −the average duration of disability cases
  - −the cost–benefit ratio per disability case.
- *Determine a budget and develop a pricing agreement.* This step would include a statement of the duration of the contract and the payment schedule. There should also be a clause to ensure that the contractor has adequate business insurance coverage.
- *Develop and distribute a Request for Proposals (RFP).* The RFP describes the organization, its core business, and its workers. It outlines the organizational needs, the service expectations and the accommodation/disability management plan. The RFP must frame questions to the bidder that will allow comparisons based on a predetermined set of criteria.
- *Analyze the RFP responses and select the external service provider that best "fits" the organization.* An interview with RFP finalists is often part of the selection process. Candidates make formal presentations to outline their strategies to meet the needs and expectations of the organization. As a matter of business courtesy, when the successful external service provider is selected, all bidders should receive a response letter, whether the bid is successful or not.
- *Quality assurance and continuous improvement strategies should be implemented.* Evaluation is based on previously determined performance measures.

The decision to use an external service provider for accommodation and disability management services should result from a well-documented and reliable process. Documentation of the process protects the employer in the case of a future dispute. The decision to continue using an external service provider should result from a comprehensive evaluation of outcomes and performance measures (see Chapter 17).

Recommended Reading and Resources

Dyck DG (2009) *Disability Management: Theory, Strategy and Industry Practice.* London, Butterworths.

Guidotti TL (2010) *The Praeger Handbook of Occupational and Environmental Medicine.* Santa Barbara CA, Praeger ABC-Clio. See Chapter 18 on "Capacity for Work."

Harder HG, Scott LR (2005) *Comprehensive Disability Management.* Philadelphia PA, Elsevier.

Office of the Law Revision Counsel, US House of Representatives. *29 USC. Sec. 791, TITLE 29 – Labor, Chapter 16 – Vocational Rehabilitation and Other Rehabilitation Services, Subchapter V – Rights and Advocacy: Sec. 791. Employment of Individuals with disabilities.* Available at: http://uscode.house.gov/uscode-cgi/fastweb.exe?getdoc+uscview+t29t32+360+0++(Handicap). Accessed October 19, 2011.

Office of the Law Revision Counsel, US House of Representatives. *42 USC Sec. 12101, TITLE 42 – The Public Health and Welfare, Chapter 126 – Equal Opportunity for Individuals with Disabilities.* Available at: http://uscode.house.gov/uscode-cgi/fastweb.exe?getdoc+uscview+t41t42+7459+0++%28%29%20%20A. Accessed October 19, 2011.

Shrey DE, Lacerte M (1995) *Principles and Practices of Disability Management in Industry.* Winter Park FL, GR Press.

Treasury Board of Canada. *Managing for Wellness – Disability Management Handbook for Managers in the Federal Public Service.* Available at: http://www.tbs-sct.gc.ca/hrh/wds-mst/disability-incapacite08-eng.asp#Toc279132220. Accessed October 19, 2011.

US Equal Employment Opportunity Commission. *The ADA: Your Responsibilities as an Employer.* Available at: http://www.eeoc.gov/employers/index.cfm . Accessed August 15, 2011.

US Equal Employment Opportunity Commission. *The Americans with Disabilities Act: A Primer for Small Business.* Available at: http://www.eeoc.gov/facts/adahandbook.html. Accessed August 15, 2011.

US Equal Employment Opportunity Commission. *Regulations to Implement the Equal Employment Provisions of the Americans with Disabilities Act.* Available at: http://www.federalregister.gov/articles/2011/03/25/2011-6056/regulations-to-implement-the-equal-employment-provisions-of-the-americans-with-disabilities-act-as. Accessed April 17, 2012.

24 Absence and Leave

Tee L. Guidotti

Perfect attendance is neither possible nor desirable in a workforce. Occupational health services support the management of absence by supervisors or human resources departments but the occupational health service is not and should never be directly responsible for managing absence. The role of the occupational health service is twofold: (1) to provide guidance on management of health issues that affect absence and the even greater problem of presenteeism (being at work but not fully engaged or capable of working due to illness or a health condition); and (2) to support the worker as well as the employer if, but only if, there is a medical issue involved. This is an area in which human resources departments often need help but often ask for it in inappropriate ways. In order to protect the occupational health service from inappropriate entanglement in absence problems, this chapter will go into some detail on issues that are actually within the domain of human resources.

Absence management has developed its own specialized vocabulary. Table 24.1 provides a glossary of terms used to describe time away from work and related issues. Absence is time away from work and is considered the opposite of "attendance." Absence can be preauthorized or unauthorized, scheduled or unscheduled. Absence may be due to sickness or injury ("sickness absence," which is usually unanticipated and not occupational), bereavement (unanticipated), need to care for a dependent person (variable), and personal needs (such as a dentist appointment or car repair; variable). "Leave" is preauthorized absence, for example pregnancy leave, jury duty, scheduled personal or dependent care time, time to recover from an injury or illness (short-term disability), or vacation. Partial absence occurs when employees arrive at work late, leave early, or take time out during the day. Workers' compensation cases are tracked separately and are not administratively counted as absence, although they contribute to a reduction in available workforce. Employer-initiated interruptions in work are never counted as absence.

Terminology is important in the human resources field as well because of the high risk of labor–management and employee–supervisor miscommunication. Occupational health professionals should be careful to use employment-related terms correctly, to avoid confusion and serious misunderstanding. "Furlough" is when employees are temporarily laid off work and not paid because they are not needed by the company, usually due to temporary interruption in supplies or funding. "Layoffs," or "redundancies" (more common in the UK), are temporary dismissals from work due to economic slowdown, corporate reorganization, or lack of business, and may be temporary or permanent. If permanent, layoffs are often called "riffs" (from "RIF," "reductions in force") and workers who are laid off are often said to have been given a "pink slip." "Firing" or "discharge" is generally understood as termination for cause. None of these terms should ever be confused with absence. Although in military usage

Table 24.1 Glossary of Terms Used in Tracking Absence and Leave

Term	Definition
Attendance	Showing up for work
Absence	Not being at work; opposite of "attendance"
Absenteeism	A pattern of repeated absence, implying possible abuse (use of the term is discouraged unless this implication is intended)
FMLA	Family and Medical Leave Act
Frequency	Number of spells of absence in a given year
Frequent absence	Frequent spells of absence above a certain criterion, e.g. ten days total in a 12-month period; the criterion is arbitrary
Leave	Absence from work that is authorized in advance
Long-term absence	Continuous periods of absence as defined by certain features, by >4 months, or multiple episodes of two or more weeks at a time in a 12-month period
LTD	Long-term disability; does not usually count as absence because worker is not expected to return to work in the near future, so tracked separately. Used when the worker will be off for an extended period of time for a non-occupational injury, and often also used when the worker will not be returning to work at all, in which case insurance benefits often hinge on clauses that specify whether the worker can do his or her usual job or any job
LTFR	Lost time frequency rate (how often employees are absent)
LTSR	Lost time severity rate (duration of absence of employees)
Presenteeism	Presence at work but functioning at low productivity
Severity	Duration of spells of absence, measured as lost time from work in days of absence in a given year
Short-term absence	Spells of absence of ≤ two weeks duration
STD	Short-term disability; counts as absence because worker is expected to return to work
Sick leave	An allocation of days of time off that can be taken by employees for sickness without special authorization
Sickness absence	Absence from work due to non-occupational illness or injury; episodes are called "spells"
Spells	Individual incidents of absence; same as "episodes"

a soldier or sailor may be relieved of duty by his or her replacement on watch, and a "relief pitcher" is commonly understood as a backup, in the civilian world the term "relieved" has become a euphemism for being fired. An occupational health professional might precipitate a serious incident by implying through careless terminology that a worker who was laid off got fired or that one who simply moved to a different position was "relieved of duty."

Absence from work is a difficult management problem for employers, since it reduces the available workforce, introduces uncertainty into the scheduling of work, and may delay a critical task that is that employee's responsibility. It is to the advantage of the employer to convert as much absence as possible, up to a practical limit, to scheduled, preauthorized leave, in order to minimize consequences for operations. That limit is reached when employees begin to feel compelled to come to work when ill and then do not work productively (a

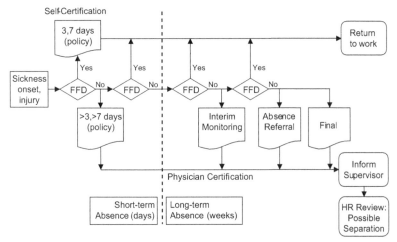

Figure 24.1 Management schema for the transition from short-term to long-term absence (FFD = fit for duty)

problem called "presenteeism") or may spread communicable disease, such as colds and flu, which results in uncontrolled absence of others in the workplace. Short-term absence and long-term absence are distinct management problems, each with separate issues and strategies. Figure 24.1 outlines a schema for managing absence as it progresses from short term to long term. Authorized leave is a separate issue, involving the Family and Medical Leave Act in the US.

Certification of time off work is customary in large employers in order to ensure that there was a valid reason for the absence and that the employee is fit to return to work. Certification involves a "note from the doctor," generally from the worker's personal or treating physician, for absences that last longer than three (sometimes as long as eight) days. It is generally not worth the expense of having supervisors or human resources departments review absences shorter than this. This practice is of limited value, however, because in the case of minor illnesses the physician usually has not seen the worker while he or she was acutely ill. Many primary care physicians confuse the validation function of certifying absence with certifying fitness to return to work (which implies that the physician has considered the implications of the illness for job duties, see Chapter 22) but they are distinct in purpose.

Unfortunately, there is often abuse of this system by personal physicians who give notes for unreasonably long periods under the circumstances (usually at the request of an employee who wants more time off). Another common problem is inappropriate return to work recommendations, usually recommending "light duty" without specifying what this means. It is often the duty of the occupational physician or nurse to contact the workers' personal physician in order to clarify just what was meant.

Absence Management

Absence is a major cost to employers. On the other hand, most absence problems can be managed with simple strategies, consistently applied, that are not onerous and that do not impugn the worker. The key point, however, is that the occupational health service should not be implementing these strategies. Personnel decisions are the responsibility of human resources managers, not the occupational health service.

Sometimes, the staff of the human resources department simply does not wish to or does not know how to handle the situation. Figure 24.1 provides a simple system for managing absence that can be proposed to an employer, but it must be implemented fairly and consistently—and by human resources.

Short-term Absence

Absence of a few days duration is an important cause of lost productivity, and is a very common precipitating cause of labor–management conflict and misunderstanding. High rates of absence and patterns of repeated absence (called "absenteeism") also trigger suspicions of abuse by employees. It does not help that the rate of sickness absence increases during major sporting events and near holidays, but insensitive management of sickness absence can make matters much worse by stoking resentment or by coercing employees to come to work sick, where they are unproductive and may spread communicable diseases such as colds and flu to other employees, making the absence and presenteeism problems worse.

There are relatively few published norms for absence in North America. This reflects the great variation in rates from employer to employer and the sensitivity of absence rates to so many factors: demographics of the workforce, seasonal trends, community health trends (such as influenza epidemics), health characteristics of the workforce (which in skilled occupations tends to be older than the community as a whole), and with the level of employment (salaried employees tend to be absent less often than wage employees, and professional and executive positions least). An absence rate of 4 percent per year is generally considered to be as low as can feasibly be achieved in any workforce without increasing presenteeism and losing productivity. An average number of five to ten days off work per employee is a more or less realistic expectation but varies widely among individuals and between employers. These statistics are not viable as targets, however, because of the high degree of inherent variability.

Older workers are absent less often but have a greater severity (total duration) of absence. Manual workers tend to take more time off than office workers and skilled labor, management and professionals much less, sometimes even to the point of coming to work while they are ill. Women tend to need more time off than men (even without taking pregnancy into account), in part because of gender roles involving family care and in part because women access health care more often than men. Even so, severity (total time off work) tends to be no greater for women than for men. Persons with chronic illnesses may or may not have frequent absences depending on how well their underlying condition is managed; often they have lower absence experience than other workers, especially if they are participating in wellness programs. These trends explain much of the absence phenomenon but it is against the law (for starters, the Americans with Disabilities Act and Equal Employment Opportunity Act) and unethical for employers to use individual characteristics to discriminate against workers in an effort to manage absence by selection.

Notwithstanding these known aspects of absence, generalizations are usually misleading and can be dangerous when setting personnel policies. Without question, the best guide for employers to expected future absence is past absence and every enterprise should use its own history as a baseline rather than attempt comparisons with other companies.

Attempts to control unauthorized absence often make matters worse. Human resources personnel often try to persuade management to take a more "objective" approach by treating the problem as one of validation and documentation. Because much of the total absence experience in industry is because of sickness and even more is claimed to be sickness, there is often a perception that absence is primarily a medical problem. It is not. Absence is a human

Box 24.1 Role of the Occupational Health Service in Absence Management

- prevention and disability management
- certification of illness during time off work, if beyond a certain threshold
- evaluation of fitness to return to work if the absence is prolonged and the job requires fitness-for-duty evaluation (but not otherwise)
- proposing accommodation for workers with disabilities
- referral for fitness for duty if employees show a pattern of absence or absenteeism suggesting an underlying illness (look for revealing patterns)
- employee assistance programs
- health promotion and wellness programs
- primary care at the worksite (to help the employee manage chronic illness)
- certific ation of early and safe return to work from occupational injuries or illness.

resources problem, and repeated absence or inability to do the job should be dealt with through personnel policies, with referral for performance-related fitness-for-duty evaluation if there is a sound reason to suspect a medical cause (see Chapter 22).

Although the occupational health service should never accept monitoring and control of absence as an operational responsibility, there are many ways by which the occupational health service can have a positive effect on the absence experience of an employee, to the mutual benefit of employer and worker. These include fitness-for-duty evaluations, proposing reasonable accommodation, wellness programs, providing supportive care on-site for employees with chronic conditions such as diabetes, certifying leave under the Family Medical Leave Act, and employee assistance. Box 24.1 lists ways in which the occupational health service can support optimal absence and attendance management. Anything else should be resisted.

It is very common for human resources departments to refer "problem" employees to the occupational health service, with the expectation that something wrong will be found that will allow the employee to be terminated on medical grounds (see Chapter 16). Sometimes there is inappropriate pressure to do so, to find anything that could be used an excuse for termination. The occupational health service must recognize, understand and resist this maneuver when it happens. It is a ploy to make the occupational health service take responsibility when human resources has failed to deal with the problem. It usually occurs when employers cannot easily fire an employee (for example, where there is a strong union or in a government agency), there is a high risk of legal action (as in cases of constructive dismissal that have not worked, or when the employee is perceived as a "troublemaker"), or where a serious mistake has been made by the human resources department. The most common mistakes are failure follow its own procedures or policies, performance evaluations that are incomplete or do not obviously justify termination, failure to plan or consider an "exit strategy" for an employee who should be terminated for cause, and an unwillingness to take responsibility for a decision.

Accepting of responsibility for absence monitoring and allowing control over retention to pass from the human resources department to the occupational health service converts a management problem into a medical and occupational health nightmare. When workers view the occupational health service as the means by which management reviews their attendance and singles them out for discipline, cooperation and goodwill promptly evaporate, and are seldom, if ever, regained. Medical judgments from the occupational health service will be viewed as untrustworthy and prejudicial to the worker. Having taken the occupational health service this far down the road, insensitive managers may then press even further for the physician to become a "team player" by siding with management on questionable policies or for violations of confidentiality.

The human resources department, on the other hand, has many tools that can be used to manage personnel issues: monitoring and tracking of trends, good policies, maintaining regular contact with absent employees, acknowledging good attendance records, flexible work organization (such as providing personal leave time), planning for major events (which can be turned into morale boosters), absence certification requirements, and "absence interviews." The latter are conferences between human resources officers and the employee, often involving the supervisor but never the occupational health service, to review the attendance record. This raises awareness on the part of the employee, allows underlying issues to be identified, and opens options for managing reasons for absence, which may result in referral for medical evaluation, but only if appropriate. If these fail, the human resources department can resort to disciplinary action in the case of abuse, consistent failure to notify the supervisor in a timely manner (usually 30 minutes after the start of the work day) without a good reason, or for a pattern (often five) of unexcused absences. If the attendance is simply inadequate, for whatever reason, the human resources department can always move to terminate on the basis of performance. Managing these issues is their job.

The frequency of spells, or identifiable episodes, of absence often reveals a pattern suggestive of a medical cause or a periodicity that could suggest a problem. For example, binge drinkers not uncommonly lose a day or so preceding or following weekends or holidays, so that their pattern of absence can be frequent but may not be severe in the numerical count of days of work lost. An individual with a severe, chronic illness may lose many days but on recovery may only have a few episodes of illness per year. Decline in the quality of work performed is also an important clue to the presence of hidden or insidious chronic illness, particularly depression.

Long-term Absence

Long-term absence is defined more by its characteristic features than by a particular time limit. It is almost always caused by a single condition, is continuous (rather than episodic, as is short-term absence), and lasts longer than a few weeks. It is less common than short-term absence but incurs greater costs. More important, however, are the issues that arise when an employee is off work for a prolonged period.

Employees who are off work for over a month have a low probability of ever returning to work. There are many reasons for this: deconditioning, loss of motivation and independence, loss of skills, anxiety or phobias over return to work, and depression, among others.

There are certain danger signs that cases with long-term absence are becoming serious management problems: human resources loses touch with the worker, active management by case managers peters out, the worker approaches retirement age, and people forget him or her in the course of turnover in human resources or in the worker's workplace. These are signs on the employer side that the worker is highly unlikely ever to return to work.

Box 24.2 is a protocol for the management of long-term absence. The occupational health service is not the unit to execute these steps but can sometimes be influential in persuading human resources to adopt such plans.

Box 24.2 A Protocol for Managing Long-term Absence

1. Stage 1
   1.1. Maintain regular contact with the employee.
   1.2. Monitor signs of recovery, active management of condition.
2. Stage 2
   2.1. After approximately four weeks, seek occupational health service evaluation.
3. Stage 3
   3.1. Establish a likely date of return.
   3.2. Assess fitness for duty just before that time.
   3.3. Ways that the employer can assist.
      3.3.1. Accommodation.
      3.3.2. Other support.
   3.4. Explain options for management action.
4. Stage 4
   4.1. Medical disability retirement.
   4.2. Termination may be an outcome. This is a decision for human resources.

Family and Medical Leave

In the US, the Family and Medical Leave Act of 1993 (FMLA), which was amended in 2008, sets the minimum allowable leave duration for employees of covered employers at 12 weeks, during which jobs are protected but the employee is not required to be paid. Employers who have more than 50 employees within 75 miles of each other (not necessarily in one place) are covered by the Act. Employees who qualify are those, with some exceptions, who have worked more than a year or a total of 1,250 hours (26 hours are granted for care of a family member in the Armed Forces) .

Under FMLA, the employer with must grant eligible employees up to 12 work weeks of unpaid leave during any 12-month period for the following purposes:

- birth and care of a newborn child
- care for a child
- placement with the employee of a son or daughter for adoption or foster care
- care of an immediate family member (spouse, child, or parent) with a serious medical condition
- medical leave when the employee is unable to work because of a serious health condition.

Employers are free to pay workers on FMLA leave voluntarily, to grant more leave, or to combine FMLA leave with sickness absence, short-term disability coverage, or other benefits. Paid annual leave or sick leave may run concurrently with FMLA, providing the employee with income, or FMLA may be taken as unpaid leave, preserving sick leave entitlements. FMLA leave may be taken as a block or as intermittent leave, for example for medical treatment. Employers are free to provide more generous policies and benefits, as long as the provisions of FMLA are complied with in full.

The occupational health service becomes involved when physicians are asked to review applications in order to certify that the medical reasons for taking leave are indeed serious, and to advise on future absences. For example, a worker asked his employer for four days of medical leave under FMLA for intraocular lens placement for simple vision correction, not for cataract. This procedure would not be covered by FMLA because the underlying problem is not a "serious medical condition." Under FMLA, the employer has the option of requiring the employee to get a second opinion from a physician of the employer's choosing, but cannot use a physician who "contracts" with or regularly provides care for the employer; a third, mutually agreed-upon physician can break the tie. That provision excludes many occupational and environmental physicians (OEM) physicians, who have relationships with employers. This is unfortunate because OEM physicians know about the workplace, possible accommodations, disability management, and fitness for duty, and could assist in reentry.

Recommended Reading and Resources

Absence as a topic in occupational health has been a particular "speciality" of the British. Many of the best resources and much of the most insightful thinking are to be found in UK titles.

Black C (2012) Sickness absence and musculoskeletal disorders. *Rheumatology* 51(2): 204–205.

Bolton T, Hughes S (2003) *Absence Management.* London, Spiro Press.

EEF and AXA. *Managing Sickness Absence: A Toolkit for Changing Workplace Culture and Improving Business Performance.* London, EEF, 2007. EEF is a federation of British companies in engineering and manufacturing. AXA is a financial services firm with an arm providing occupational health services directly in the UK. This publication is considered the state-of-the-art in absence management.

Guidotti TL (2010) *The Praeger Handbook on Occupational and Environmental Medicine.* Santa Barbara CA, Praeger ABC-Clio. See Chapter 18 on "Capacity to Work."

Hussey L, Turner S, Thorley K, McNamee R, Agius R (2012) Work-related sickness absence as reported by UK general practitioners. *Occup Med* (London); E-publication ahead of print. 62(2): 105–111.

MacDonald LAC (2001) *The Blackhall Guide to Managing Employee Absence.* London, Blackhall Publishing.

Occupational Health Advisory Group to the Electricity Industry. *The Role of Occupational Health in the Management of Absence Attributed to Sickness.* Guidance Note 1.2, 2008. Available at: http://www.energynetworks.org/modx/assets/files/electricity/she/occ_health/OHAG_guidance_notes/OHAG_1_2.pdf. Accessed January 5, 2011. Note that the UK Disability Discrimination Act of 1995 is similar to the US Americans with Disabilities Act.

Reed Group. MDGuidelines™. Westminster CO, The Reed Group. Information at: http://www.reedgroup.com/mdguidelines.htm. Accessed January 5, 2012.

UK Health and Safety Executive. *Working Together to Prevent Sickness Absence Becoming Job Loss.* 2010. Available at: http://www.hse.gov.uk/pubns/web02.pdf. Accessed January 5, 2012. Describes the use of the "fit note" in Britain and other measures to optimize absence.

US Department of Labor. Family and Medical Leave Act. Available at: http://www.dol.gov/whd/fmla/. Accessed January 5, 2012.

25 Independent Medical Evaluation

David G. Lukcso

An "independent medical evaluation" (IME) is an evaluation performed by a physician who reviews the circumstances of a case and provides a written opinion report regarding an individual subject but who does not provide care for that subject. The IME takes place outside of the physician–patient relationship and is characterized by a search for independent, objective judgment and opinion. The duty of the physician is to provide accurate, impartial, and complete information and an independent opinion solely to the party who requested the evaluation, not to provide a clinical consultation. The evaluating physician must not treat the subject of the evaluation and may never recruit the subject as a patient, but may, under limited circumstances and with approval, order limited additional tests without which the evaluation cannot be made.

The evaluating physician has no physician–patient relationship with the subject of an IME, and so that individual should never be called a "patient." The evaluating physician, in order to be truly independent, must not have any ongoing obligation as the treating physician or as a consultant in the care of the subject. The evaluating physician of course continues to have an ethical obligation to the subject to be impartial, fair, professional, and honest. There is no treating relationship. In the rare occasions when acute issues arise, the evaluating physician should share with the subject knowledge of any serious health condition that is uncovered of which the subject is unaware, and must manage any medical emergencies that may arise during the evaluation (see Chapter 3). Otherwise, the evaluating physician not only has no duty to assume medical care but would breach the duty of an IME if he or she attempted to do so.

The party (parties) who requests the evaluation is called the "client" or "referral source." The client is most commonly an attorney for the plaintiff or for the defense, a workers' compensation claimant or the insurance carrier, a motor vehicle or other insurance claimant or carrier, a disability evaluation agency, or a self-insured employer. Sometimes, an IME is requested from one physician by both sides in a dispute, a process known as an "agreed medical evaluation" in California, when that physician is trusted and considered objective by both parties. The evaluating physician, in order to be truly independent, must not have any ongoing obligation to or employment relationship with the referral source, in order to ensure against bias. The evaluating physician owes a responsibility to the client requesting the evaluation to be accurate, impartial, fair, honest, and complete within the context of what has been requested.

IMEs are performed for many purposes, most often to clarify unclear issues in the case, to confirm disputed facts, to determine if treatment was medically necessary, to assess causation of an injury or illness, to estimate how long a temporary impairment may continue, to determine if a subject has improved as much as they are likely to (which is called "maximum medical improvement" or being "at permanency," depending on the system), and to assess permanent impairment (see Chapter 26).

IMEs are used in different systems and settings, each of which has its own expectations, rules, and specialized vocabulary, including: parties to a legal action; state, provincial, or federal workers' compensation claims; Social Security Administration claims; motor vehicle insurance claims; short- and long-term disability evaluations; lawsuits; and return to work evaluations. The examination may be requested by many different representatives on behalf of clients, representing different degrees of expertise: claims adjustors, occupational health nurses, rehabilitation nurses, representatives of self-insured employers, and attorneys.

Increasingly, IMEs are arranged by professional IME scheduling services, who maintain rosters of suitable physicians for the most commonly used specialties (orthopedics, psychiatry, internal medicine, rehabilitation medicine, occupational medicine). Sources for physicians qualified to conduct IMEs are listed at the end of the chapter.

Most, but not all, IMEs will include a physical examination of the subject as well as a review of medical records. Some systems, confusingly, restrict the use of the acronym IME to mean "independent medical examination" by which nomenclature they mean an evaluation that includes a physical examination. Other organizations use one of several other terms such as "independent medical record review" or "peer review" to describe "chart-review" evaluations for which no physical exam is performed. In this text, and in common usage, the term IME will be used to describe independent medical evaluations either with or without physical exams because the process is otherwise the same.

An IME is performed and the report is generated by the evaluating physician in response to a request from the client, the referral source, which should specify the information that is to be obtained and the questions that the opinion should address. It is essential that sufficient information be obtained from the referral source to allow the IME physician to address all the necessary questions. It is the responsibility of the referral source to define the scope of the report; this will usually be done in the form of a letter, sometimes a standardized form. The referral source should identify the reason for the IME clearly and without ambiguity. For example, the physician will need to know whether an IME has been scheduled to address appropriate duration of care and medical necessity, determination of the subject's status with respect to maximum medical improvement, or to determine causation. Certain components will be the same regardless of the purpose (such as understanding the medical issues) but the emphasis placed on other components, such as prognosis, may be quite different. The referral source should always provide any specific questions they desire to be answered as this will allow the physician to obtain the data necessary to fully answer each area of inquiry and thereby provide the highest quality report. If it is not supplied in the referral letter, the IME physician should always request this information prior to performing the IME.

The basic components are the same or similar among IMEs but there is no "one size fits all" IME or report format. Which component is included in any particular IME and how it is presented is dictated by the purpose of the examination and the needs of the referral source. The basic components of an IME include:

1   the record review (which should be performed prior to the physical examination)
2   current history taken through interview
3   physical examination
4   the opinion report, including the responses to specific questions posed by the referral source.

Each of these areas is critical to providing the highest quality report and will be discussed in turn. Sometimes there is a section on "general causation" or the literature on the problem, but usually not.

Record Review

All relevant records should be sent to the IME physician prior to the scheduled exam, with ample time to review them in detail before the day of the IME. Some evaluating physicians review the record first and then write the report as a second step. Others begin a draft by writing the chronology as they go along, which is risky because a wrong assumption may not be corrected until the final record, and then the entire draft may have to be revised. Care must always be taken to prevent paraphrasing or incomplete quotes that may distort the intent and meaning of the original records.

At a minimum, medical records should cover the date of the onset of the condition in question until the present or the date that the condition resolved. For simple status exams, or questions of whether the individual can return to work, a simple review of the medical records and summary of treatment may be enough for the record review component. IMEs that are performed for more complex issues, such as questions of appropriateness and medical necessity of prior treatment or a question of diagnosis and causation, require a more in-depth review of the records. For assessing causation, medical records predating the onset of the condition are usually also required, in order to identify pre-existing conditions or to assess evidence for the presence of a condition that made the subject susceptible. Emergency room records are particularly valuable because they are the first report of an injury and are therefore more likely to be "uncontaminated." For conditions related to occupational exposures or the environment, exposure assessment may be an important part of the evaluation. The evaluating physician should be prepared to review safety data sheets of agents to which the individual was exposed, industrial hygiene monitoring reports providing documentation of exposure levels, or environmental sampling data. In matters involving a motor vehicle accident or incidents involving the responses of public safety personnel, important information may be obtained by reviewing the reports created by police, fire, emergency medical technicians, or hazardous materials (hazmat) team reports.

During the record review, the IME physician should document all the records received in a master list or check the records against a list that has been provided. If there are conspicuous gaps, the evaluating physician should determine if they could be important and is entitled to ask for more documentation. In a court case, this may mean that additional records have to be subpoenaed, but even if there is nothing noteworthy in them it is useful to know that and that there is no important information missing. Sometimes the omission of information from a record is revealing, for example if a visible or disabling condition is not mentioned when it would be expected. Small errors are common but entirely contradictory statements may be revealing.

The number of records and the depth of review will be dependent on the type of IME and the questions to be answered. Once all the records have been obtained, a thorough review of the records in chronological order should provide significant insight into how the incident/injury/illness occurred and how the subsequent medical injury or illness has developed and progressed. If it does not, supplementary information may often be found in depositions. The evaluating physician should always ask for any missing records that might alter the findings and conclusions. Unless the issue is one of medical liability, treatment records are seldom critical in causation cases and are of interest mostly for any additional details of prior history they might provide in passing.

If the record is evidence in a lawsuit or administrative legal action, it usually comes already paginated. The page numbers are stamped on each page of the record, in sequence, and is called a "Bates number" (named after the person who invented a sequential page stamping device). Referral to a document by Bates number is a convenient way of keeping track of relevant passages and guiding others to the information in the record. Providing a Bates number, or at a minimum the date and title or description of the report, also implies that the IME physician is not taking the information out of context, because any reader can find it quickly and see for themselves.

Missing records can be identified by looking for diagnostic studies that have been ordered but for which reports are missing. Medical notes may also indicate a referral to another medical provider or contain a consultation note that may be addressed to or indicate the name of the referring medical provider. The role of each treating professional should be clearly identified and tracked as the record is reviewed. Nursing and social-worker's notes from hospital emergency department and in-patient admissions will often list medical providers who have treated the individual.

It is essential to include a specific list of all the records reviewed in the final IME report, thereby eliminating any uncertainty regarding the source of the information on which the opinion and conclusions are based. It is often helpful as well to prepare a written chronology of the records to attach to the final IME report. Some evaluating physicians have the entire medical record transcribed into a searchable database which also allows for sorting entries based on subjective issues, physical findings, exposures, testing data, diagnoses, treatments, or other specific items. This, of course, is very expensive but may be necessary for complicated legal cases. Other evaluating physicians dictate a chronological summary including verbatim sections of text to be used as the basis for opinions and conclusions, and attach PDF copies of specific medical encounters as an appendix to the report. The final chronology must be a complete, accurate, and objective summary of the records.

Consent

When the subject arrives at the physician's office, the physician should introduce him- or herself to the individual as the evaluating physician who will be conducting the IME. The physician must review the IME process with the subject and ensure that he or she understands that the IME process is very different from most other physician encounters that the subject has experienced. It is essential, for the protection of all parties, that the IME physician verbally review each of the points with the subject and answer any questions the individual may have, taking as much time as necessary. Most physicians who frequently conduct IMEs have a consent form that contains all of the pertinent information for review and signature. This can be mailed to the subject ahead of the examination date, together with a questionnaire to facilitate the history and review of systems (see Exhibit 25.1 at the end of the chapter).

The evaluating physician must always:

1   *Advise the subject that the purpose of the independent medical examination is to evaluate a specific medical issue/incident.* An IME is not conducted as part of the subject's health care. There is no expectation of confidentiality and the information obtained will be shared with the referral source and may become available to all parties involved. No medical advice will be provided to the subject or recommendations for treatment. The physician will not render an opinion to the subject regarding the medical issue/incident. As this is not medical care, no doctor–patient relationship will be established. The subject should be informed that any medical questions that arise will need to be addressed with their treating health care provider. (The physician does have an obligation to inform the subject of any health-threatening conditions discovered during the examination. The subject should then be advised to seek appropriate medical attention and this should be documented in the record.)

2   *Advise the subject of the name of the referral source, that the assessment is being done at their request and that the IME report is their property, not the property of the patient or the provider.* The subject should be advised that if he or she wishes to obtain a copy of the IME report, they or their authorized representative (usually a lawyer) will need to request a copy from the referring source.

3   *Advise the subject that he or she may take a break at any time during the process.* Additionally, if they feel that the IME must be stopped because of health, discomfort, or any other reason, they should immediately notify the physician and the IME will be terminated. However, if the IME is terminated, it may affect their case or claim in ways the physician cannot and is not authorized to predict. The referral source will be notified of the reason that the IME was terminated.

4   *Finally, the IME physician should ask the subject if they have any questions and if they are willing to proceed with the IME.* A written consent form should be signed and dated by the individual undergoing the IME. Some physicians conducting an IME in cases involving high stakes for the parties (as in some highly visible lawsuits) or high risk (for example, when a subject has been litigious against health care providers in the past) require witnesses to sign to attest that the subject did so freely and after being given this notification.

Current History

Depending on the nature of the IME, physicians may have the subject complete a history form designed for the purpose. At a minimum, the history form should request the subject to provide a description of the incident/injury/illness that led to the current medical issues, along with a list of all symptoms associated with or ascribed to the medical issue and the names and addresses of all health care providers (physicians, chiropractors, physical therapists, etc.) involved in treating the symptoms, manifestations, complications, and impairments associated with the medical issues. Additionally, the history form may, depending on the nature of the IME, include past medical history, current medications, and occupational, environmental, social, and family histories (which in this context is not restricted in the US by the Genetic Information Nondiscrimination Act). Obtaining this information in the individual's own handwriting can be particularly useful, in the event of dispute or conflicting data reliability later.

The physician should then take a comprehensive history from the subject, organized chronologically from the date of the incident/injury/illness through the present. It is invaluable to hear the subject's description of the incident/injury/illness and subsequent treatment in the subject's own words. As is true in all of medicine, an accurate history is critical in determining the etiology of most medical conditions and most of the time the diagnosis can be determined based on history alone. It is equally valuable, in disputed cases, to hear the description of events from the subject him- or herself, in order to assess credibility and to clarify contradictory or obscure issues. The use of standardized, well-validated instruments for evaluation of pain and depression are especially helpful in making the IME more reliable and objective (see Box 25.1).

The history should be obtained systematically, in greater or lesser detail depending on the nature of the case, as outlined in Box 25.2.

Physical Examination

Before beginning the physical examination, the evaluating physician should again inform the subject that he or she may take a break at any time during the process and that if they feel that the IME must be stopped they should immediately notify the physician. The physician should

Box 25.1 Pain Scales, Pain Diagrams and Behavioral Inventories

These standardized instruments may improve the reliability and objectivity of an IME.

Borg's Perceived Exertion and Pain Scales
http://chestjournal.chestpubs.org/content/116/5/1208

Visual Analogue Scale (for pain)
http://www.ncbi.nlm.nih.gov/pubmed/11733293

Ransford Pain Diagram
http://www.ncbi.nlm.nih.gov/pubmed/2937007

Oswestry LBP Disability Questionnaire
http://www.ncbi.nlm.nih.gov/pmc/articles/PMC2647244/pdf/rcse9006-497.pdf
http://ajp.physiotherapy.asn.au/AJP/vol_51/4/AustJPhysiotherv51i4Clinimetrics.
pdf

Roland Morris Disability Questionnaire
http://www.rmdq.org/
http://www.rmdq.org/downloads/English%20(original).doc
http://www.ncbi.nlm.nih.gov/pubmed/6222487

SF-36 Questionnaire (a multipurpose short-form health and function survey)
http://www.ncbi.nlm.nih.gov/pubmed/11784274
http://www.shcdenver.com/LinkClick.aspx?fileticket=Ayz%2B5NDL6io%3D&tab
id=9523

McGill Pain Questionnaire
http://www.ncbi.nlm.nih.gov/pubmed/1235985
http://www.ama-cmeonline.com/pain_mgmt/pdf/mcgill.pdf
http://www.uofapain.med.ualberta.ca/ReadingDocuments/McGillPain
QuestRevisited2005.pdf

Beck Depression Inventory
http://www.ncbi.nlm.nih.gov/pubmed/21197365
http://thecenterforcreativeevolution.com/wp-content/sitefiles/~public/test-
beck%20depression%20inventory.pdf

Box 25.2 Content of a Standard IME Interview

Depending on the scope and complexity of the case, not all items may be necessary or additional items may be required.

1. Chief complaint
    1.1. Current symptoms related to the incident/injury/illness.
    1.2. Date of onset of each symptom.
    1.3. Current treatment regimen for each symptom, along with the name of the health care provider providing the treatment.
    1.4. Pain (should be described in detail: location, frequency, radiation, aggravating and alleviating factors).
    1.5. Factors that reliably exacerbate or aggravate the condition.
    1.6. Factors that reliably relieve or ameliorate the condition.
2. History of present injury/illness
    2.1. Describe in detail the incident/injury/illness: when it occurred, how it happened, and what happened to the subject (obtain as much detail as possible; a detailed description of the mechanism of injury is one of the most important aspects of causation analysis).
    2.2. Chronology of events from date of incident/injury/illness including:
        2.2.1. Onset of symptoms.
        2.2.2. Complete information on all treatment received: date of evaluations, names of providers, findings for all diagnostic testing performed, treatment, and the subject's response to the treatment provided. (The names of additional medical providers will often be discovered; their medical records can then be requested.)
    2.3. Complications and secondary effects, such as drug side effects or surgical misadventures.
3. Past Medical History
    3.1. Prior episodes of similar complaints or conditions should be documented in detail, including dates, mechanism of injury, treatment, and outcomes.
    3.2. All other conditions should be documented (none should be omitted but those that are clearly not relevant do not need to be described in detail).
    3.3. Conditions that may confer unusual susceptibility (such as allergies and asthma, or past injuries resulting in impairment).
4. 4. Occupational and Environmental History
    4.1. Chronology of employment with job duties should be noted. (This should be more extensive in workers' compensation matters, issues where exposures may be of importance in the etiology of the current condition, and in long-term disability determinations and planning for vocational rehabilitation.)
    4.2. Circumstances of exposure to an environmental, consumer, or a vocational hazard (most commonly in toxic tort litigation).
    4.3. Housing quality, structural integrity, and maintenance (most commonly in construction defect and mold cases).
5. Social and Family History
    5.1. History of tobacco, alcohol, and drug use.
    5.2. Family history of same or similar conditions to the subject's current condition (many illnesses are genetic, or heritable conditions, or reflect inherited states of susceptibility).

6. Current Status
  6.1. Comprehensive symptom inventory including whether the subject had similar or the same symptoms before the incident/injury/illness.
    6.1.1. Symptom inventory before and after the incident/injury/illness.
    6.1.2. If the individual had no symptoms before the incident/injury/illness it should be appropriately documented, being alert to predisposing, pre-existing conditions, and indications for treatment.
    6.1.3. Information obtained from the subject during the interview should be compared with data from the records and physical examination.
  6.2. Current functional status (include how the subject's current condition and symptoms are affecting activities of daily living, work, sports, hobbies, and social functioning).
  6.3. Pain diagrams, scales and/or behavioral inventories may be beneficial (see Box 25.1).

observe closely for signs of discomfort and ask whether a particular test or maneuver is painful. Allegations that a physician has harmed a subject during an examination are often used in contentious cases to disqualify an IME report.

Usually the only individuals present during the examination are the examinee, the examiner, and, when appropriate, a chaperone of the appropriate gender. The subject should be provided appropriate gowns or draping for modesty as necessary. The subject must always be treated with dignity and respect, as a matter of professionalism. Also, allegations of disrespect on the part of the physician are a significant source of complaints by subjects of IMEs and are often used in contentious cases to disqualify an IME report.

The physical exam should focus primarily, but not exclusively, on evaluation of the medical issues that led to the IME. The IME physical examination is a one-time examination for the purpose of objective documentation of the subject's medical and functional status and will not be repeated. Therefore, the examination is focused, detailed, and must be thoroughly and precisely documented. It usually takes much longer than a "normal" medical evaluation.

The examination notes should include the information outlined in Box 25.3, recorded in legible handwriting, in the event that notes are later subpoenaed. Standardized survey instruments and scales are very helpful in obtaining objective and reliable information and strengthen the IME (see Box 25.1).

Upon completion of the physical examination, subjects should be given the opportunity, through an open-ended question, to provide any additional information they believe to be pertinent to their current condition. The individual should then be thanked for their time and cooperation. The answer to the inevitable question of whether the subject will receive a copy of the report from the physician is no, as this report will be the property of the referral source.

The results of the physical examination must be precisely and objectively documented including all pertinent objective signs, both positive and negative, as well as any objective signs indicating a non-physiologic component. "Not thoroughly documenting the exam" is one of the ten biggest mistakes evaluating physicians make in writing their reports, according to Steven Babitsky, Esq., whose firm SEAK is a major trainer in the field. The examination section should include any objective data such as spirometry, radiographs, or other functional testing performed during the physical examination. The physical examination section should

Box 25.3 Content of a Standard IME Examination

Depending on the scope and complexity of the case, not all items may be necessary or additional items may be required.

1. Names of all persons present during the examination (including family member, advocate, chaperone, translator, other).
2. General appearance and behavior, including overall attitude (pleasant, hostile, cooperative, etc.).
   2.1. Grooming and appearance (evidence of personal neglect).
   2.2. Observations relevant to the individual's reliability and/or credibility.
   2.3. Responsiveness to queries.
3. General posture, gait, and the use of any ambulatory aids or braces.
   3.1. Objective difficulty with sitting, standing, walking, or changing positions (consistency with claimed injury).
   3.2. Consistency of gait (whether the subject's gait changes when they walk into the waiting room, walking toward the room where the IME is conducted, when exiting the building, and when getting into their vehicle, if this can be observed unobtrusively).
4. Vital signs, including height and weight as appropriate.
5. Detailed clinical examination of findings focusing on the medical issues that led to the IME, including all pertinent positive and negative findings, and any non-physiologic findings, to include as appropriate:
   5.1. Musculoskeletal examinations should include:
      5.1.1. Range of motion using goniometry if appropriate.
      5.1.2. Strength findings and whether weakness or abnormal functions are accompanied by objective evidence of atrophy.
      5.1.3. Sensory findings and whether the findings are consistent with anatomical distribution of nerves.
      5.1.4. Tenderness and muscle spasms.
      5.1.5. Atrophy.
   5.2. Pulmonary examination should include:
      5.2.1. Breathing rate.
      5.2.2. Visual inspection, chest shape, use of accessory muscles.
      5.2.3. Auscultation.
      5.2.4. Spirometry and or chest radiograph if preapproved by the referral source.
   5.3. Cardiovascular examination should include:
      5.3.1. Arterial pulse (rate and rhythm).
      5.3.2. Blood pressure.
      5.3.3. Palpation of chest wall documenting point of maximal impulse (PMI).
      5.3.4. Visual inspection of jugular venous pulse and lower extremity edema.
      5.3.5. Auscultation.
      5.3.6. Electrocardiogram, if preapproved by referral source.

5.4.   Neurological examination should include:
  5.4.1.   General observations: mood, affect, posture, and gait.
  5.4.2.   Mini-mental status.
  5.4.3.   Strength findings and whether weakness or abnormal functions are accompanied by objective evidence of atrophy.
  5.4.4.   Sensory findings and whether the findings are consistent with anatomical distribution of nerves.
  5.4.5.   Depression survey (if indicated) such as the Beck Depression Inventory (see Box 25.1).

not include any opinions or inconsistencies between the history and clinical exam; these items should be addressed in the opinion report.

Opinion Section

The opinion section is written later, after the subject has left, taking into account what has been learned from the record review and the examination. The IME report must be an objective, evidence-based evaluation. Therefore all opinions must be based on facts and should be supported by objective evidence in the medical record, physical examination, or reference to the current medical or scientific literature.

The data collected in the IME is used to identify and/or confirm diagnoses. The first component of the opinion section is a listing of all medical diagnoses specifying which are related to the incident/injury/illness, which are pre-existing but related, and which are unrelated. Any pre-existing diagnosis that was worsened by the incident/injury/illness should be noted. Subjective symptoms mentioned in the medical record or reported by the subject in interview that are not supported by objective findings should also be noted.

The content of the discussion section is dictated by the reason for the IME and the specific questions posed by the referral source. An IME scheduled to determine whether the subject is capable of returning to some level of work may only need to discuss current status and the subject's current physical and mental capabilities within the workplace. An IME to review past treatment and medical necessity, most often retrospective reviews, should discuss other treatment options and cite published practice or treatment guidelines as well as published disability duration guidelines.

Most other IMEs will require a more comprehensive discussion of the diagnoses, whether the subject has attained maximum medical improvement (see below), and causation analysis. The evaluating physician is asked to determine, to a reasonable medical certainty, whether there is a cause and effect relationship between the incident/injury/illness and the medical condition of the subject. All causal opinions must be fully explained and supported by objective data in the history and examination. In many states' workers' compensation system, the physician is also required to "apportion" (estimate the degree of contribution, as a percentage) that each factor or cause may have contributed to the outcome.

The basis for each diagnosis should be thoroughly discussed including history, physical examination, and diagnostic testing data to support or refute the diagnosis. It is sometimes appropriate in this section to explain the diagnoses/symptoms and sometimes the mechanisms of disease in lay terms in order to educate the reader, especially in a legal action.

The IME physician is often asked to determine if the individual is at maximum medical improvement (MMI), which is sometimes called "permanency." MMI is defined as occurring when the individual is not expected, as a result of medical intervention, to demonstrate a significant change in his or her objective findings, subjective complaints, or both. The determination that an individual is at MMI does not rule out the possibility that the subject may improve independently of treatment, nor that he or she will get worse with age. It simply means that he or she is not likely to get significantly better for the foreseeable future.

All inconsistencies in the data should be discussed; for example, if the history the subject has provided is not consistent with that contained in the medical records, a discussion of the reliability of the respective sources should be included. Most often the history provided at the time of the incident/injury/illness onset will be deemed more credible and given more weight in the analysis, especially in a court case. Inconsistencies between the symptoms described and the physical examination performed as well as the physical examinations contained in the medical record should be discussed. Additionally, if the IME physician's diagnoses differ from that of other medical providers, a discussion of the basis for the disagreement should be included, along with supporting data and citations from the current medical literature. If the apparent disagreement is strictly a matter of terminology and vocabulary, with no fundamental differences, this should be made clear.

Specific questions posed by the referral source must be answered as definitively as possible. This often includes the question of causation and sometimes calls for informed speculation, as whether one factor or another has impeded recovery.

The conclusion is a separate section, which is the final summation of the opinion and an expression of the confidence (in terms of certainty) of the physician in that opinion. If not properly worded, the strength and value of even a very thorough and comprehensive IME report can be greatly diminished. IME reports are often used as evidence in hearings or in court even when they were not written for this purpose, so it is imperative that the IME physician understand the law's perception of vocabulary in the IME report and the concept of certainty that applies.

The standard of certainty for causal association in the legal community is very different than that in medicine and science. In the legal community, the rule is "the weight of evidence" or "balance of probabilities." Causal association is accepted when the chance that the two events are causally related is greater than 50 percent, or "more likely than not." This is very different than the 95 percent probability that is used in medical and scientific research. Often the IME physician is asked to opine "within reasonable medical certainty" or "reasonable medical probability." These statements have essentially the same meaning within the legal community; they are understood to mean that the chance the two events are causally related is greater than 50 percent, or "more likely than not." Using terms such as "it could," "it appears," "I think," "I believe," or "possibly" implies less than a 50 percent probability and therefore signals that the IME physician is not sure. This diminishes the weight of the conclusion and if the IME report were written for a legal action it could be excluded from a legal proceeding.

IME Report

In order to provide the maximum value to all parties, the IME report should be well organized and written in a clear and concise manner for a non-medical reader. With the understanding that the IME report is often used as evidence in hearings and other legal proceedings, the IME physician should avoid using complex medical terminology, instead explaining the key issues so they are understandable to the lay reader. The conclusions should be to a level of greater than 50 percent or "more likely than not." There is no expectation of scientific certainty in an IME.

The exact format of the report will vary, depending on the reason for the IME and therefore the information to be included. The length and detail of the report should be consistent with the complexity of the medical issues that lead to the reason for the IME. Every report should include a specific listing of the medical records reviewed, the results of the physical examination and testing (if performed), the diagnoses, and opinion/conclusion supported by objective evidence from the medical records and physical examination. An IME to assess causation may require a review of the scientific literature on general causation before the opinion about specific causation in the case is presented. Some IME reports will be supported by citations from the current scientific and medical literature. Others may have an appended list of "documents relied upon." The opinion/conclusion section must address the specific questions asked by the referring source.

Above all else, the IME report must be fair, accurate, and unbiased; otherwise it will have no value.

Recommended Reading and Resources

American Board of Independent Medical Examiners (ABIME). *Guidelines of Conduct.* Available at: http://www.abime.org/node/21. Accessed August 17, 2011.

American College of Occupational and Environmental Medicine (ACOEM). *ACOEM Code of Ethics.* Available at: http://www.acoem.org/codeofconduct.aspx. Accessed August 17, 2011.

American College of Occupational and Environmental Medicine (ACOEM). *Occupational Medicine Practice Guidelines 3rd Edition.* Available at: http://www.acoem.org/practiceguidelines.aspx. Accessed August 18, 2011.

Babitsky S. *The 10 Biggest Mistakes Physicians Make in Writing their IME Reports.* Available at: http://www.seak.com/10biggestmistakesphysician.html. Accessed August 18, 2011.

Brigham CR, Babitsky S, Mangraviti JJ Jr. (1996) *The Independent Medical Evaluation Report: A Step-by-Step Guide with Models.* Falmouth MA, SEAK.

Guidotti TL, Rose SG (2001) *Science on the Witness Stand: Evaluating Scientific Evidence in Law, Adjudication, and Policy.* Beverly Farms MA, OEM Press.

Kleinfield, N.R. *A World of Hurt – Exams of Injured Workers Fuel Mutual Mistrust, The New York Times.* Available at: http://www.nytimes.com/2009/04/01/nyregion/01comp.html. Accessed August 17, 2011.

Official Disability Guidelines. *ODG Treatment 2011.* Available at: http://odg-disability.com/treatment.htm. Accessed August 17, 2011.

Official Disability Guidelines. *Official Disability Guidelines 2011.* Available at: http://odg-disability.com/duration.htm. Accessed August 17, 2011.

The Reed Group. *MD Guidelines.* Available at: http://www.reedgroup.com/mdguidelines.htm. Accessed August 17, 2011.

Sources for Physicians Qualified to Conduct IMEs

American Academy of Disability Evaluating Physicians: http://www.aadep.org/

American Board of Independent Medical Examiners (ABIME) http://www.abime.org/node/19

Canadian Society of Medical Examiners http://www.csme.org/

SEAK, Inc. http://www.imenet.com/search?search%5Bspecialty%5D=266&search%5Blocation%5D=21

There are many commercial enterprises managing IME referrals. Some have national networks and others focus on referrals to local physicians. Most will contact the physician on behalf of the client, schedule the appointment, convey the questions to be answered, deliver records, manage payment, remind and monitor attendance by the subject, and sometimes arrange transportation for the subject.

Exhibit 25.1 Consent form and expedited review of systems for IMEs

IMPORTANT NOTICE – PLEASE READ CAREFULLY

You have been referred for evaluation by Dr. [Insert Name], a medical doctor. This evaluation is what is called an "independent medical evaluation" (IME), which is performed for a specific purpose that does not involve treatment or on-going medical care. Dr. [Insert Name] is acting for the party who requested this evaluation in the first place, not on your behalf. The party who requested this evaluation is [Insert Name(s) of Client here] There is no patient – physician relationship created by this appointment, as there would be if you were seeing Dr. [Insert Name] as a consultant specialist. Dr. [Insert Name] will not become your regular doctor and is not serving as a consultant for treatment of your condition. Dr. [Insert Name] will take reasonable care to keep your medical information private but you are hereby informed that your records may be requested, subpoenaed, or produced to parties to a legal action involving your health. Please sign below if you wish to proceed with the evaluation. *The evaluation cannot go forward without your signature here.*

_____ Date:_____

I consent for Dr. [Insert Name] to share my information with the party who initiated this evaluation. *The evaluation cannot go forward without your signature here.*

_____ Date:_____

Party who initiated this evaluation: _____

Case or Claim to which this evaluation refers: _____

INTAKE QUESTIONNAIRE
Your full name:_____
Your address: _____ Phone:_____
_____ E-mail:_____
Male Female (Circle)   Marital status (current): Single Married (Circle)
Your date of birth: _____
Your current occupation: _____
Place of birth (country or state): _____
Have you traveled recently outside North America or Europe? If so, where:

_____
Please fill out the following medical information completely and accurately. If you are unsure, put a question mark next to the item and ask Dr. [Insert Name] at the time of the interview and examination.

Past Medical History

Please circle any condition or diagnosis that you have had in the past or have currently.

Heart disease	Pneumonia	IV drug use
Stroke	Tuberculosis	Psychiatric disorder
Cancer	Pleurisy	Substance abuse issues
Diabetes	Hay fever (allergies)	Anemia
Asthma	Sinusitis	Hepatitis
Emphysema	Eczema as a child	HIV/AIDS
Bronchitis	Goiter	Arthritis

Current Medications and Treatments

Please list the medicines or treatments that you are currently taking. Continue on reverse side of page if necessary.

Name of drug or device	Dose/How often	What for? (Your understanding.)

Are you allergic to anything you know of? Yes No (Circle)
If Yes, please list what you know you are allergic to, including drugs, animal dander, plants, mold, foods:

_____

_____

Do you or have you ever smoked cigarettes? No Yes (Circle) If yes:
Answer the following questions only if you have ever smoked.
Do you currently smoke? No Yes (Circle): Number of packs per day: _____
For how many years? _____years. How many packs, on average?: _____
Do/did you smoke pipes, cigars, or sheeshah (hookah)? No Yes (Circle)
Do you use / have you used oral tobacco products (snuff, snuss): No Yes

Family History

Please indicate blood relatives in your immediate family who have the following conditions:

	Father	Mother	Brother	Sister	Grand-mother*	Grand-father*
Heart disease						
Stroke						
High blood pressure						
Asthma						
Allergies						
Lung disease						
Cancer						

* Please mark M for "Mother's side" and F for "Father's side".

General Review of Systems

Please circle any symptoms that you are currently experiencing or have experienced since the onset of your problem (the reason for this evaluation).

General
Weight loss
Weight gain
Fatigue
Fever
Sweats
Chills
Loss of appetite

Skin
Rash
Sores
Itching
Easy bruising
Changes in nails/hair
Change in mole or growth

HEENT
Head
Headache
Head injury
Dizziness

Syncope (lightheaded)
Vertigo (spinning)

Eyes
Sudden change in vision
Double vision
Photophobia (light
bothers your eyes)
Blurry vision
Flashes of light or dark
spots in vision

Ears
Hearing loss
Discharge
Tinnitus (ringing)
Dizziness
Loss of balance

Nose/Sinuses
Runny nose
Stuffiness

Discharge
Nose bleeds
Frequent colds

Mouth/Throat
Sores
Hoarseness
Dry mouth

Neck
Pain
Swollen glands
Stiffness
Change in range of motion

Respiratory
Cough
Coughing phlegm
Coughing blood
Wheezing
Shortness of breath
Last chest x-ray

CV
Chest pain
Palpitations (irregular
heartbeats)
Loss of consciousness
Heart murmur
Fingers turn blue
Rheumatic Fever

GI
Abdominal pain
Difficulty/pain with
swallowing
Heartburn
Nausea
Vomiting
Vomiting blood
Black colored stools
Bloody stools
Hemorrhoids

GU
Difficulty/pain on
urination
Blood in urine
Excess urination

Endocrine
Hot/cold intolerance
Tremor
Excessive sweating
Change in voice
Increased food
consumption

MSK
Joint pain
Back pain
Swelling
Redness
Stiffness in morning

Neurologic
Loss of consciousness
Dizziness
Seizures
Room spinning around
Change in memory

Psychiatric
Anxiety
Depression
Panic episodes
Suicidal thoughts

Women's Health
Number of pregnancies
Number of live births
Menstrual irregularity

Note: Because of the nature of Dr. [Insert Name]'s practice, it is rarely necessary for us to ask about breast, genital or sexual health. If you have experienced problems with any of the following, and believe that it is relevant to the condition for which Dr. [Insert Name] is evaluating you, please tell him at the time of the examination:

Breasts: Lumps, discharges from nipple, pain, tenderness, size change. Sexual History: Increased/decreased sexual desire (libido); level of satisfaction, orgasmic/potency problems or ejaculatory problems, frequency. Negative impact of illness on sexual functioning. Problems with the use of contraceptives. Number of lifetime partners, same sex partners, use of condoms, STD history including HIV/Hepatitis B. Female Reproductive System: Menarche, menses, frequency, duration, amount, dysmenorrheal (difficult periods); menopause, age, symptoms, contraception; irregular periods; vaginal discharge, pregnancy complications, abnormal vaginal bleeding, infertility. Male Reproductive System: Erectile disorder, inability to achieve orgasm or ejaculate, discharge, pain in the scrotum.

26 Impairment Assessment

David G. Lukcso

The physician practicing occupational medicine is often tasked with performing impairment assessments or disability evaluations. Such exams are requested by many clients, including attorneys, case managers, insurance representatives, and agencies, who work in many different venues: compensation benefits, including workers' compensation, Social Security Administration disability, state temporary disability, long-term disability insurance, self-insured employers, and personal injury insurance. In a few jurisdictions the same system used to evaluate occupational impairment is used to adjudicate claims arising from motor vehicle accidents. They are a very common reason for requesting "independent medical evaluations" (IMEs), as discussed in Chapter 25. They are usually not requested by patients or injured workers themselves, but sometimes their lawyers or the workers themselves will have them done in anticipation of a future claim or to counter an adverse or unfavourable rating by another expert.

Impairment assessments are often complicated but it is essential that they be performed consistently and follow recognized standards. There is a well-developed system for assessing impairment from occupational injuries and illness that must be mastered. To minimize mistakes and professional liability, training in impairment assessment and the use of standard references, such as the American Medical Association's *AMA Guides to the Evaluation of Permanent Impairment* (referred to as the *AMA Guides* or simply the *Guides*, always in the plural among knowledgeable physicians who do this work), is essential for physicians who plan to engage in this practice. (See the end of chapter for selected resources.)

At the same time, there are variations among the systems that depend on impairment assessment. Depending on the venue, the terminology and procedures of the exam, report, and the rating system may be different. The most common is that different states require different editions of the *AMA Guides* to be used in workers' compensation. The physician who conducts impairment assessments must become familiar with the requirements of the specific venue or system for which the evaluation is conducted.

Definitions

It is not uncommon for the client who requests such evaluations to use the terms "impairment assessment" and "disability assessment" interchangeably, and different systems do use the same words differently. To ensure that the results of the assessment are consistent with the requestor's needs, precise understanding of the terminology is essential because impairment and disability are actually not the same at all.

In an impairment assessment, the evaluator is charged with defining an individual's health status in comparison to normal physiology or to the individuals' prior health status, and quantifying the amount of change. The examiner determines what the individual cannot do and measures the deviation from normal or from the individual's pre-existing baseline, if the individual already had an impairment. In practice, impairment is measured against normal physiology by the use of guidelines, of which the most important for workers' compensation are outlined in the *AMA Guides*. The most important guidelines for impairment that is not related to workplace injury are provided in *Disability Evaluation under Social Security* (the "Blue Book"). (Canada Pension Plan has no similar resource because evaluations are done by the program.)

The *Guides* define impairment as "an alteration of an individual's heath status, a deviation from normal in a body part or organ system and its functioning that interferes with an individual's activities of daily living." This is consistent with the World Health Organization's (WHO) definition: "An impairment is a problem in body function or structure." The Social Security Administration (SSA) further defines impairment in its "Blue Book": "A medically determinable physical or mental impairment is an impairment that results from anatomical, physiological, or psychological abnormalities, which can be shown by medically acceptable clinical and laboratory diagnostic techniques. A physical or mental impairment must be established by medical evidence consisting of signs, symptoms, and laboratory findings—not only by the individual's statement of symptoms."

Impairment assessments provide quantification of the difference between the individual and the normal as defined by the guidelines or from the examinee's baseline (if known). In many venues this quantification is then translated into an "impairment percentage" or rating. The *Guides* describe the rating as "an informed estimate of the degree to which an individual's capacity to carry out daily activities has been diminished." The purpose of the rating is usually to determine a financial remuneration by a third party to an individual who suffered a measurable loss. The third party may be an employer in the case of workers' compensation claims, an entity that caused the impairment as in personal injury, or an insurance carrier, such as the SSA and long-term disability carriers.

Disability is a determination based in part on the impairment assessment that interprets the implications of the impairment for participation in activities of daily living and work. Disability evaluations require the conceptual understanding that disability is the gap between what the individual can do and what the individual needs or wants to do, and is a complex analysis of how an impairment affects activities of daily living, social functioning, play, enjoyment of life, and work life.

The *Guides* define disability as "an alteration of an individual's capacity to meet personal, social, or occupational demands, or statutory or regulatory requirements, because of an impairment. Disability refers to an activity or task the individual cannot accomplish. A disability arises out of the interaction between impairment and external requirements." The WHO defines disability as "a complex phenomenon, reflecting an interaction between features of a person's body and features of the society in which he or she lives." The evaluating physician must ensure that he or she understands what is actually meant by these terms by the client requesting the evaluation.

Impairment Assessments

The evaluating physician must know which rating system is required to be used in the matter's specific venue and must become familiar, if he or she is not already, with that system. The various venues also have varying rules about the content of the report, as well as the required rating system.

Workers' Compensation

Impairment assessments for workers' compensation (see Chapter 2) are the most common type of impairment assessment that a physician practicing occupational medicine is called on to perform. Impairment assessments in workers' compensation are based on a deviation, loss, or loss of function of use of any body structure or body function.

The physician practicing occupational medicine who performs impairment assessments must determine which version of the *Guides* is used in the jurisdiction, as not all use the most current version, and must master the several variations that are used in some states. At present, 16 states mandate the sixth edition (2007), which is the latest as of this writing: Alaska, Arizona, Connecticut, Illinois, Indiana, Louisiana, Massachusetts, Mississippi, Montana, New Mexico, North Dakota, Oklahoma, Pennsylvania, Rhode Island, Tennessee, and Wyoming. Connecticut, the District of Columbia, Indiana, and Massachusetts do not stipulate which edition of the *Guides* to use and only specify use of the latest available edition. Although the fifth edition (2000) was not well received when it appeared, 11 states mandate this edition: Delaware, Georgia, Hawaii, Idaho, Iowa, Kentucky, Nevada, New Hampshire, Ohio, Vermont, and Washington. In part because the fifth edition did not win general acceptance, the fourth edition (1993) is still mandated in eight states: Alabama, Arkansas, Kansas, Maine, Maryland, South Dakota, Texas, and West Virginia. (Maryland also requires additional consideration of "five factors": pain, weakness, atrophy, loss of function, loss of endurance.) Colorado still uses the third edition, in a revised version (published in 1990). Seven states use their own state specific guidelines: Florida, Minnesota, New York, North Carolina, Oregon, Utah, and Wisconsin; most recently, California adopted its own system on a temporary basis. Six states do not mandate any specific guideline at all: Michigan, Missouri, Nebraska, New Jersey, South Carolina, and Virginia. The Utah state system has received much attention because it was developed to decrease inter-rater variability. The *Guides* are also used under the Federal Employees Compensation Act, and the Longshore and Harbor Workers' Compensation Act, which either mandate or recommend using the *Guides* (see Chapter 2). Canadian provinces and Australian states also use the *Guides* in workers' compensation claims.

The *Guides* describe impairment ratings as a "consensus-derived percentage estimate" of loss of capacity, reflecting severity for a given health condition, and the degree of associated limitations in terms of activities of daily living (ADLs) rather than work activity. The same impairment in two individuals will more uniformly affect ADLs, yet may cause very different levels of disability in the two individuals with different jobs.

Disability is therefore a complex issue that takes more factors into account than impairment. The *Guides* state explicitly that they are "not intended to be used for direct estimates of work participation restrictions." Interpreting what an impairment rating means in terms of disability for an individual is not the task of the examining physician. In theory and in practice, it is the task of the agency or insurance carrier that receives the impairment rating to determine what a given impairment rating means for that individual, based on their usual occupation, what they are trained for or the prospect for retraining, what jobs they can still do, and what jobs are available in the community. For example, the loss of use of an index finger may totally disable a weapon-carrying law enforcement officer or a surgeon or a violinist, but may have only minimal effect on a lawyer, an internist, or a general laborer. The *Guides* are intended for "impairment assessment ... [which] is a first step toward disability assessment." In practice most states' workers' compensation systems treat impairment ratings as direct measures of disability for purposes of matching with job requirements but not for calculating benefits.

Impairment ratings are only determined after the injured worker has reached maximum medical improvement (MMI) or has become permanent and stationary. The *Guides* indicate that the physician practicing occupational medicine performing the assessment must first determine that the medical condition is static and well stabilized. An individual is determined to be at MMI when "further formal medical or surgical intervention cannot be expected to improve the underlying impairment." The term "at permanency" is often used interchangeably and is regarded as when recovery or deterioration is not anticipated despite medical treatment. Additionally, the *Guides* do not permit the rating of future impairment. The rating is strictly based on the status of the injured worker at the time of assessment, given that the individual is at MMI.

The *Guides'* approach to impairment assessment is based on impairment of the "whole person," which is the degree to which a person's overall capacity to function is limited. An individual with no loss, no functional deficit, and no limitations on ADLs would be rated at 0 percent impairment of the whole person. A person who is completely impaired and cannot perform ADLs for themselves due to their impairment would be at 100 percent. Notwithstanding frequent allusions in the casual literature to the contrary, this rating does not imply that they are in a coma or dead; it simply means that they cannot function independently at home or at work. No impairment may exceed 100 percent impairment of the whole person.

The *Guides* provide impairment ratings based solely on whole-person impairment for most organ systems. However, the musculoskeletal system and hearing system ratings provide regional impairment ratings (for example, percent impairment of use of the upper extremity) that must then be converted to impairment of the whole person, which is done using relational value charts in the respective chapters.

Certain types of cases are particularly difficult. Claims for psychological illness or impairment as a result of work-related psychogenic stress (which are called "mental-mental" claims in the jargon of workers' compensation) are hard to rate in the absence of objective criteria and it is hard to prove causation, and so insurance carriers tend to be resistant to such claims. Claims involving chronic pain, sometimes with a question of opioid dependency, are notoriously difficult to rate, despite increasing attention to subjective symptoms and pain in later editions of the *AMA Guides*. Some states allow ratings to be enhanced by the addition of percentage points for other factors. Maryland, for example, allows additional points to be added to the rating for each of the "Maryland five factors", which are pain, weakness, atrophy, loss of function, and loss of endurance. Where this is allowed, the enhanced ratings may be given quite freely by some practitioners and not by others.

Many injuries and illnesses affect more than one body part or organ system. The process outlined in the *Guides* requires determination of impairment for each specific body part or organ system. Since no individual may have more than 100 percent impairment of the whole person and some impairments overlap in functional capacity, the specific impairments for each body part are not simply added together. Rather, they are "combined," using the principle that a second, third, and subsequent impairment rating applies to the residual functional capacity of the person after earlier impairments are taken into account, not to the original 100 percent capacity.

In the *Guides*, multiple impairments are combined using a combined values chart provided in the book, beginning with the largest impairment and successively incorporating the next largest impairments into the combined value. For example, if an individual has two separate impairment ratings of 30 percent and 25 percent, he or she is not really 55 percent impaired but rather 48 percent impaired. The process begins with the 30 percent impairment, which leaves only 70 percent of the individual unimpaired (residual functional capacity after the first impairment) and available to be affected by the second impairment. Therefore the second impairment rated at 25 percent affects only 70 percent of the person, resulting in 17.5 percent additional impairment. When the 30 percent and 17.5 percent impairment ratings are added, the individual has a 47.5 percent impairment of the whole person. The *Guides* recommend rounding to whole numbers, therefore the individual has a 48 percent impairment of the whole person. The same number can be more conveniently obtained from the combined values table in the *Guides* by finding the first impairment rating in the row and the second in the column in the table at the back of the book, without making this calculation.

Workers can and do have multiple injuries and illnesses over a working lifetime. Subsequently, evaluating physicians are often asked to perform an impairment assessment of a workers' body or an organ system that was previously impaired, usually a musculoskeletal re-injury. In performing these impairment assessments it is critical to determine if the second injury or illness has caused any permanent decrement to the function of the body or organ system.

"Exacerbation" or "flare-up" are terms used to imply a temporary worsening of condition which subsequently returns to baseline. An injury or illness that does not cause a permanent decrement in function does not qualify for an additional impairment rating. For example, a worker who has asthma and suffers an exposure that precipitates an acute asthma attack but returns to baseline after treatment has suffered an exacerbation. Since there is no permanent worsening of the condition the individual would not qualify for an additional impairment rating.

A worker whose condition is permanently worsened by a second injury or illness which makes their existing condition permanently worse is considered to have sustained an "aggravation" and would therefore qualify for a new additional impairment rating. For example, a worker with a shoulder impairment characterized by limited range of motion who re-injures the shoulder ultimately experiences further restriction on his or her range of motion. The individual is now at a new reduced level of function and has sustained a second ratable impairment, which is calculated as the difference between the final whole-person impairment rating and the baseline impairment rating before the second injury.

The evaluating physician may also be asked to apportion (allocate) impairment to either specific injuries or to various causes of a single injury or illness. In apportioning impairment the physician may have to determine the impairment rating of the pre-existing impairment as well as determining the impairment rating at the current point in time. The difference in the two impairment ratings is allocated to the intervening injury or illness. In the case of a single injury or illness with multiple causes the physician is often required to estimate the amount of the resulting total impairment related to each, a process known as "apportionment of impairment." (Unlike apportionment of causation, as discussed in Chapter 25, apportionment of impairment can be quite accurate.)

Upon completion of the analysis, the evaluating physician must compile the information and final impairment rating into a report. For jurisdictions using the *Guides*, sample impairment assessment reports are provided in the *Guides*. In other jurisdictions, the evaluating physician must ensure that he or she knows the specific report requirements, if any. (For a discussion of record review, consent, exam performance, and report content in independent medical evaluations see Chapter 25.)

Social Security Administration

SSA administers two programs that provide benefits based on disability: the Social Security Disability Insurance (SSDI) program for disabled individuals and dependents who paid into the trust fund through employment (Title II) and the Supplemental Security Income (SSI) program for disabled individuals (including children under age 18) who are disabled and have limited income and resources (Title XVI).

The rules for determining whether an individual's impairments are disabling take into account age, education level, work history, work skills training prospects, and job markets. The SSA defines disability "as the inability to engage in any substantial gainful activity by reason of any medically determinable physical or mental impairment(s) which can be expected to result in death or which has lasted or can be expected to last for a continuous period of not less than 12 months." In September 2011, the SSA reported that just under 8,500,000 qualifying disabled workers (persons who had worked and paid into the system) were receiving SSDI benefits.

The SSA requires that documentation of the existence of a claimant's impairment must come from "medical professionals defined by SSA's regulation as acceptable medical sources." The SSA prefers that medical documentation come from the treating physician, but if the evidence provided by the claimant's own medical sources is inadequate, additional medical information may be sought by arranging for a consultative examination.

With their extensive experience in workers' compensation impairment evaluations, physicians practicing occupational medicines are very well suited to perform SSA disability examinations. The SSA publishes two documents to assist physicians in performing these exams: *Consultative Examinations: A Guide for Health Professionals* (the "Green Book") which provides basic information about the process and the essential elements of the report, and disability evaluation under SSDI; and *Disability Evaluation Under Social Security* (the "Blue Book") which contains the rating guides as the Adult and Childhood Listings of Impairments.

Canada Pension Plan

The Canada Pension Plan (CPP) is the Canadian social insurance program for retirees and the disabled. In order for an individual to qualify for CPP disability benefits, the impairment must cause a disability that is "severe" (preventing the individual from performing any gainful employment) and "prolonged" (of at least 12 months duration). The CPP requirement of inability to perform any gainful employment does not have to be permanent. Under the CPP, the benefits are all or nothing and are not tied to financial need, because the amount of the benefit is based on contribution to the system. The process for CPP is streamlined (information is available online) and focused on reviewing the medical information provided by the treating physician rather than having an examining physician conduct an impairment assessment.

Other Programs

State Disability Plans

These are provided by several states (California, Hawaii, New Jersey, New York, Rhode Island) and Puerto Rico. They provide cash payments during temporary disability for individuals unable to work. For example, an individual who becomes temporarily unable to work after involvement in a motor vehicle accident would be eligible to receive benefits. California's program, which covers disability not related to employment, is funded through a payroll tax.

Long-Term Disability Insurance

These are commercial insurance policies developed to pay cash benefits, which are paid monthly, to an individual who becomes permanently disabled and is unable to work in either their own occupation or any occupation (more common). These policies exclude employment-related disability. The criteria for determining disability are contained within the policy which often includes a waiting period (period of disability during which the individual is ineligible to receive payment). Another requirement of many of these policies is that the disabled individual must apply for SSDI benefits, which are deducted from the policy benefit.

Personal Injury Claims

Personal injury claims are another venue in which impairment examinations are often performed. In the US and Canada (and also Australia) the *Guides* are often used to quantify the impairment after automobile and other personal injury matters. The resulting impairment rating is used by both insurers and attorneys in settling personal injury claims.

Veterans' Disability Compensation Benefits

These benefits are administered by the Department of Veterans' Affairs (VA) in the US. It is the second-largest federal department, after the Department of Defense, with which it interacts closely. Veterans who are more than "10% disabled" under VA guidelines or who are unemployable due to impairment as the result of or made worse by active-duty military service may be eligible for compensation, pension, health care, and, if homeless, permanent domiciliary benefits, depending on need and eligibility criteria. These impairment determinations are conducted by a panel of VA physicians. There were an estimated 2.9 million disabled veterans in 2009 (according to a CBS News story on the topic). This has increased substantially in recent years because of medical advances that increase survival after combat injuries.

Physician's Role and Responsibility

The evaluating physician's role when tasked with performing an impairment assessment or disability evaluation is to perform a through independent medical evaluation (see Chapter 25) and to provide an unbiased assessment of the subject's health conditions, the resulting impairment, and its effect on function and any limitations on the activities of daily living.

The evaluating physician has an ethical duty to provide an independent and accurate report and fair impairment rating. Physicians who are also treating physicians are naturally expected to act compassionately and always in the best interest of their patients, although physicians examining claimants solely for the purpose of independent medical evaluation do not have a physician–patient relationship (see Chapters 3 and 25). While it may at first glance appear to be in the best interest of the claimant to be given a high rating, it is unethical for an examiner to provide a rating that is not honest. The American College of Occupational and Environmental Medicine (ACOEM) Code of Ethics and the AMA Code of Ethics both incorporate the ethical value of justice: the ACOEM Code requires that occupational health physicians "behave honestly and ethically," and the AMA Code requires physicians be "committed to evaluating cases objectively and to providing an independent opinion."

Inflating impairment values may also have profoundly negative consequences for the claimant. An inequitable monetary outcome from a purposely-biased impairment assessment may adversely affect a person as profoundly as a false diagnosis made during a routine medical examination. An inflated impairment rating can ruin prospects for future employment and impede the injured worker's social adjustment from an injury.

Recommended Reading and Resources

American College of Occupational and Environmental Medicine. ACOEM Code of Ethics. 2010. Available at: http://www.acoem.org/codeofconduct.aspx. Accessed January 2, 2012.

American Medical Association. AMA Code of Ethics. 2008. Available at: http://www.ama-assn.org/ama/pub/physician-resources/medical-ethics/code-medical-ethics.page?. Accessed January 2, 2012.

American Medical Association (2009) *Guides to the Evaluation of Permanent Impairment.* Chicago IL, 6th ed.

Demeter, SL, Andersson GBJ (2003) *Disability Evaluation.* St. Louis MO, Mosby, 2nd ed.

Guidotti TL (2010) *The Praeger Handbook of Occupational and Environmental Medicine.* Santa Barbara CA, Praeger/ABC-Clio. See Chapter 18 on "Work Capacity."

Holmes, EG, Lorenzo CT. *Impairment Rating and Disability Determination*, August 19, 2011 Medscape Reference. Available at: http://emedicine.medscape.com/article/314195-overview. Accessed January 2, 2012.

Social Security Administration. *Consultative Examinations: A Guide for Health Professionals* ("Green Book", November 1999) Available at: http://www.ssa.gov/disability/professionals/greenbook/index.htm. Accessed January 2, 2012.

Social Security Administration. *Disability Evaluation Under Social Security* ("Blue Book", 2008). Available at: http://www.ssa.gov/disability/professionals/bluebook/index.htm. Accessed January 2, 2012.

Available Training in Impairment Assessment

American Academy of Disability Evaluating Physicians (AADEP). http://www.aadep.org/

American Board of Independent Medical Examiners (ABIME). http://www.abime.org/

American College of Occupational and Environmental Medicine (ACOEM). http://www.acoem.org/courses.aspx

American Medical Association. http://www.ama-assn.org/ama/pub/physician-resources/clinical-practice-improvement/clinical-quality/resources-publications/guides-to-evaluation-permanent-impairment.page

Canadian Society of Medical Examiners. http://www.csme.org/

27 Drug and Alcohol Testing

David G. Lukcso

This chapter outlines the many factors that must be considered in developing and introducing a workplace drug and alcohol screening program. It also presents a stepwise process which can be used as a guideline for planning for employers.

Much drug testing done today in the US is required ("mandated") under the regulations of the US Department of Transportation (DOT) and its various agencies, particularly for "commercial driver medical certification," because truck drivers are so numerous (regulated by the Federal Motor Carrier Safety Administration, FMCSA), and pilots (Federal Aviation Administration, FAA). Most employers in major high-risk industries extend drug testing to safety-sensitive positions in general. However, almost 80 percent of workplace testing in the US performed by employers is not required by regulation.

Because the American system of drug and alcohol testing is unique and extensive, most of this chapter pertains to the US, with only brief notes on Canada.

Impact in the Workplace

Drug abuse and drug trafficking have been called the great plague of modern society, and not without reason. Substance abuse and addiction have been a problem in societies for millennia and we do not have an effective solution. Unfortunately, with recent technology and ever-increasing potency of drugs, it is easier to fall prey to addiction than ever. The Substance Abuse and Mental Health Services Administration (SAMHSA) documented in its *2009 National Survey on Drug Use and Health* that an estimated 22.5 million people in the US (8.9 percent of the population aged 12 or older) were classified with substance dependence or abuse in the past year. Americans comprise only 4 percent of the world's population but consume two thirds of the world's illicit drugs. A staggering US$250 billion dollars of the nation's yearly health care dollars can be related to substance abuse, addiction, and the human afflictions they cause. Alcohol and drug abuse is involved in most violent and property crimes, with about 80 percent of inmates and juvenile arrestees committing their offenses in relationship to their substance abuse. The cost in terms of human suffering, diversion of scarce financial and professional resources, and loss to national productivity is staggering.

The workplace is not exempt from this phenomenon. The prevalence of substance abuse is higher among unemployed persons than among full-time workers. However, because about two thirds of Americans aged 18–64 are employed full-time, most substance abusers are also employed full-time. SAMHSA documented that the prevalence of past-month substance abuse among full-time workers aged 18–64 was estimated to be 8.2 percent for illicit drugs and 8.8 percent for heavy alcohol use; an estimated 3.1 percent of employed adults used illicit drugs before reporting to work or during work hours at least once in the preceding year; 1.8 percent of employed adults consumed alcohol before coming to work; and 7.1 percent drank alcohol during the workday.

Substance abuse in the workplace results in lowered productivity, increased absence, increased turnover, endangered security, and increased accident rates. Workers reporting heavy alcohol use or illicit drug use are more likely to have skipped work more than two days in the previous month. They are more likely to have worked for more than three employers in the previous year. Studies (see Larson et al., 2007) have reported that workers reporting illicit drug and alcohol use and/or dependency were more likely to have missed two days of work due to illness or injury. Co-workers are also negatively affected; they report being put in danger, having been injured, or having had to work harder, to redo work, or to cover for a co-worker as a result of fellow employee's substance use or abuse.

In Canada, the Canadian Centre on Substance Abuse reported similar impacts in the workplace, including poor job performance (e.g. lower quality products, redone work), increased job turnover (e.g. loss of experienced employees/corporate memory, severance, recruitment and orientation costs), legal liabilities associated with accidents and injuries, increased sick leave or other employee health benefit costs, disruptive behavior and declining work relationships, pilfering and vandalism, and grievances and arbitrations. However, the extent of the problem in Canada and the Canadian response to the problem have been quite different from the US and similar to policies in Germany. Programs that are typical for the US will usually not be suitable for Canada and may be against the law.

Drug Testing

In an attempt to respond to these problems, an increasing number of employers in the US introduced employee drug testing programs. The majority of the Fortune 500 companies screen job applicants for drug use. In a survey by SAMHSA, 48.8 percent of full-time workers reported that their employer conducted drug testing.

Studies carried out by the US Navy and Army, and by companies that have screened their employees for drug use have found that a carefully planned screening program is associated with significant accident rate reductions. Statistics from one large drug testing lab revealed that in 1987, 18.1 percent of all drug tests were positive; by 1997 the positive rate was down to 5.4 percent. Drug experts debate whether this means that drug use has fallen, or that drug abusers simply avoid employers that test and instead apply at firms that do not test. Nevertheless, many people believe that the evidence confirms that employee drug screening does have the capability of making a particular employer's workplace safer and more secure.

The Americans with Disabilities Act

The Americans with Disabilities Act (ADA) protects qualified individuals with disabilities from employment discrimination (see Chapter 23). This has several implications with respect to alcohol and drug-free workplace programs. The ADA states that drug and alcohol testing are not considered a medical examination and therefore they may occur prior to the offer of employment. Therefore such testing does not fall under the requirement for preplacement evaluation to be "post-offer, pre-hire." The ADA specifically excludes "any employee or applicant who is currently engaging in the illegal use of drugs" from coverage as a qualified disabled applicant or employee, and therefore permits an employer to discipline or discharge an employee for current illegal drug use. Individuals who have undergone treatment for drug or alcohol dependency or have a history of past drug use are covered by the ADA if the individual is no longer engaging in such use.

Drug Testing in the US Federal Government

Federally mandated drug testing in the US began with the "War on Drugs" in 1986, when President Ronald Reagan signed Executive Order (EO) 12564, declaring all federal agencies drug-free workplaces and prohibiting federal employees from using illegal drugs. EO 12564 required the Department of Health and Human Services (HHS) to develop guidelines and procedures for the federal drug testing programs. In 1988 HHS published the National Institute on Drug Abuse Guidelines. This was followed in 1989 by the Department of Transportation (DOT) with promulgation of 49 CFR Part 40 *Procedures for Transportation Workplace Drug Testing Programs*. Drug testing programs have also been implemented by the Department of Defense for both civilian and military personnel, the Department of Energy, and the Nuclear Regulatory Commission. The various federal agencies periodically update their guidelines on the process and procedures for workplace drug testing. Many of the guidelines eventually got incorporated into rules through rulemaking processes. Rules are more authoritative than guidelines, in that rules are legal requirements.

Instituting an Alcohol and Drug Screening Program

The first and most important step is to define clearly why the organization is instituting an alcohol and drug screening program, if it is not to meet a US federal government requirement. Drug and alcohol testing should only be undertaken for clearly defined operational reasons. Some companies have, with little or no planning, introduced mandatory drug screening of the entire workforce and in so doing have created another set of problems for themselves.

Employers who are covered must comply with applicable federal safety regulations that require drug testing. However, most workplace alcohol and drug testing programs are implemented by employer choice and are not federally mandated. Employers choose to conduct drug tests for various reasons, including deterrence of illicit and abusive drug use, to improve safety, to avoid liability, to increase productivity, or to identify individuals who are not in compliance with substance abuse policies. The employer's philosophy will dictate why alcohol and drug testing programs are implemented and will greatly influence the scope and processes of the programs.

Whether or not to test randomly is the next big issue. Scheduled testing allows employees who are casual drug users to be clean on the day of the test or to plan evasions, and so may have limited effectiveness. Pre-employment testing qualifies the candidate for hire but can be anticipated. Random testing, to catch employees unprepared, signals mistrust and is widely resented, but because it is increasingly used for public employees as well as DOT-regulated employees, workers are getting used to it. (The American Civil Liberties Union has argued that it is an unlawful search and seizure in violation of the Fourth Amendment.) Random testing works best when it is truly statistically random (which is a defense against discrimination or allegations that some workers are singled out), when the time between notification and test is very short (the employee should go straight to the testing facility), and the process is meticulously documented (protecting both the employee and the employer). It does not need to cover all employees, if it can be justified as a bona fide job requirement for safety-sensitive employees.

An employer's philosophy concerning alcohol and drugs sets the tone for its drug-free workplace policy and program. Some employers focus on detection, apprehension, and discharge, and apply a strong law enforcement model that treats employees who use drugs as criminals. Other employers focus on performance and emphasize deterrence and employee assistance (see Chapter 28), because they view alcohol and drug use as a health issue causing impairment of otherwise capable employees. The most effective drug-free workplace programs strike a balance between these two philosophies. They send a strong, clear message of zero tolerance for use and at the same time encourage employees to seek assistance if they are struggling with alcohol or drug problems.

Programs that are not required by regulation are often referred to as "non-regulated" testing programs. However, the implications of that term are not strictly accurate, as even the programs that are not federally mandated are subject to state laws and are also subject to the ADA, although drug testing procedures are not prescribed in the ADA Act. The federal guidelines have prevailed against legal challenges and thereby provide a standard against which employers can base their non-regulated programs.

Coverage of Employees

Employers with employees in any aspect of the transportation industry are covered by DOT regulations and are required to participate in the employer's DOT testing program. Who is covered by a federally-mandated employer's alcohol and drug testing policy varies with the regulation for the industry. Each DOT agency regulation states who is subject to testing in that particular transportation industry. (See Box 27.1 for list of DOT agencies.) An employer in the industry may have both a DOT program for covered employees, and a non-regulated program for other employees. The employer's philosophy will determine which employees of the organization will also be covered in "non-regulated" (more accurately, non-mandated) programs. An organization with both programs may elect to include or exclude the DOT-covered employees from the non-regulated program.

In non-regulated programs, the determination of who should be covered by the policy is constrained by a number of ethical and legal obligations. An employer may elect to include everyone from the chief executive officer down to front-line employees. Such a policy would demonstrate that the organization believes that a drug-free workplace is an important issue and that the program has the full support of management, which is prepared to lead by example.

Box 27.1 Agencies Overseeing Part 40 Procedures and Industries Regulated

US Department of Transportation
- Federal Motor Carrier Safety Administration (FMCSA): Commercial motor carriers.
- Federal Aviation Administration (FAA): Aviation industry.
- Federal Railroad Administration (FRA): Railroad industry.
- Federal Transit Administration (FTA): Public transportation.
- Pipeline and Hazardous Materials Safety Administration (PHMSA): Pipeline industry.

US Department of Homeland Security
- United States Coast Guard (USCG): Maritime industry. (USCG was a DOT agency, but was moved to the Department of Homeland Security in 2003. The USCG continues to follow Part 40 procedures for drug testing.)

Such a universal policy preempts claims of unfair or unjust implementation and some owners and managers may see it as a moral statement. Other employers may choose to perform only pre-employment (not preplacement, as explained) tests on applicants, or only on those employees who are directly involved in hazardous operations that could endanger the health or safety of co-workers or the public. Such a policy may limit the direct costs, but the employer must consider the possible consequences to workforce morale should drug screening be applied in what employees interpret to be an unjust manner. Far from improving or maintaining productivity, a poorly applied drug screening program could well have the opposite effect.

In a unionized workplace, implementation of a non-regulated alcohol and drug policy will be subject to collective bargaining, which may limit who is covered by the policy. DOT regulations override any collective bargaining agreement for covered employees in transportation. However, even when testing is required by federal or state regulations, certain aspects of how it is implemented must be agreed upon through collective bargaining.

Drug Screening in Canada

The approach to drug testing in Canada is quite different and closer to European models, especially Germany, than to the US. However, the North American Free Trade Agreement and extensive trading links, including cross-border transport, involve many employers in both systems, often with requirements for testing the same employees, such as truck drivers. Managers involved in cross-border transportation therefore need to know not only the system they are working in but the details of both systems and may need to test Canadian drivers if their duties require them to cross the international border.

The emphasis in Canada is on actual performance on the job, not on drug testing. Levels of drugs in body fluids are considered in Canada only to demonstrate use and not to serve as reliable indicators of impairment, with the exception of alcohol. In the case of alcohol, impairment and blood level are proven to be closely correlated. Alcohol or other substance addiction is considered a disability in Canada and is covered as are other disabilities for accommodation. Overall, the frequency of positive tests has been lower in Canada and there is a greater emphasis on rehabilitation when a positive result is found.

In Canada, the burden of proof is on the employer to demonstrate why drug screening is a "bona fide occupational requirement" (BFOR). Employees cannot be dismissed or disciplined for a positive drug test, alone, unless drug screening can be rigorously demonstrated to be a BFOR. However, it is recognized that for cross-border drivers, drug screening to comply with US DOT regulations may be a BFOR. A Canadian employee who is affected by a US requirement that does not apply in Canada has grounds to file a complaint within Canada on grounds of real or perceived disability.

The Canadian approach to drug testing in the workplace is derived from the Canadian Charter of Rights and Freedoms, the Canada Labour Code, the Canadian Human Rights Code, and provincial human rights codes. The Canadian Human Rights Code and provincial human rights codes consider drug and alcohol addictions to be physical or mental disabilities and specifically prohibit employers from discriminating against disabled workers and job applicants. The Canadian Human Rights Commission's policy states: "In accordance with current case law on the issue of drug and alcohol testing, and consistent with the Act's prohibition of discrimination on the ground of real or perceived disability, drug and alcohol testing are *prima facie* discriminatory."

The Canadian Human Rights Act specifically prohibits pre-employment drug or alcohol testing and random drug testing of employees in non-safety-sensitive positions. The Canadian

Human Rights Commission (CHRC) does allow for random testing of employees in safety-sensitive positions and post-accident testing if the accident occurred due to impairment. Additionally, the Code requires that positive drug test results must be used to direct workers to rehabilitation and that the employer make reasonable accommodation for the worker's needs, including reassignment if necessary.

Random testing of employees for alcohol in safety-sensitive positions is permitted, again because alcohol level directly correlates with performance and safety. Testing for cause, or after an incident, is permitted as long as it is part of a broader medical evaluation for fitness for duty. Mandatory disclosure of a drug or alcohol problem can be required for employees in safety-sensitive positions. Random drug testing may be allowed for employees as part of a rehabilitation or probationary program.

Employer Policies and Support

For mandated programs, sanctions are prescribed and out of the control of the employer. Non-regulated programs have more flexibility and should always be governed by an explicit written policy. This policy should not only be freely available but should be given out to all employees both as new hires and periodically. The policy is a very sensitive document and must be crafted with the assistance of lawyers with experience in alcohol and drug testing programs, but at the same time the language must be clear and easy to understand.

The policy and all procedures should be reviewed regularly and its performance tracked over time. This review will require input from operational supervisors, occupational health and safety staff, and employee representatives. Although the basic policy on drug use will probably not change much, the specific procedures may need revision from time to time and it is generally useful to determine trends in the workforce. This information can be used for preventive programs and to set priorities for the employee assistance program (EAP).

Employers are encouraged to design a drug-free workplace program in a way that deters drug and alcohol use but encourages rehabilitation. Ideally, a drug screening program is designed to encourage anyone who uses drugs or abuses alcohol to seek help early, prior to use becoming a problem. Employees who have had a problem with alcohol and drugs may have special protection under the ADA or Rehabilitation Act (see Chapter 23) during the period of their rehabilitation. Careful and painstaking attention to this part of the process will go a long way toward obtaining cooperation from employees and avoiding misunderstandings.

All suspected violations should be investigated following regulated requirements and standardized procedures which aim for proof. This is generally the duty of a designated physician called the "Medical Review Officer" (MRO), whose responsibilities will be described below. The supervisor, however, may become involved if there is a question of work performance related to drug use.

Supervisory personnel need to be trained and educated in some depth, not only on employer policies and procedures but on drug issues broadly. They will be faced with many challenges, some of them very uncomfortable, and they need to have a deep understanding of the issues in order to respond. The drug screening program cannot solely respond to drug test results. It will involve the cooperation of supervisors in confronting and referring employees for assessment and assisting in their rehabilitation. Supervisors must follow uniform disciplinary guidelines, basing their actions firmly on unsatisfactory performance or violation of rules, not personal beliefs, making no individual or group exceptions. At the same time, the punishment should be proportional to the offense in non-mandated programs. By being as fair as possible, the employer can keep labor–management relations on an even keel.

Testing Procedures

Federal agencies and private sector employers covered by federal DOT regulations must follow standardized procedures established by SAMHSA, known as the *Mandatory Guidelines for Federal Workplace Drug Testing Program* (referred to as the National Institute on Drug Abuse (NIDA) Guidelines). The objective of the NIDA Guidelines was to establish scientific and technical procedures for the analytical methods, sample handling procedures, and quality assurance aspects of testing. In 1988, the HHS chose urine as the required specimen rather than other types of specimens because laboratories were already in existence that were capable of testing high volumes of urine samples reliably. HHS required the use of testing laboratories certified by SAMHSA and included confirmation testing by gas chromatography/mass spectrometry (GC/MS), which was the gold standard for accuracy, in order to eliminate earlier concerns of cross-reactivity and false-positive results.

HHS then established, for federally-mandated testing, a standard five-drug panel of primary concern, called the "NIDA 5": amphetamines (amphetamine and methamphetamine), cocaine, marijuana, opiates (mainly for heroin), and phencyclidine (PCP). They established initial screening cut-off levels for each drug. Any sample above the screening threshold requires confirmation testing by GC/MS using specific metabolites with confirmation cut-off level differentiating negative and positive. (See Table 27.1 for the screening and confirmation levels for each of the five drugs in the NIDA panel.) The NIDA 5, it should be noted, does not include alcohol.

However, the NIDA 5 is by no means the entire universe of possible drugs of abuse. There are many other drugs in circulation, new "designer drugs" being introduced, and legal or "legitimate" drugs that are available over the counter or by prescription that can be abused. Employers establishing a non-regulated program now have the ability to test for any number of illicit drugs beyond the NIDA 5, as well as a choice of specimen type and cut-off thresholds. Employers may also test for drugs that employees may use legitimately under the prescription of a health care provider, knowing that many of these are also common drugs of illicit abuse (see Table 27.2).

Alcohol and drugs are detectable for a period of time after ingestion. Drug testing determines a specified amount or presence of a drug or its metabolite in the specimen. Drugs are eliminated from the system at different rates and thus detectable for different periods of

Table 27.1 The NIDA 5 Drug Panel: Cutoff Thresholds for Substance Class and Individual Substance

Substance	Screening (ng/ml)	Screening (ng/ml)
Amphetamine and Methamphetamine	500	
Amphetamine		250
Methamphetamine		250
Cocaine metabolites	150	
Benzoylecgonine		100
Marijuana metabolites	50	
THC		15
Opiates (Codeine/Morphine)	2000	
Codeine		2000
Morphine		2000
6-Acetylmorphine	10	10
Phencyclidine	25	25

Table 27.2 Drugs Commonly Screened for in the Workplace

Substance	Commercial and/or street names	Detectable time in urine specimens	Acute Effects/Health Risks
Ethanol (ethyl alcohol)	*Alcohol*: any alcoholic beverage (numerous street names)	1.5 oz for 1.5 hours	Euphoria, mild stimulation, lower inhibition, drowsiness, slurred speech, loss of coordination, loss of consciousness
Stimulants			
Amphetamine	*Dexedrine*: bennies, black beauties	48 hours	Increased heart rate, blood pressure, temperature. Increased energy; mental alertness, irritability, anxiety, paranoia, violent behavior.
Methamphetamine	*Desoxyn*: meth, ice, crank, crystal	2–3 days	Cocaine: also nasal damage
Cocaine	Cocaine hydrochloride: coke, crack	2–4 days	Methamphetamine: also severe dental problems
Cannabinoids			
Marijuana	*Marijuana*: blunt, dope, ganja, grass, joint, Mary Jane, weed	2–3 days with light use. Up to 10 days with heavy use	Euphoria, relaxation, slowed reaction time, impaired balance, increased appetite, impaired memory, anxiety, panic attacks
Opiates			
Heroin	*Diacetylmorphine*: smack, horse, H, brown sugar	Metabolites < 1 day	Euphoria, drowsiness, impaired coordination, dizziness, confusion, nausea, sedation, slowed breathing, respiratory arrest
Morphine	Morphine	1–3 days	
Codeine	*Codeine*	1–3 days	
Oxycodone	*Oxycontin, Oxycodone, Percocet, Percodan*	Up to 24 hours	
Hydrocodone	Lortab, *Vicodin, Oxycodone*	1–3 days	
Methadone	*Methadone*: amidone, fizzies	1–3 days	
Hallucinogens			
Phencyclidine	*Phencyclidine*: PCP, angel dust	3–7 days occasional use Up to 14 days chronic use	Hallucinations, excessive salivation, combativeness, severe paranoia, psychosis, flashbacks, vomiting, amnesia

LSD	*Lysergic Acid Diethylamide*: acid, cubes, sunshine, blue heaven	2–3 days	Increased heart rate and blood pressure, dilated pupils. Hallucinations, dry mouth, insomnia, tremors, paranoia, anxiety, flashbacks
CNS Depressants			
Benzodiazepines	*Valium, Librium, Xanax*	3 days for short acting 3 weeks for long acting	Drowsiness, impaired motor functions, nausea
Barbiturates	*Phenobarbital, butalbital*/downers, tranqs, barbs	2 days for short acting 14 days for long acting	Drowsiness, slow heart beat, slurred speech, weakness
Methaqualone	*Methaqualone:* quaaludes, ludes, sopor	2–4 days	Euphoria, drowsiness, reduced respiration, increased sexual arousal, respiratory depression, slurred speech, headache, delirium, vomiting, respiratory failure
Other Drugs			
Anabolic steroids	*Anadrol:* roids, juice, gym candy	2–3 days for short acting steroids >30 days for long acting steroids	No intoxication. Hypertension, livery cysts, hostility and aggression, shrunken testicles in males, menstrual irregularities in females

time, often long after the drug's effect has worn off. Aside from alcohol testing, where the blood concentration is directly related to current impairment, drug testing does not reliably determine impairment or even necessarily indicate current drug use.

While employers can develop their own list of drugs to include in a non-regulated program, laboratories usually have predetermined panels available. Although employers are not required to follow SAMHSA's guidelines in their non-federally mandated programs, doing so will help them stay on safe legal ground. Court decisions have supported employers who followed the guidelines and tested for only those drugs identified in them and for which laboratories are certified. As a result, many employers choose to follow them. A listing of laboratories that are certified by SAMHSA may be found on their website.

A cut-off level is determined in advance, at the onset of the testing program, for each drug. The cut-off point is the minimum amount of a drug or its metabolite above which the sample is reported as positive, and is always greater than the detection limit, to prevent challenges based on analytical uncertainty. Setting cut-off levels requires thinking through the implications of an apparently positive result. If a cut-off level is set low, test results will come back with more "false positives," because some "passive users" who are in close proximity to the drug, but did not actively use it, could test positive. Conversely, a high cut-off level will result in more "false negatives," and thus some active users may go undetected. Generally, a high cut-off level lessens the likelihood of taking action against someone who did not actively use drugs but was around them knowingly or inadvertently, and for this reason SAMHSA's guidelines set cut-off levels on the high side. Any employer electing to select their own drug panel and cut-off levels should work closely with their occupational health provider and the chosen laboratory to achieve goals consistent with their alcohol and drug testing philosophy and policy.

After collection, the specimen is labeled and its handling and transportation is documented at each hand-off and transition to ensure that it was secure at all times and could not have been tampered with, switched with another sample, or lost. This is called the "chain of custody" (COC). Documentation of the chain of custody must demonstrate control of the specimen from the time of collection to laboratory analysis. An intact or unbroken COC establishes that the original sample provided by the employee is one and the same as that which was analyzed by the laboratory. Any break in the COC may end up as the basis for a legal action and may compromise crucial evidence in court.

Employees who wish to beat the system may become very familiar with testing procedures in order to identify weaknesses that could allow them to pass despite active drug use. There are many websites and sources of information to help them, and many underground vendors willing to sell unadulterated urine or products that supposedly interfere with tests. Such scams are well known and understood by testing laboratories and are easily countered. It has been said often that drug screening, particularly pre-employment, functions less as a method for detecting risky substance abuse behavior than as an intelligence test.

Specimen Types and Collection

Different bodily fluids and excretion pathways could be tested to detect evidence of recent drug use. Urine is the most commonly used medium for testing for illicit drugs and breath is the most common for alcohol. Some state laws dictate which types of tests can be used as well as when testing can be performed. (The Department of Labor provides a general overview of each state's regulations: http://www.dol.gov/asp/programs/drugs/said/StateLaws.asp .)

Diagnostic urine testing should never be combined with drug testing. In part, this is because the COC must be maintained for drug testing but mainly it is because the practice would create mistrust. It would lead to resentment among employees toward the occupational health service and resistance to other health-related tests. Many employees already have latent suspicions that periodic health surveillance and other tests are diverted for drug screening.

The specimen used in the test, which is also called the "matrix," has technically important characteristics as noted below.

Urine

Urine tests show the presence or absence of drug metabolites in a person's urine. Urine testing has been challenged in the courts and its accuracy has been upheld. Metabolites remain in the body for some time after the effects of a drug have worn off. It is important to note that a positive urine test does not necessarily mean that a person was under the influence of drugs at the time of the test.

Employees are not directly observed providing their urine sample unless there is evidence of substitution of samples or adulteration. There is a brisk trade in adulterants and clean urine marketed to employees who hope to take drugs and still beat the system. A urine sample can be adulterated in two ways. One is by ingesting a product that is intended to mask the presence of the drug or the metabolite. The second is to add something to the sample such as bleach, water, or vinegar. Most laboratories now routinely perform adulteration tests, looking for substances that have been introduced into the sample. Urine samples can also be substituted or diluted, which is why their temperature and specific gravity are recorded at the time of collection.

Occupational health services that collect urine for drug testing must have a suitably equipped restroom to avoid dilution. Valves controlling water to the sink should be outside the room so that they can be turned off during collection. The toilet should have bluing agent in the water.

Expired Air

Breath-alcohol testing is most often used to determine the alcohol level because expired air accurately reflects the concentration of alcohol in the blood. The employee blows into an "evidentiary breath-testing device" (EBT) which has been calibrated to ensure accuracy. The results show the level of alcohol in the blood at the time of the test and are usually reported as the Blood Alcohol Concentration (BAC). BAC levels correlate closely with impairment. A legal limit of 0.08 percent (as g/dl) for driving has been set in all states, and 0.05 percent across Canada (except Quebec, where the limit is 0.08 percent). Saliva testing is sometimes used to screen for alcohol, but confirmation by breath testing is preferred.

Blood

Blood alcohol tests measure the concentration of alcohol or other drugs in the blood at the time of the test. Blood testing is believed to produce the most accurate results, but venipuncture is also the most invasive of procedures required to obtain body fluids for testing and is not acceptable for screening employees. Additionally, the detection period for most drugs is shorter in the blood than in other drug testing specimens. Blood has its place in forensic and medical evaluations but not in screening tests.

Hair Analysis

Hair analysis provides a much longer drug-use history and provides longitudinal data as far back as 90 days. Like urine testing, hair testing does not provide evidence of current impairment, only past use of a specific drug. Hair testing is considered the least invasive form of drug testing, therefore privacy issues are decreased. Unlike trace element analysis, where contamination is a major issue, hair testing for drugs is considered reliable.

Saliva

Saliva, or oral fluids, collected from the mouth also can be used to detect traces of drugs and alcohol. They are easy to collect (a swab of the inner cheek is the most common collection method), harder to adulterate or substitute. The detection period for most drugs is shorter in oral fluids than in urine.

Employer Notification and Confidentiality

All information received by the employer through the drug and alcohol workplace program is confidential personal health information. Access to this information is limited to those who have a legitimate need to know in compliance with relevant laws and regulations (see Chapter 3). Employees often are reluctant to discuss problems with alcohol and/or drugs due to the stigma attached to the illnesses, and the denial and minimization that are part of the problem. If employees feel that their confidentiality will not be protected, they will not seek help from an employee assistance program (see Chapter 28).

In federally-mandated testing, laboratories must report results only to the employer's designated MRO. The MRO is a licensed physician who functions as the gatekeeper between the laboratory and the employer. The MRO is required to have passed a nationally recognized MRO certification examination (sponsored by the Medical Review Officer Certification Council, MROCC, or the American Association of Medical Review Officers, AAMRO). The first MRO duty is to review the COC. The second duty of the MRO is to receive and review the laboratory results. Some positive laboratory results could be due to legitimate medications. The MRO provides the employee an opportunity to provide evidence that the positive result is not the result of abuse. If the employee can provide this evidence, the MRO then reports the result as negative to the employer's designated management representative.

An employer who is considering or developing a non-mandated workplace drug and alcohol testing program should review state laws regarding review and reporting of results. Several states require a certified MRO for non-regulated drug test review; others simply require physician review of laboratory results. While some state laws allow direct reporting to the employer, this practice is not recommended. If the employer does elect to directly receive laboratory results, employee confidentiality must absolutely be maintained. This can be very risky with respect to liability and labor–management relations and the occupational health service may wish to consider very carefully whether it should get involved in such a situation. On the other hand, non-regulated programs that resemble regulated programs have not encountered such problems.

Employers with non-regulated programs are encouraged to institute a process similar to DOT-mandated programs, in which analytical laboratory results are directly communicated to the occupational health service within their organization or to an independent certified occupational health physician who agrees to serve as their MRO. (See "Recommended

Reading and Resources" at end of the chapter for assistance with locating a certified MRO.) The physician serving as MRO can assess the results with knowledge of the job safety factors and can then alert the employer to fitness-for-duty or safety issues. The physician–MRO is an advocate for the accuracy and integrity of the drug testing process and ensures employee confidentiality.

The goal of any alcohol and drug-free workplace program is deterrence of the illicit use of drugs and substances, not the detection of valid medical issues. Health issues that are discovered as an incidental finding during drug testing should be treated as confidential health information and dealt with by the employee's personal physician. Management has no right to this information.

Employee Notification and Referral

Once the company policy and procedures have been developed in detail and agreed upon at all levels, resources must be allocated to support it: a budget, personnel, a contract with a qualified analytical laboratory, an MRO (if not the occupational physician associated with the employer), and an EAP (see Chapter 28). The role of the EAP is to receive referrals from positive tests. Initiation of the alcohol and drug testing program and policies should be announced in advance, well before it is implemented. The announcement must be absolutely clear and must reach every employee in the organization.

Published material on the program should be written simply and clearly, and describe every aspect. Employees should be given the opportunity to ask questions. They will want to know everything but especially the following:

- who is going to be tested
- how they will be tested
- when, how often, and where
- who is going to analyze the samples
- what drugs will be tested for
- who will receive the results and who will have access to the records
- the rules about drug use and possession at work and whether they have changed (i.e. become even stricter)
- what will happen if they refuse to be tested
- their rights and whether they can appeal a determination
- what will be offered to or required of them in the way of treatment and rehabilitation
- the consequences of violating the drug-free workplace policy.

Under DOT regulations, 49 CFR, Part 40 Subpart O, an employer must refer a covered employee with a verified positive drug test, a breath alcohol concentration of 0.04 or greater, or any other violation of the prohibition on the use of alcohol or drugs under a DOT agency regulation to an outside "substance abuse professional" (SAP). A SAP generally has the same requirements as an EAP counselor (see Chapter 28), but has completed special training with an emphasis on public safety in transportation. (There are many organizations in the US that provide this training.) Treatment in an employer's EAP may also be undertaken but evaluation by the SAP must take place separately from the EAP. The SAP is not an advocate for the employer nor for the employee, rather the SAP's function is to represent the public's interest in safety by professionally evaluating the employee and recommending appropriate education and/or treatment, follow-up tests, and return to duty recommendations.

Recommended Reading and Resources

Califano J (2008) High society: how substance abuse ravages America and what to do about it. *On The Brain – The Harvard Mahoney Neuroscience Institute Letter*, Fall, 14(3).

Canadian Centre on Substance Abuse. Working to Reduce Alcohol and Drug Related Harm. Available at: http://www.ccsa.ca/Eng/Topics/Populations/Workplace/Pages/WorkplaceOverview.aspx. Accessed January 3, 2011.

Canadian Human Rights Commission. Policy on Alcohol and Drug Testing. 2009. Available at: http://www.chrc-ccdp.ca/legislation_policies/padt_pdda/toc_tdm-eng.aspx. Accessed January 3, 2011.

Hartenbaum N, Hegman K, Wood E (2010) *The DOT Medical Examination: A Guide to Commercial Driver's Medical Certification*, Beverly Farms MA, OEM Press, 5th ed.

Holmes N, Richer K (2008) *Drug Testing in the Workplace*, Ottawa, Parliamentary research paper. Available at: http://www.parl.gc.ca/Content/LOP/researchpublications/prb0751-e.htm. Accessed January 3, 2011.

Larson SL, Eyerman J, Foster MS, Gfroerer JC (2007) *Worker Substance Use and Workplace Policies and Programs*. DHHS Publication No. SMA 07-4273, Analytic Series A-29, Rockville MD, Substance Abuse and Mental Health Services Administration (SAMHSA), Office of Applied Studies. Available at: http://www.oas.samhsa.gov/work2k7/work.pdf. Accessed January 3, 2011.

Medical Review Officer Certification Council (2008) *MRO Code of Ethics*. Available at: http://www.mrocc.org/Code.htm. Accessed April 18, 2012.

National Institute of Drug Abuse (2004) *Drugs of Abuse Information*. Available at: http://www.nida.nih.gov/drugpages/. Accessed January 3, 2011.

Ropero-Miller J, Goldberger BA (2008) *Handbook of Workplace Drug Testing*, AACC Press, 2nd ed.

Swotinsky RB, Smith D (2010) *The Medical Review Officer's Manual: MROCC's Guide to Drug Testing*, Beverly Farms MA, OEM Press, 4th ed.

Transport Canada (2009) *The History of the Testing Debate in Canada*. Available at: http://www.tc.gc.ca/eng/railsafety/publications-ontrack-206.htm. Accessed January 3, 2011.

US Department of Health and Human Services, Substance Abuse and Mental Health Services Administration (SAMHSA) (2004) *HHS Mandatory Guidelines*. Available at: http://workplace.samhsa.gov/FedPgms/Pages/Mand_Guid_04.html. Accessed January 3, 2011.

US Department of Health and Human Services, Substance Abuse and Mental Health Services Administration (SAMHSA) (2010) *Results from the 2009 National Survey on Drug Use and Health: Volume I. Summary of National Findings*, Office of Applied Studies, NSDUH Series H-38A, HHS Publication No. SMA 10-4586 Findings, Rockville, MD. Available at: http://oas.samhsa.gov/nsduh/2k9nsduh/2k9resultsp.pdf. Accessed January 3, 2011.

US Department of Health and Human Services, Substance Abuse and Mental Health Administration (SAMHSA) (2011) *National Survey on Drug Use and Health*. Available at: http://www.samhsa.gov/data/NSDUH/2k10NSDUH/2k10Results.htm. Accessed January 3, 2011. This is the current survey. Note the "2k10" for 2010, "2k9" for 2009 for finding the current version in future years.

US Department of Labor. Drug-Free Workplace Advisor. Available at: http://www.dol.gov/elaws/drugfree.htm. Accessed January 3, 2011. Assists users to build tailored drug-free workplace policies and provides guidance on how to develop comprehensive drug-free workplace programs. It also provides information about coverage and requirements of the Drug-Free Workplace Act of 1988.

US Department of Transportation, Office of Drug and Alcohol Policy and Compliance. Available at: http://www.dot.gov/odapc/. Accessed January 5, 2011. Includes text of 49 CFR 40.

US Department of Transportation. The Substance Abuse Professional Guidelines. Available at: http://www.dot.gov/odapc/testingpubs/SAP_Guide_200403.pdf. Accessed January 5, 2011.

Sources for Professional Services Required for Drug Screening Programs

Laboratories

A list of SAMHSA certified laboratories can be found published in the Federal Register. The most recent at the time of this writing:

Federal Register. Vol. 76, No. 133, *Current List of Laboratories and Instrumented Initial Testing Facilities Which Meet Minimum Standards To Engage in Urine Drug Testing for Federal Agencies*. This list is accessed through their website at: http://www.workplace.samhsa.gov/DrugTesting/pdf/FR071211.pdf. Accessed April 18, 2012.

Medical Review Officers

There are two organizations that certify Medical Review Officers:

American Association of Medical Review Officers (AAMRO) maintains a list of Medical Review Officers who have been certified through AAMRO. The list is accessed through their website at: http://www.aamro.com/locate/. Accessed April 18, 2012.

Medical Review Officer Certification Council (MROCC) maintains a list of Medical Review Officers who have been certified through MROCC. The list is accessed through their website at: http://www.mrocc.org/portal.htm. Accessed April 18, 2012.

28 Employee Assistance Programs

David G. Lukcso

Approximately half of Americans at some time in their life, 25 percent in any given year, have mental health or substance abuse problems according to a 2011 survey by the Centers for Disease Control and Prevention (CDC), imposing a cost of over US$300 billion for mental illness alone. An additional number of neighbors and co-workers face short-term life adjustment issues involving family and finances. Such personal problems interfere with their work, attitude, and enjoyment of life, and they can be found in any community and in any workplace. The business community in the US has recognized that everyday life stresses can negatively affect employee attendance and concentration, the general workplace morale, and an employee's ability to perform well on the job.

In the workplace, particularly, personal problems cause conflict, interfere with performance, and may even cause an otherwise valued and productive worker to lose his or her job. If serious problems are identified early, before they cause the worker to break down, to fail in performance, or to be dismissed from the job, an enlightened employer can intervene to help the worker and in so doing avoid the loss of a valuable employee who may have many productive years ahead.

Employee assistance programs (EAPs) are employer-sponsored counseling services designed for personal or family problems, including mental health, substance abuse, various addictions, marital problems, parenting problems, emotional problems, and financial or legal concerns. They are designed to assist employees in getting help for these problems so that they may remain on the job and effective. EAP services are provided by an employer to the employees, usually under contract with an EAP provider. EAPs have always had an emphasis on rehabilitating valued employees rather than terminating them for their substance problems. Over the years, the scope of EAP services has expanded beyond alcoholism, drugs, and mental health issues to include health and wellness and work/life balance concerns. EAP services are oriented toward the individual employee and their family members; however, they also provide population health services to the organization. This may include prevention, training, consultation, and organizational development.

Programs designed to help employees who have personal problems that interfere with their work performance and enjoyment of life have been widespread in business since the 1940s. It was not until the 1950s, when the American Medical Association sanctioned the concept that alcohol abuse was a treatable medical condition, that the foundation for modern EAPs was established. Since the 1980s, Federal agencies have been required by Title 5 Code of Federal Regulations Part 792 to establish appropriate prevention, treatment, and rehabilitative programs and services for alcohol and drug abuse problems for Federal civilian employees. This provided a model for the private sector. Today, according to the

EAP Professional Association, over 97 percent of employers with more than 5,000 employees have EAPs, 80 percent of companies with 1001 to 5000 employees, and 75 percent of companies with 251 to 1000.

The design and implementation of an EAP depend upon the perceptions and attitudes of the various stakeholders, the nature of the industry, the characteristics of the community, the background of professional consultants, and the availability of local agencies to receive referrals. If an EAP is to succeed, key players must not only accept the initiative but participate in its design and implementation: management, the union or other employee representatives, the occupational health service, and the human resources or personnel department.

Certain underlying principles must be in place for an EAP to succeed:

- Alcohol and drug abuse and stress-related behavioral disturbances must be accepted as legitimate, treatable illnesses.
- The program must not be used as a substitute for usual disciplinary procedures, as a means of constructive dismissal, or to compromise rules, regulations, contracts, or binding agreements.
- Strict confidentiality must always be held inviolate, with no executive or human resources officer entitled to access to an employee's EAP record, but only authorized professionals and staff of the occupational health service.
- In the case of voluntary self-referral, not only must the nature of the problem be kept in strictest confidence but the fact of the referral itself and the employee's participation must never be disclosed.
- In the case of a directed referral, the fitness-for-duty procedure described in Chapter 22 should be followed. This procedure ensures confidentiality for the worker, while at the same time giving the supervisor and others who need to be involved sufficient information to manage the employment situation.
- The employer, through regular reports that disclose no confidential information, monitors the progress of the employee and guarantees return to the same job or one involving similar work.

These principles must be articulated in a company EAP policy that is known and understood by all employees. The policy should outline these underlying principles, describe the program content, identify the key players, describe their roles and responsibilities, and specify the EAP's relationship to other employment policies. (A sample EAP Policy appears as Exhibit 28.1 at the end of this chapter.)

EAPs should be widely advertised, but in a nonthreatening way. All publicity regarding the EAP should emphasize strict confidentiality and professionalism, and provide a phone number outside the workplace and not under the employer's control so that the employee can call from a private phone. It is absolutely necessary that the office of the EAP be off-premises or concealed from view in some way, within a larger unit, such as the occupational health service, with an entrance that is not visible to other workers.

In development and implementation of an EAP, there are several different management models of EAPs to consider: "internal," "external," "blended," and "free" EAP models:

- Internal EAP programs are delivered by a team that is staffed from within the organization by the occupational health service or by the human resources department.
- External EAP services are purchased from an EAP provider outside of the organization, which is the most common practice among employers today.

- Blended EAPs may use internal staff, within the occupational health service, for triage and conventional counseling or follow-up, but may rely on contract providers for rehabilitation and specialized services.
- "Free EAPs," the newest model, are bare-bones versions of the external model that are embedded in other insurance offerings and usually offer only minimal levels of service, including immediate access to counseling or crisis event response services.

The choice of a suitable program is determined by the scope and breadth of services an employer's working population is likely to need, the degree of integration and onsite contact of the EAP with the workplace, the kinds of counseling modalities used to provide EAP clinical services, and their ability to support the workplace for critical incidents and other difficult situations. (Resources for selecting contract services are included in the "Recommended Reading and Resources" at the end of this chapter.)

Most employers that choose an internal approach deliver EAP services using their occupational health team, through the human resources department (which may cause obvious concern), or by an EAP counselor working as an employee of the company. Often these internal EAP programs limit services to those relating to alcohol and drug abuse education and training as well as short-term counseling services delivered to individual employees at the organization. Core services include conducting crisis event management, clinical case assessments, providing short-term problem solving and counseling, making referrals, suggesting educational resources for self-help, and ensuring follow-up.

In outreach population health and educational sessions, employees receive information on how to avoid or to cope with alcohol, drugs, and stress, and how the overall program works. Supervisor training encourages the supervisor not to speculate on the meaning of a worker's behavioral problems at work but rather to watch for and react to early signs of trouble—irritability, tardiness, chronic or "Monday morning" absence, sloppy work habits, and any unusual changes in behavior on the part of the worker. Supervisors are taught to refer workers who may be exhibiting these signs to the occupational health program or EAP even before the problem leads to failing job performance.

Employees who are experiencing difficulties may also enter the EAP through self-referral. In self-referral, the employee, for whatever reason, has decided to get help before work performance has deteriorated to the point where it is necessary for a supervisor to become involved. In the directed situation, job performance has already deteriorated such that, if improvement does not occur, discipline or dismissal is likely.

Most EAPs, including both internal and external models, do not attempt to provide ongoing in-house counseling, treatment, or rehabilitation. Rather, they provide the necessary framework for case identification, management, and follow-up, and provide liaison with community treatment and resources for rehabilitation. The counselor should be familiar with the resources available in the local area, their suitability for different people and situations, their fees, criteria for enrollment, and treatment approaches. Not every treatment center is suitable for every worker. Some people respond to intensive residential programs away from home and work; others do better in a visiting setting, such as Alcoholics Anonymous. Sometimes referral to a special counselor is required; the EAP counselor should have on hand a roster of practicing professionals in the area and extensive knowledge about the ones used.

The counselor is the key to an effective EAP. Alcohol rehabilitation counselors have a special rapport with alcohol abusers and many have themselves had and overcome drinking problems. The EAP counselors should be licensed and/or certified professionals such as physicians, nurses, "Licensed Clinical Social Worker," "Licensed Psychologist," "Licensed

Professional Counselor," or "Certified Employee Assistance Professional". Whatever the credentials of the counselor, an employee must feel at ease and confident in his or her presence. For this reason the demeanor and attitude of the counselor is critical, as is the counselor's ability to relate to workers of different ages and social classes.

The EAP counselor closely monitors the progress of the worker through treatment (and after returning to work, if time off is required), thereby reinforcing treatment and increasing the likelihood of successful recovery. By providing assistance before a worker's performance deteriorates to the point of dismissal, the EAP preserves an important part of the worker's life. In many cases the worker's family has been so negatively affected that the job remains the only point of stability in a chaotic life. By stepping in before the worker's job performance goes the way of his or her family life, the EAP gives the worker a foundation from which to work toward recovery. Both employer and employee gain as the employee's job performance returns to normal.

Employees covered under DOT regulations with a positive breath alcohol or urine drug test are also referred outside the EAP to designated evaluation professionals, known as "substance abuse professionals" (SAPs). A SAP generally has the same requirements as an EAP counselor, as listed above, and has undergone special training. The SAP has a role different than the traditional EAP counselor. The SAP's function is to protect the public interest in safety by professionally evaluating employees who have violated a DOT-mandated drug and alcohol program regulation and recommending appropriate education and/or treatment, follow-up tests, and return to duty recommendations. EAP professionals can be SAPs but not at the same time for a particular worker or employer.

Recommended Reading and Resources

Employee Assistance Professionals Association (EAPA): An international organization of EAP professionals in 35 countries providing training, the CEAP credential by examination, and professional development. http://www.eapassn.org/. Accessed April 18, 2012.

Employee Assistance Society of North America (EASNA): A tri-national membership association (Canada, US, and Mexico) of employee assistance professionals, organizations, and employers advancing knowledge, research, and best practices toward achieving healthy and productive workplaces. http://www.easna.org/. Accessed April 18, 2012.

EASNA (2009) *Selecting and Strengthening Employee Assistance Programs: A Purchaser's Guide.* Available at: http://www.easna.org/wp-content/uploads/2010/08/EASNA-PURCHSERS-GUIDE-TO-EAPs-FINAL-102209.pdf. Accessed January 5, 2011.

Reeves WC, et al. (2011) Mental illness surveillance among adults in the United States. *Morbidity and Mortality Weekly Report*, 2 September, 60(03 Suppl.): 1–32. Available at: http://www.cdc.gov/mmwr/preview/mmwrhtml/su6003a1.htm. Accessed January 5, 2011.

Substance Abuse and Mental Health Services Administration (SAMHSA). *Provide Assistance: Employee Assistance Program.* Available at: http://www.workplace.samhsa.gov/wpworkit/eap.html. Accessed January 5, 2011.

US Department of Labor. Employee Assistance Programs for a New Generation of Employees: Defining the New Generation. Available at: http://www.dol.gov/odep/documents/employeeassistance.pdf. Accessed January 5, 2011.

US Department of Transportation. The Substance Abuse Professional Guidelines. Available at: http://www.dot.gov/odapc/testingpubs/SAP_Guide_200403.pdf. Accessed January 5, 2011.

Exhibit 28.1 Sample Employee Assistance Program Policy

(The following is an example of a corporate policy on employee assistance that may serve as a model for management.)

Purpose

To provide employees and their families with opportunities to obtain assistance for a variety of personal problems that may affect their continued functioning as productive members of the organization or society at large.

The Employee Assistance Program (EAP) is a confidential counseling and referral service with professionally certified employee assistance providers who are experienced in a wide range of issues including relationship, conflict, family concerns, and alcohol or drug dependence.

Policy

1. Personal problems of employees which result in unacceptable behavior or which affect or may affect the workplace, are a legitimate concern of the organization. Further, the organization encourages all employees of the organization to live in a responsible and healthy manner.

2. Research supports the conclusion that the majority of unacceptable workplace behavior is related to drug or alcohol abuse and other treatable medical/behavioral problems. Employees with these problems are responsible for most absenteeism, injuries, inferior work, unsound decisions, conflict with co-workers, thefts from employers, poor public relations and many other job performance shortcomings that result in direct costs to the organization and which serve as an imposition on co-workers and those the organization serves.

3. The Employee Assistance Program encompasses education, treatment, and rehabilitation.

Scope

This policy applies to all operations, subsidiary, and affiliated organizations.

The organization offers EAP services to its employees and their families. Examples of issues addressed by this program include, but are not limited to:

- Alcohol and Drug Dependency Problems
- Anxiety Disorders
- Depression and Mood Changes
- Family Conflicts
- Job Crisis
- Eating Disorders
- Adolescent Behavioral Problems
- Marital Problems
- Stress at Home and Work
- Threatening and Destructive Behaviors
- Financial Concerns

General Procedures

1. Voluntary Self-Referral

Employees who believe they have a health problem that is affecting or could affect work performance may voluntarily seek confidential assistance through the organization's EAP or occupational health services. In this circumstance, no other member of the organization or any other employee will be informed of the referral unless authorized by the employee or where the employee's life or the lives of others are in imminent danger.

2. Employer-Initiated Referral

Although contact with EAP providers is usually voluntary, referral to the occupational health services or EAP provider may sometimes be required. If an employee's work performance is inadequate or deficient; his or her behavior is aberrant or otherwise outside commonly accepted standards of conduct or if there is reason to believe a threat of violence exists or may exist, that employee may be directed to participate in an evaluation. Following the confidential evaluation, the employee may be required to obtain rehabilitative counseling, treatment, or assistance to resolve the problem. Failure or refusal by an employee to complete the conditions of an administrative referral to the occupational health services or EAP will result in the implementation of the appropriate disciplinary process.

Responsibilities

1. Supervisor

Organization administrators and supervisors attempting to have employee behavioral problems addressed should consult with <Human Resources> for assistance with specific procedures required for administrative referral. It is essential that supervisors and administers deal only with acceptable workplace behavior and avoid giving advice to employees regarding specific medical, emotional or substance abuse problems.

   If work performance is unacceptable and health reasons are given as or suspected to be the cause, the supervisor will direct the employee to the occupational health services and to human resources to discuss accommodations under the ADA or Rehabilitation Act.

2. Employee

Employees have a responsibility to maintain a satisfactory standard of work performance. Employees have a responsibility to seek assistance and participate in appropriate treatment programs when health conditions are affecting or could affect adversely their work performance.

3. Human Resources

<Human Resources> will provide direction to supervisors and employees on the various options available when dealing with deteriorating work performance.

4. Occupational Health Services/Employee Assistance Program

- Voluntary Self-Referral: The occupational health services staff will evaluate the employee's situation and, where appropriate, coordinate treatment and/or rehabilitation. Except under defined situations (where the employee's life or lives of others are in imminent danger) the fact that the employee sought help will never be revealed to any other employee or member of the organization.
- Employer-Initiated Referral: The occupational health services staff will objectively evaluate relevant information and determine fitness to work and may arrange referral to an appropriate internal resource or community agency. The occupational health services staff will coordinate the treatment and/or rehabilitation plans between the organization and any outside health professionals and will maintain complete confidentiality of health information.
- Education and Training: The occupational health services staff will develop and assist in the delivery of educational material and training programs for management and employees.

Questions concerning the Employee Assistance Program should be referred to <*Insert correct contact, i.e.* **the EAP Coordinator or the Occupational Health Service.**>

29 Psychological Health and Safety

M. Suzanne Arnold and Ian M. F. Arnold

The links between working productively and good mental health are well documented. Rewarding, meaningful work enhances mood and mental health, and sound mental health makes workers more productive. Psychological issues within the workforce and workplace can affect the business of the organization and it employees, and must be dealt with effectively using a strategic and sustainable approach. Employee assistance programs (EAPs, see Chapter 28) are invaluable for dealing with disorders and serious problems of addiction and mental health in the individual worker. However, broader interventions are required to deal with the larger problem of psychological safety and health in the social environment of the workplace.

Psychological health issues fall on a continuum from mild psychological problems (negative moods, sleep disorders, excessive worry) to severe mental disorders (bipolar disorder, schizophrenia, deep depression). The former occur far more often in the work environment, and so in their totality may have a more significant negative impact on workers and on the workplace than the latter. Occupational health and safety recognizes psychogenic and social hazards and risks in the workplace (see Chapter 21).

All business organizations, large and small, have a de facto obligation towards corporate social responsibility, which extends to the well-being of employees and their families, the broader community, shareholders and other stakeholders. Top corporate leaders in small and large businesses, unions, governments, and courts and tribunals are recognising that the prevention, mitigation, and management of psychological issues in the workplace has become, in the words of Dr. Martin Shain (2010), a "must do" rather than a "nice to do."

Some indicators that psychosocial health may be at risk include the following:

- Denial of (dis)stress amongst employees, including management staff, until they reach a breaking point or become mentally or physically ill.
- Failure to achieve targets and meet deadlines.
- Conflict among and between employees.
- Loss of good employees—quitting or transferring.
- Excessive time off—that is, more than seems reasonable.
- Difficulty in returning people to work from short-term or permanent partial disability.
- Prolonged or repeated disability absences, in the context of unresolved workplace tensions.

Psychological health and safety (PH&S) is a new way of looking at psychogenic hazards in the workplace. In the formulation of Samra and Gilbert (2011), "*Psychological health* consists of our ability to think, feel and behave in a manner that enables us to perform effectively at work, at home, and in society at large. *Psychological safety* is a bit different – it deals with the risk of injury to mental well-being that a worker might experience." Improving workplace psychological safety means recognising hazards (often associated with how the workplace is organized or related to employees' own issues) and lowers the associated risks of adverse effects to employees' mental health.

The active involvement of occupational health professionals is a critical ingredient for a successful workplace approach to PH&S. Effective integration of mental health strategies in an occupational health practice can have a positive impact in the areas of professional and social responsibility, cost-effectiveness, and risk management.

Estimates for the number of workers who have psychological health conditions or experience distress vary greatly, because stigma and negative perceptions within the workplace culture lead to a reluctance to disclose this kind of information. Self-reporting surveys usually underestimate the scale of the problem. Even so, conservative estimates from the UK (Secretaries of State for the Department of Work and Pensions and the Department of Health, 2009) suggest that at any one time:

- One in six people of working age experience symptoms of distress (sleeplessness, irritability, worry) which do not meet the criteria for medical diagnosis of a mental illness, but which can affect the person's ability to function and to work.
- An additional one in six of the working-age population experiences symptoms of a nature, severity and/or duration that do meet the criteria for medical diagnosis, such as anxiety or depression.
- Approximately 1 in 100 adults of working age has severe mental health conditions such as bipolar disorder or schizophrenia.

Cost and Losses from Impaired Mental Health

The cost of mental illness is staggering, both in terms of economic impact and loss of productivity. In the US, mental health conditions are reported to be the second leading cause of workplace absence. On any given day, according to Mental Health America (2011) approximately 1 million workers miss work due to (dis)stress. The overall costs for mental illness amount to US$150 billion in annual lost productivity—US$44 billion of these costs are paid by businesses. Improvement is possible: three out of four workers who seek help for workplace issues or mental health conditions experience significant improvements in work performance after treatment.

Annual costs are also significant in Canada: 7.2 percent of total government health expenditures go to mental health, according to the Institute of Health Economics, and mental health issues lead the list for causes of long- and short-term workplace disability. Across the European Union, work-related stress affects more than 40 million employees and costs approximately €20 billion annually in lost time and medical expenditures (Institute of Work, Health and Organization, 2008).The total cost to UK employers for mental illness among their workers is over £25 billion, equal to £1,035 per employee in the workforce (Business in the Community, 2009)

Disability management (essentially a tertiary care and prevention approach) is also becoming an increasingly costly factor for all workplaces. Professional programs and training tend to focus on physical causes of disability not related to mental health and psychological issues, even though psychological issues may account for 40 to 45 per cent of all long-term disability (LTD) and short-term disability (STD). Disability duration is also often related to psychological health regardless of the primary cause of the disability and may be further influenced by the worker's lack of skills in developing and implementing effective strategies for coping with workplace stressors. When the return to work process (see Chapter 22) ignores employee psychological health or coping strategies and lacks a process for resolving workplace issues, the chances for success are significantly reduced.

It is clear that increasing costs associated with psychological issues in the workplace (including legal judgements against employers) require the development and implementation of risk management principles for PH&S in the same way that physical health, safety, and environmental factors are integrated into the business agenda of the workplace.

A Process for Managing Psychological Health

There is a growing international movement to develop standards for workplace PH&S, most notably in Canada and the UK (most recently the BSI PAS 1010 (2011)), but the issue has not achieved as much prominence in the US. A number of related management standards are familiar to workplaces, primarily the International Organization for Standardization (ISO) series for quality (ISO 9000 series), environment (ISO 14000 series), and the Occupational Health and Safety Assessment standards (OHSAS 18000 series).

Many workplaces, and workers, are familiar with the ISO process and management model. To date only one ISO standard (ISO 10075-3:2004) refers to "mental workload" and only in a general way. However, the ISO elements can also be applied to the management of psychological health. These basic elements derive from the Hazard Identification/Risk Assessment/Risk Control (HIRARC) paradigm and the Plan → Do → Check → Act approach (also known as the "Deming Cycle"; see Chapter 17). In brief, these ISO elements are, in order:

1 *Obtain commitment and develop policies*, from organizational management.
2 *Plan*, including needs analysis, hazard identification, and risk assessment.
3 *Implement and operate* risk control strategies to address the organization's identified needs.
4 *Evaluate and institute corrective action*—evaluate the program's effectiveness through planned auditing, and recommend changes to improve the outcomes.
5 *Review and improve*—implement recommendations and re-evaluate.

Obtain Commitment and Develop Policies

A clear commitment from senior management to improve mental health/PH&S in the workplace is key to addressing these issues. This commitment starts with an endorsement from the Board of Directors (whose role at the highest level is to set policy, provide direction—and resources—and evaluate results) of a workplace policy statement on PH&S risk management. Identification of a champion to drive the process forward is another key element for success. Dissemination throughout the organization, by a process of discussion, can assist in building commitment and fostering the engagement of all employees. The provision of adequate resources also provides evidence of senior management commitment. The Policy Statement on Mental Health may be: (1) a stand-alone policy with its own framework; (2) part of the organization's health (or health and safety, or environment, health, and safety) policy; or (3) a key component of the human resources policy.

While the Policy Statement may be deliberately short and to the point, the larger policy document should include:

- Clear definitions of psychological hazards and related risks.
- A statement of goals and objectives, as well as the policy's link to health and safety legislation.
- Links to other company policies and practices.
- Implementation, including roles and responsibilities of key personnel, and a schedule of ongoing policy evaluation.
- Ethical issues relevant to confidentiality for employees at all levels.
- A statement of support for return-to-work strategies.

A model policy statement is presented as Exhibit 29.1 and can be found at the end of the chapter.

Plan

Needs Assessment and Analysis

All initiatives in workplaces today, including health and safety programs, once there is leadership commitment to move forward, begin with a process to decide whether there is a need for further action.

The needs analysis examines the psychological hazards identified, along with their adverse potential health effects, in relation to the prevalence of the hazard and the degree of relative harm (risk), and the number of workers affected. The needs analysis helps to identify baseline measures (a key performance indicator) against which improvements can be made. It also serves to identify the hazards and assess the risks so the organization can respond with the right resources. Four key areas should be addressed: legal requirements, key organizational and structural issues that can affect workplace PH&S, financial analysis, and the impact of mental health issues in the organization's own workforce.

LEGAL REQUIREMENTS

While few jurisdictions have legal requirements specifically related to an overall approach to workplace PH&S, many other aspects of the law apply. These include but are not limited to accommodation for employees with disabilities, labor relations laws, employment standards, human rights legislation, the law of torts (negligence), health and safety regulations, workers compensation, and employment contract obligations (detailed in the Shain Reports, 2010). Organizations must determine where their legal liabilities exist as a first step to understanding their overall minimum requirements to adequately address PH&S in their specific workplaces.

ORGANIZATIONAL AND STRUCTURAL ISSUES

These are known to be primary sources of psychological hazards and risks. Several tools exist to assess organizational and structural factors that affect workplace PH&S. One of these, Guarding Minds at Work (Samra and Gilbert, 2011; produced by Simon Fraser University), assesses 12 factors considered scientifically necessary for a good workplace environment. While the factors are similar to those described by the World Health Organization (WHO),

Table 29.1 Psychogenic and Psychosocial Hazards Recognized by the World Health Organization

Job content	Lack of variety or short work cycles, fragmented or meaningless work, underuse of skills, high uncertainty, continuous exposure to people through work
Workload and work pace	Work overload or underload, machine pacing, high levels of time pressure, continually subject to deadlines
Work schedule	Shift working, night shifts, inflexible work schedules, unpredictable hours, long or unsociable hours
Control	Low participation in decision making, lack of control over workload, pacing, etc.
Environment and equipment	Inadequate equipment availability, suitability or maintenance; poor environmental conditions such as lack of space, poor lighting, excessive noise
Organizational culture and function	Poor communication, low levels of support for problem solving and personal development, lack of definition of, or agreement on, organizational objectives
Interpersonal relationships at work	Conflict, lack of social support, bullying, harassment
Role in organization	Role ambiguity, role conflict, and responsibility for people
Career development	Career stagnation and uncertainty, under promotion or over promotion, poor pay, job insecurity, low social value to work
Home–work interface	Conflicting demands of work and home, low support at home, dual career problems

Source: Leka and Cox, 2008

additional information and assessment forms are included in the Guarding Minds at Work website. Table 29.1 presents a list of recognized psychological hazards in the workplace, but this list is not comprehensive.

FINANCIAL CONSIDERATIONS

Financial considerations address the cost impact of PH&S issues in the workplace. Much of this information is available through analysis of insurance costs, absenteeism (direct and indirect costs) due to mental health concerns, group health care costs, EAP costs (see Chapter 28), and short- and long-term disability costs (see Chapter 24). Box 29.1 provides a template for estimating the cost of losses due to impaired mental health in the workplace.

DETERMINING THE ADVERSE IMPACT OF PH&S ISSUES ON EMPLOYEES

This is the fourth important area to help define employee and organizational needs. To ensure confidentiality, all data must be aggregated and anonymous. Useful sources of information are summarized at the end of this chapter.

Planning for Change

Planning should begin with a review of what already exists to address the psychological health issues of workers, because there is a wealth of information, much of it international.

Box 29.1 Template for Assessing Costs of Losses Associated with Impaired Mental Health in the Workplace

1. Extended/Group Health Care Costs
2. Drug claims
    2.1. Total, by major drug category
    2.2. Total claims per covered active employee
    2.3. Mental illness-related drug claims as a percentage of total drug claims
    2.4. Mental illness-related drug claims per covered active employee
    2.5. Number of mental illness-related drug claims plus those where a second drug is also being claimed for another ailment (co-morbidity)
3. Employee Assistance Costs
    3.1. Number of employees using the program for mental illness-related disorders
    3.2. Utilization as a percentage of total program users
    3.3. Number of cases referred to community-based treatment programs
    3.4. Number of high-risk mental illness cases
4. Absence Costs
    4.1. Lost workdays (paid and unpaid) per active employee
    4.2. Lost workdays (paid and unpaid) for mental illness-related disorders
    4.3. Lost workdays (paid and unpaid) as a percentage of total lost workdays per active employee
    4.4. Absence rates by type of ailment/disorder
    4.5. Average duration of absence
5. Replacement Worker Costs
    5.1. Number of replacement workers (fulltime equivalent) used per reporting period
    5.2. Total cost of replacement workers
    5.3. Cost of replacement workers as a percentage of total active payroll costs
6. Employee Turnover Rates Relating to Mental Health Disorders
7. Short and Long Term Disability Costs
    7.1. Number of short term disability claims related to mental health disorders
    7.2. STD claims as a percentage of total short term disability claims
    7.3. Number of long term disability claims related to mental health disorders
    7.4. LTD claims as a percentage of total long term disability claims
    7.5. Average duration of short/long term disability claims relating to mental disorders
    7.6. Cost per claim of short and long term mental health related disorders
8. Presenteeism Costs
    8.1. Actual output per worker as a percentage of targeted output per worker
    8.2. Quality of output (e.g., defect rates, customer feedback, etc.)
    8.3. Actual vs. targeted worker output percentage times the total active payroll cost
9. Other Useful Financial Metrics
    9.1. Health-related costs as a percentage of payroll
    9.2. Productive capacity measures

Source: "CFO Framework for Mental Health and Productivity", The Global Business and Economic Roundtable on Addiction and Mental Health. http://www. mentalhealthroundtable.ca/nov_07/CFO_Report_FINAL%20Nov%202007.pdf

Box 29.2 Template for Assessing Nonfinancial Adverse Impacts on the Organization

1. Audit results, if the audit includes questions on psychological health and safety.
2. Aggregate statistics from the organization's EAP provider.
3. Data on absence from the human resources department.
4. Aggregate statistics on the causes of worker visits to the occupational health centre.
5. Trade union grievances, reports, incidences, records of concerns, employee relations committee reports.
6. Joint health and safety committee reports, investigations, etc. (see Chapter 6).
7. Worker surveys, for example:
   7.1. Health risk appraisals, especially if the document referenced has sections related to depression, such as the Patient Health Questionnaire 9 (PHQ-9) and the Stress Satisfaction Offset Scale (SSOS) (both referenced at the end of this chapter).
   7.2. Job satisfaction surveys
   7.3. Stress surveys, targeting stress at work and at home.
8. Insurance company data, focusing on aggregate descriptions of the organization's disease profile, and relevant medications and pharmaceutical costs.
9. Workers' compensation records, especially frequency of "mental-mental" claims (see Chapter 26).

The experience of other countries in implementing effective remedial action should not be ignored. This review should include local and accessible (including online) programs and initiatives available to employees to assist them in coping with psychological hazards, work-related stress, and other issues of mental health, and the strategies in place to support workers with mental health problems.

A needs analysis needs to be performed for the specific workplace. The mental health aspects of the specific workplace, including policy, jobs, culture and values, current organizational changes, and access to mental health support and job accommodation, must be examined honestly, objectively, critically, and from the point of view of the worker rather than management. This task is usually very difficult for management. A consultant may be required for objectivity. Input from employees is, of course, essential.

These data from the needs analysis are then applied to the development of an action plan for risk reduction. The plan should set appropriate objectives and priorities given identified risks and hazards. They must be realistic, in keeping with the organization's concerns, resources, and priorities. The plan and its priorities should be reviewed and modified as changes occur within the workplace environment and processes, and as the workplace PH&S situation improves. The process should drive continuous improvement, while at the same time reaching out to offer assistance to workers experiencing concerns related to mental health.

A PH&S Program Committee, consisting of members from senior management, worker and union representatives, and "champions" of mental health issues (often workers who have experienced psychological health issues themselves) can be a key ingredient for success. The role and functions of the program committee include:

• Establishing, implementing, and maintaining effective strategies to identify psychological hazards and assess/reduce related risks.

- Consulting and communicating with stakeholders regarding the:
  - identification and elimination of work-related psychological hazards
  - assessment of related risks and implementation of reduction and control strategies.
- Communicating risk analysis results, program performance, and planned interventions to top management, workers, and worker representatives.
- Encouraging participation of employees in the Program.

Implementation: Intervention and Risk Reduction

Box 29.3 provides broad, general guidance for the basic elements of a psychologically healthful workplace.

The PH&S Program Committee (if the organization uses this modality) has the responsibility for overseeing and facilitating the risk management process. Prior to the implementation of the PH&S program, a company-wide awareness strategy is of great importance to ensure transparency of the process and recruit widespread involvement (engagement) of the workforce.

The PH&S program must be fully integrated into the overall culture of the organization and its daily operations, and not be just another "add on." Training for management personnel should include awareness of legal requirements, basic knowledge about PH&S and mental illness, the development of interpersonal skills, coaching and mentoring strategies, and access to resources within the organization and the community.

Initial implementation strategies should describe:

- Introduction to the program as part of the orientation of new employees and training for current employees.
- Crisis prevention and protective measures, including strategies for allowing employee input and warning (whistle-blowing) regarding issues such as discrimination, harassment, unfair treatment due to mental illness, etc.
- Emergency preparedness, and response.
- Competence and training for in-house emergency responders, peer support personnel, and program committee members.
- Communication and awareness initiatives:
  - within the organization, to ensure ongoing transparency of the program within the workplace.

Box 29.3 Psychological Elements Recognized to be Critical to the Mental Health of the Workforce

- Respect and appreciation
- Being listened to
- Freedom to speak up
- A sense of confidence and self worth
- Absence of chronic feelings of hostility and anger
- A sense of belonging to a meaningful and supportive work group
- Absence of chronic symptoms of distress, anxiety and depression
- Periods of relative calm and peace of mind.

Source: Health Canada, 2011

- with relevant emergency response services within the community and government authorities as appropriate.
- Management of change within the organization and the program.
- Documentation and records, including methodology and confidentiality.

Workplace primary prevention programs may include: confidential psychological health risk assessments, including the provision of referral advice; safe return to work programs that recognise the vulnerability of returning workers to psychological injury and stress; (dis)stress reduction programs; and management and workforce mental health awareness and training programs.

Strategies targeting workforce needs could include (as outlined in Great West Life, 2011):

- Facilitated access to mental health professionals and professional advice.
- Training of designated peer supporters within the workplace.
- Flexible work scheduling practices.
- Designation of a safe workplace advocate (ombudsman).

Existing mental health issues need to be addressed through initiatives such as:

- Training of line supervisors and management to identify and to approach workers who may be struggling with psychological issues.
- Appropriate accommodation and effective return-to-work strategies that acknowledge the vulnerability of all returning workers to potential psychological injury.
- Referral to peer support programs, either in-house or off-site, such as EAPs (see Chapter 28), Alcoholics Anonymous, post-traumatic stress disorder peer support groups, etc.

Implementation of interventions and initiatives is the crucial step in reducing risks. The action plan for risk reduction must be carefully and thoughtfully managed—its progress systematically monitored, recorded, and discussed within the Program Committee to identify when corrective action and changes need to take place. Ownership and active participation of managers, workers, and other stakeholders are essential for the success of the implementation process.

Evaluation and Corrective Action

The next step in the risk management process is the evaluation of the organization's status with respect to PH&S compared to the previous baseline evaluation and the objectives of the action plan. The goals of the evaluation are to determine both what has changed (whether the intervention had any impact on the concerns identified in the risk assessment) and whether the intervention was implemented effectively according to the plans developed to address specific, identified needs. This evaluation benefits the program and the organization in a number of ways: it drives continual improvement; it measures the effectiveness of the policy and the program; it promotes regular review to identify gaps and new opportunities for improvement; and it facilitates integration of the psychological health program into the organization's overall approach to occupational health and safety.

Any of the many available methodologies used to evaluate the PH&S program should relate to the initial assessment, the targets, and the objectives. Several evaluation tools can be used:

- Internal audits to identify strengths, ongoing challenges and gaps, and opportunities for improvement.
- Comparative review of documents used in risk assessment, as well as investigation and analysis of incidents, to gauge the progress.
- Surveys of management and workers, including those questionnaires used in the risk assessment process (pre-test/post-test methodology) to measure changes in workers' perceptions of mental health and well-being.

The evaluation tools should yield important information on the level of awareness of mental health, participation in and reaction to planned interventions, and the impact of the intervention on the health of employees. The determination of direct and indirect financial benefits, if feasible, will add strength to the evaluation process.

This process of evaluation feeds into a cycle of continuous improvement within the workplace. A secondary benefit is organizational learning through discussion during the evaluation process as well as communication of the results by the Program Committee to the management and employees. The organization should use the evaluation report as a basis for discussion and communication of recommendations, for incorporation into future risk management protocols, and for the (re)design of work organization and changes in workplace culture as part of the normal continuous improvement process.

Review and Continuous Improvement

Review is the final element of the systematic approach used by many standards. The review should articulate with cycles of audit and review for continuous improvement (see Chapter 17). It should cover the responsibilities and accountability of senior management and the program's conformity to the original policy approved by the Board of Directors.

Initiatives to address PH&S risks and work-related stress should not be viewed as stand-alone activities, but should be incorporated into daily business practices. In so doing, a continuous improvement cycle promoting a better psychological work environment will be supported.

Ongoing Challenges

PH&S is relevant to the core values underpinning organizational practices, and also represents an ethical responsibility for employers. Workplace mental health is a legal imperative, a proven business strategy, and demonstrates good corporate social responsibility. Leaders who recognize this can take advantage of the opportunities and benefits that arise from truly leading their organization towards a psychologically safe and mentally healthy workplace. Psychological risk management needs to be an integrated, systematic, and ongoing process that complements, and may be included within, the comprehensive occupational health program and the larger business context of the organization so that risks to workers' health can be monitored and managed effectively. This approach is especially important, given its relevance to subjective perceptions and the dynamic nature of the work environment that makes the ongoing assessment a critical necessity. It is also imperative that the assessment and management of psychological risks be considered when new processes are introduced to the workplace and/or when significant organizational change occurs (mergers, acquisitions, devolutions, lay-offs, closure). A healthy, productive workforce, a safe work environment, and a reputation as a great place to work all contribute to the bottom line results for which leaders are held accountable.

Recommended Reading and Resources

Risk Assessment Tools

Guarding Minds @ Work, *The 12 Psychosocial Risk Factors*. Available at: http://www.guardingmindsatwork. ca/info/risk_factors. Accessed May 2, 2011.

Guarding Minds at Work, *Psychosocial Risks – Employee Survey* (PSR-12). Available at: http:// www.viha.ca/NR/rdonlyres/BCA23E92-223A-4A86-A07C-D45B37B5815E/8564/ PHQ9PatientHealthQuestionnaireforDepression.pdf . Accessed April 18, 2012.

University of Washington, *Patient Health Questionnaire* (PHQ-9). Available at: http://steppingup. washington.edu/keys/documents/phq-9.pdf. Accessed May 2, 2011.

Strategic resources

American Psychological Association, *Workplace Mental Health*. Available at: http://www.apa.org/topics/ workplace/index.aspx. Accessed May 2, 2011.

American Psychiatric Foundation (2011) *Partnership for Workplace Mental Health*. Available at: http:// www.workplacementalhealth.org/. Accessed May 2, 2011.

Great West Life Insurance Company (Toronto), *Workplace Strategies for Mental Health: Accommodations that Work*. Available at: http://www.gwlcentreformentalhealth.com/display.asp?l1=175&l2=6&d=6. Accessed May 2, 2011.

Great West Life, *Workplace Strategies for Mental Health: 5 Elements of a Standard Management Approach*. Available at: http://workplacestrategiesformentalhealth.com/mhcc/5Elements.aspx. Accessed May 2, 2011.

Readings

Americans with Disabilities Act of 1990, as Amended. Available at: http://www.ada.gov/pubs/ada. htm. Accessed May 2, 2011.

Arnold, IMF. *A Leadership Framework for Advancing Mental Health*. 2009 presentation. The Mental Health Commission of Canada Leadership Initiative, http://www.mhccleadership.ca/. Accessed May 2, 2011.

Baynton MA (2010) Return to work: Strategies for engaging the employee in the return-to-work process when mental health is a factor. *Ontario Occup Health Nursing Assoc J*, Winter, pp. 16–20

British Standards Institute (2011) PAS 1010. *Guidance on the Management of Psychosocial Risks in the Workplace*, University of Nottingham, UK.

Business in the Community (2009) *Emotional Resilience Toolkit*. London UK, Department of Health.

Canadian Human Rights Commission (2008) *Policy and Procedures on the Accommodation of Mental Illness*. 2008. Available at: http://www.chrc-ccdp.ca/pdf/policy_mental_illness_en.pdf. Accessed May 2, 2011.

Centers for Disease Control and Prevention (CDC) *Workplace Health Promotion: Depression*. Available at: http://www.cdc.gov/niosh/programs/workorg/risks.html. Accessed May 2, 2011.

Funk M, Saraceno B (2005) *Mental Health Policies and Programmes in the Workplace*, World Health Organization. Available at: http://www.who.int/mental_health/policy/workplace_policy_ programmes.pdf . Accessed May 2, 2011.

Great West Life (2011) *Workplace Strategies for Mental Health*. Available at: http:// workplacestrategiesformentalhealth.com. Accessed May 2, 2011.

Great West Life. *Workplace Strategies for Mental Health: Elements and Priorities for Working Toward a Psychologically Safer Workplace*. Available at: http://workplacestrategiesformentalhealth.com/mhcc/5Elements. aspx. Accessed May 2, 2011.

Hardman TJ (1997) *Psychiatric Disabilities, Employment, and the Americans with Disabilities Act Background Paper*, Office of Technology Assessment. Available at: http://earthops.org/ada_ota.html. Accessed May 2, 2011.

Health Canada (2011) *Best Advice on Stress Risk Management in the Workplace*. Available at: http://www.hc-sc.gc.ca/ewh-semt/pubs/occup-travail/stress-part-1/foreword-avant_propos-eng.php.   Accessed May 2, 2011.

Industrial Accident Prevention Association. Strees and Satisfaction Offset Score. Available at www.iapa.ca/pdf/fd_ssos.pdf

Institute of Health Economics. Mental Health Economic Statistics. *Gaining a competitive edge Through Mental Health: The Business Case for Employers*. Available at www.ihe.ca/documents/AMHB_Statistics_pktbk07_eng.pdf   Accessed 20 January 2012

Institute of Work, Health and Organization (I-WHO) (2008) *Towards the Development of a European Framework for Psychological Risk Management at the Workplace*. Nottingham UK, I-WHO Publications.

Leka S, Cox T (eds) (2008) *PRIMA-EF / WHO: Guidance on the European Framework for Psychosocial Risk Management: A Resource for Employers and Worker Representatives*. Nottingham UK, I-WHO Publications.

Leka S, Cox T (eds) (2008) *The European Framework for Psychosocial Risk Management*, PRIMA-EF. Nottingham UK, I-WHO Publications. Available at: www.prima-ef.org. Accessed May 2, 2011.

Mental Health America (2010) *Workplace*. Available at: http://www.mentalhealthamerica.net/go/information/get-info/workplace. Accessed May 2, 2011.

Mental Health America (2011) Available at: www.mentalhealthamerica.net. Accessed May 2, 2011.

Mental Health Round Table (2007) *CFO Framework for Mental Health and Productivity*. Available at: http://www.mentalhealthroundtable.ca/nov_07/CFO_Report_FINAL percent20Nov percent202007.pdf . Accessed May 2, 2011.

Samra J, Gilbert M (2011) *What is Psychological Safety & Health?* Guarding Minds at Work. Available at: http://www.guardingmindsatwork.ca/info/safety_what. Accessed May 2, 2011.

Secretaries of State for the Department of Work and Pensions and the Department of Health (2009) *Working Our Way to Better Mental Health: A Framework for Action*. London UK, HM Stationery Office

Shain M (2010) *Tracking the Perfect Legal Storm*. The Shain Reports. Mental Health Commission of Canada. Available at: http://www.mentalhealthcommission.ca/SiteCollectionDocuments/Key_Documents/en/2009/Stress percent20at percent20Work percent20MHCC percent20V percent 203 percent20Feb percent202009.pdf. Accessed May 2, 2011.

US National Institute for Occupational Safety and Health. *Program Portfolio: Work Organization and Stress-Related Disorders*. Available at: http://www.cdc.gov/niosh/programs/workorg/risks.html. Accessed May 2, 2011.

Exhibit 29.1 An Example of a Corporate Policy Statement for Psychological Health

[Insert Employer, e.g. ABC Corporation] considers the psychological health and safety of its employees to be as important as all other aspects of health and safety. [Insert Employer] is committed to the prevention and resolution of psychological health and safety issues in its workplaces through the fair and equitable use of appropriate programs to assist employees towards the overall improvement of all aspects related to mental health in the workplace.

Source: Based on British Standards Institution, Publicly Available Specification (PAS) 1010:2011.

30 Health Promotion

Joel Bender and Sami A. Bég

Occupational health services typically begin by providing individual medical services for injured workers and then expand their scope of services (see Chapter 8). The next logical step in development of occupational health service lines (see Chapter 16) is the design and provision of health promotion or wellness programs that benefit the entire workforce and that benefit the employer through improved productivity, reduced health care and compensation costs, and enhanced employee well-being. These programs are centered on wellness, rather than illness, and so are complementary to employer-sponsored health insurance. However, their benefits go far beyond savings on health care costs because they directly affect the health, morale, and productivity of employees both on and off the job. These programs can yield a striking return on investment (see Chapter 18).

There are three basic elements to these programs:

- Prevention services, which include protection against disease risk (for example, by helping employees quit smoking) and screening for disease (secondary prevention).
- Health promotion, which is an approach to changing health-related behavior through education, psychological motivation, and support in the social environment.
- Case management, which is an approach to supporting employees with health issues through on-site monitoring (for example, blood pressure checks), facilitating and providing support for adherence to medical treatment (as by diabetes care), and education.

The most popular name for these programs in the private sector has become "wellness," supplanting "worksite health promotion," which was popular in the 1990s when the emphasis was more narrowly on fitness and health education. However, some self-insured companies use "wellness" as a euphemism for case management, so it is important to look beyond the name at the actual program components.

Health promotion is quickly becoming one of the primary defenses for employers against rising health care costs. Health insurance premiums have been rising 8 to 14 percent per year since 2000, and at least prior to the recent recession, inflation and changes in workers' earnings had been increasing around 3 to 4 percent. In addition, an increasing proportion of the cost of health care has been shifted onto employees in the form of copayments, uncompensated services, and out-of-pocket expenses. Both employees and their employers are being squeezed by the price of health care, creating a favorable, even enthusiastic, environment for the initiation of health promotion programs. The right worksite strategies can be very effective and lead to real cost savings for businesses. Some worksite health promotion programs have been shown to reduce absence, health care costs and disability/ workers' compensation costs by more than 25 percent.

However, the value of health promotion and wellness programs is not universally accepted. Employees are often cautious about participating in such programs offered by employers, particularly with respect to confidentiality. Organized labor may view such programs as a diversion to gain the support of workers without making concessions on fundamental issues such as wages, hours, working conditions, and autonomy on the job. Managers wonder whether supporting them is an effective use of company resources. Occupational health professionals understand their importance for an individual's health, but are reluctant to see support for them getting in the way of programs to ensure worker health and safety. Health services researchers point out that fitness programs, in particular, are generally most popular with employees who need them the least and are usually unavailable to or unpopular with the workers who need them the most.

Even so, where such programs have been successfully implemented, employees and employers alike have generally come to believe that they are very helpful and appropriate. Today, the views of organized labor are changing because health care costs have now become a competitive issue in the survival of employers. They have also become very popular among employees themselves, since they promise a better quality of life and the benefits of a healthy lifestyle. What the employer perceives as increased productivity and the insurance carrier perceives as demand reduction is perceived by the employee as an improved quality of life, less illness, and feeling better.

Health Promotion Planning

The aim of a health promotion program is to influence the health attitudes of individual employees so they will make personal choices each day that will lead to a more positive and healthy lifestyle. This necessarily requires that the organization change, too, and commit itself to a long-term program to support behavior change among its employees.

Specific objectives should be clearly stated and made known to all potential participants. These may include:

- Support the organization in creating a healthful environment in which employees are supported in making safe and healthy choices.
- Help employees to adopt and maintain a more physically active lifestyle.
- Help employees to adopt and maintain proper eating habits that optimize nutritional status and weight.
- Help employees to stop smoking.
- Help employees to eliminate or dramatically decrease alcohol and drug abuse.
- Help employees cope with ordinary and unexpected life stresses.
- Help employees learn about common diseases and how to prevent or minimize their impact.
- Provide comprehensive medical assessments.
- Help employees learn important health-related skills, such as cardiopulmonary resuscitation (CPR) and first aid.
- Empower employees with knowledge, a positive attitude toward health change, tools to change their personal disease risk, and health-related habits that they can take home and do for themselves.

Successful health promotion programs have the support of senior management and take a comprehensive approach to wellness. Such an approach starts with an understanding that the lifestyle behaviors of individuals need to be viewed from within the prevailing culture in the organization. For any health promotion program to be successful, individual efforts to improve health need to be supported by a culture that values wellness within the organization. Without this culture, improvements in behaviors are not sustainable. Creating a culture of wellness within an organization supports employees in making better choices and adopting behaviors that will improve their health, vitality, and productivity in the short and long term. Nothing is more important to creating this culture than commitment from executives to make this an integral part of the organization's mission and sharing this vision with all the employees. There should be a written policy regarding health of employees and the operations of the health promotion program, which includes protection for confidential health information.

Along with dedicated leadership from executives, success of a health promotion program depends on its design and implementation. There is a logical sequence to implementing a health promotion program:

Start with an Assessment of the Organization

A worksite assessment is a prerequisite to all other steps necessary to building a comprehensive, successful health promotion program. A worksite assessment is necessary in order to understand the existing strengths and weaknesses of the organization and its capacity to create a culture of wellness. Assessments can be longer or shorter, as needed, and cover various topics depending on the exact needs of the organization. In addition to gathering information about the challenges facing an organization, it also helps identify potential opportunities for the organization to improve the health and well-being of its employees. Comparing the responses from senior leadership, mid-level management, and other classes of employees can provide insights into the current level of commitment at all levels of the organization and the challenges that are coming. For example, management may think there are clearly defined wellness policies while the rest of the organization may not even be aware of their existence. Table 30.1 is an example of a short assessment that can provide insight into an organization.

Planning

There are numerous books and articles in the literature on how to plan health promotion programs. The most universally accepted template is the so-called "PRECEDE/PROCEED" model developed by health education specialist Lawrence Green in the 1970s, which was part of the revolution in thinking that led to health promotion. This model proposes eight sequential phases in every health project, from assessment to evaluation. These phases are outlined in Box 30.1.

In planning for health promotion programs, sustainability is key. They cannot be so expensive, onerous, or staff-intensive that they will be cancelled or cut back at the first sign of fiscal restraint. A health promotion program that only lasts for a short time creates frustration and loses trust with employees, and fosters an attitude among managers that "we tried that and it didn't work."

Table 30.1 A Short Organizational Assessment for Assessing the Culture of Health

#	Question	Yes	No
	Points	1	0
1	There are official health and wellness policies		
2	Management actively supports and participates in wellness programs and initiatives		
3	Supervisors are required to support wellness programs and initiatives		
4	Senior leadership briefs the staff on wellness initiatives at least twice a year		
5	There is an official wellness committee that meets at least monthly		
6	Employees are encouraged to volunteer as "wellness champions"		
7	Worksite is tobacco free indoors		
8	Worksite is tobacco free outdoors on company premises		
9	Company provides incentives for non-tobacco users or those who quit tobacco		
10	Employees are granted use of at least 15 minutes of work time/flex time per day for participation in wellness activities		
11	Worksite formally supports physical fitness by such things as promoting stair use, walking clubs, through signage, announcements etc.		
12	Job related ergonomics program is available		
13	Company offers onsite, indoor exercise facilities or offers discounted memberships to off-site exercise facilities		
14	Company coordinates a company-wide intramural sports activity at least once a year		
15	Worksite offers healthy choices in its cafeteria and/or in vending machines		
16	Healthier items are clearly labeled/identified for employees		
17	Worksite has a microwave and a refrigerator to encourage employees to bring their own lunch		
18	Company offers healthy food choices at meetings and functions		
19	Worksite has a monthly company-sponsored or brown-bag group luncheon which involves short talks and presentations from employees or invited guests		
20	Company makes water available at no cost to office and field workers		
21	Hand washing is encouraged and promoted		
22	Job-related occupational health and safety training is provided		
23	Employee Assistance Program is available to employees		
24	Worksite has bike racks or storage and/or encourages car pooling		
25	The company offers a health promotion program, including labs and biometrics, to all employees at no cost		
	Total		

If your worksite scored:
20+   You are well on your way to a culture of health and prevention
11-19   There is room for improvement
10 or less Get busy!

Implementing the Plan

Once the assessment is complete and the data have been analyzed, the staff or consultants tasked with designing the health promotion program can start developing goals, allocating resources, and adopting the most appropriate strategies and interventions. Customizing the program to address the specific needs of the employees and the employer helps ensure that the program is built on a strong foundation that is widely accepted and self-sustaining.

Box 30.1 Outline of the PRECEDE/PROCEED Model for Health Promotion Planning

PRECEDE (Assessment and Planning)

1. Social "diagnosis" (assessment of the culture of wellness).
2. Epidemiological, Behavioral, and Environmental "diagnosis" (health issues and needs assessment)
    2.1. Epidemiological "diagnosis" (what data exist on the health of the workforce and the communities from which they come; from these data, what are the principal health problems in terms of prevalence, disability, absence from work, chronic disease, health care costs).
    2.2. Behavioral surveys (what health-related behaviors are related to these health issues: e.g. tobacco use in young men in a given community might not be adequately reflected by smoking rates, because of the high prevalence of snuff dipping).
    2.3. Environmental "diagnosis" (what factors in the consumer or personal environment affect these health issues: e.g. availability of nutritious foods at the food service, access to fitness facilities).
3. Educational and Ecological "diagnosis" (what knowledge or motivation does the employee need to commit themselves to a healthier lifestyle; what social factors impede or facilitate such commitment).
4. Administrative and policy "diagnosis" (what organizational structures, barriers, policies or procedures are impediments to healthy living and working).

PROCEDE (Implementation and Evaluation)

5. Implementation (there may be various subphases of implementation, such as "roll out" when the program begins, maintenance, successive waves of innovation and novelty to create new interest, additional services or features, and "wind-up" when the program is over).
6. Process evaluation (measures whether the steps and procedures in the program are being implemented as planned, consistently, and at a high level of quality).
7. Process evaluation based on leading indicators (measures impact on intermediate steps, such as quitting smoking, adherence to medication, fitness).
8. Outcome evaluation (measures changes in outcomes in the longer term, such as frequency of hospital admissions, new health conditions, health care costs).

This PRECEDE/PROCEED model is only a template, adapted from Green and Kreuter (2005). Persons with responsibility for health promotion planning are advised to familiarize themselves with the extensive literature on the subject.

Sources: Adapted, with modifications, from: Green LW, Kreuter M (2005) *Health Promotion Planning: An Educational and Ecological Approach.* New York, McGraw Hill.

Creation of a "wellness committee" to oversee the program is an effective way for an employer to create a culture of health and wellness. Senior management can create the initial policies and then recruit individuals for this new leadership role in the organization. The exact number on the committee is determined by the size of the organization and results of the organizational assessment. Effective wellness committees generally meet at least monthly and are comprised of individuals from different sections of the organization (human resources, management, frontline employees, etc.). Having the committee rotate new members in every 12 months helps to broaden support, prevent fatigue, and contribute to creating a culture of health and wellness at the worksite.

As the program is launched, employees are asked to fill out an individual health assessment to determine adverse lifestyle risks, level of knowledge about wellness, readiness to change, and personal engagement. A health risk assessment (HRA) together with early detection/screening through basic biometrics (body mass index, blood pressure, lipid profile, and glucose), are recommended for a comprehensive health promotion program. Once individual health risks are identified, programs to maintain or improve health can be instituted. Although organizations may emphasize different action plans, core components of a well planned health promotion program include: tobacco cessation, physical activity, nutrition, stress management, and preventive screenings.

Given that four of the top ten most expensive health conditions to US employers—heart disease, cancer, pulmonary disease, and diabetes—are largely preventable, each wellness initiative needs to pay close attention to weight management, nutrition, exercise, and smoking cessation to address the high cost drivers. A comprehensive program should also address topics such as ergonomics and back pain prevention and management, substance abuse, and even maternal and infant health topics.

Responsiveness and Programming

Over time, new services can be phased in either as part of a master plan or in response to the desires or needs of employees. The health promotion program should therefore be a living, dynamic institution. Most employers find it easiest to begin with simple measures, such as lunchtime educational sessions, health fairs, and one-on-one screening tests. Over time, services can be expanded in scope and sophistication. The best way to describe this is by an example.

Figure 30.1 summarizes a proposed plan for expansion of a health promotion program serving a group of 10,000 workers involved in the banking industry at three sites, all close together and mutually accessible by van service. The in-house occupational health program already offered a health screening service for cardiovascular risk factors and individual consultation on diet and risk modification. An on-site fitness center at the headquarters location was not integrated into this program. The plan proposed to phase in services over five to eight years, starting with a health risk assessment (HRA) using one of many questionnaire instruments, most of them proprietary, for assessing individual health. This would be combined with the Work Limitations Questionnaire, a standard tool for measuring presenteeism and health-related impediments to productivity. The two together would provide data on individual progress, allow analysis of productivity changes by disease or risk category, and support program evaluation.

Over the next few years, the program was proposed to expand incrementally, as staff became available, first into the major cardiovascular and behavioral risk factors, and later diabetes, and then to individualized wellness programs targeting non-cardiovascular conditions known to cause the most ill health and greatest loss of productivity among working populations (migraine, depression, asthma and allergies, irritable bowel syndrome, and arthritis). Eventually it was expected that this program would save more than enough in health care costs to fund its own operations.

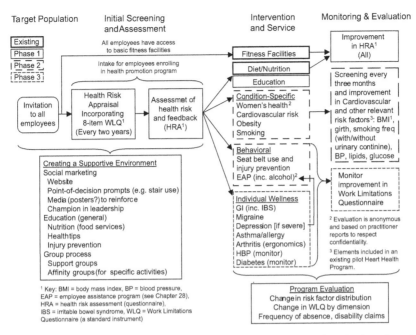

Figure 30.1 Plan for the development of a health promotion program, showing phasing of services and use of health risk assessment for both individual and program evaluation

Health Promotion and Wellness Program Components

Health promotion programs may choose to emphasize one or a few program components. Those serving very large employers may incorporate all of the major components and may initiate specialized programs for their particular workforce. Box 30.2 lists many of the typical components of a health promotion program.

Box 30.2 Typical Components of a Health Promotion Program

Health education	Smoking	Pulmonary function testing
Cancer prevention	Occupational hazards	Weight control
Common minor illnesses	Back care (prophylactic)	Weight monitoring
Heart disease	Health fairs	Stress reduction
Cardiopulmonary resuscitation	Preventive medicine	Breast cancer
Mental health	Screening activities	Prescriptive exercise regimes
	Intervention	Colon cancer
Diabetes	Activities	Referral to physician
Nutrition	Hypertension screening	Physical conditioning
Allergies	Smoking cessation	Aerobic activity
Stress	Diabetes screening	Fitness center
Family health	Dietary interventions	Strength and stretch
Substance abuse	Cardiovascular risk factors	Sports medicine
Automotive safety	Back care (rehabilitation)	Depression

Programs need to address the needs of all employees at a given workplace, regardless of age, gender, ethnicity, culture, and physical capacity. For example, young and hip workers in creative industries may be concerned with the (very real) health risks of piercing. Some immigrant groups (for example, Chinese recently arrived from rural areas) may wish to approach health-related behavior within their own health care traditions. Certain ethnic groups may prefer nutrition education pertinent to the foods they actually eat. Some, for example Arab women from traditional backgrounds, may enthusiastically embrace programs relevant to their needs but only when provided by culturally acceptable providers (other women). Individuals with disabilities should not be defined by their disability, and their needs and issues should be included in these programs; many nondisabled employees have disabled family members.

Some health promotion programs rotate messages and in so doing keep health education fresh. Box 30.3 is an example of a program that rotated messages on a daily basis to maintain employee engagement.

Health Education

Health education forms the backbone of the health promotion program and each program component. It is concerned with teaching employees the essentials of a healthy lifestyle, such as walking or running, sound nutrition practices, relaxation exercises, and the consequences of smoking and alcohol abuse. This process can start with something as simple as designating a health theme to each workday. These practices emphasize the importance of prevention to the organization, serving as a simple reminder to practice the culture of health and wellness on a regular basis. Box 30.3 provides some examples.

Employees should also learn about common medical problems, how to keep themselves and their families healthy, and how to prepare for a visit with their physician or other care giver. Content should cover basic knowledge on how the health problems are detected, how they develop, and how conditions can be prevented or at least controlled. Topics of most consistent interest include cancer (all forms), heart disease, back and other musculoskeletal problems, sports medicine, diabetes, HIV/AIDS, psychological stress, and mental disorders (especially depression). Different topics may appeal to different groups.

At the time of a general educational session, or later as a special event such as a health fair, it is often useful to conduct screening tests for hypertension, diabetes, and other conditions easily detectable in a health fair setting.

Beyond the informative aspect of health education, attention must be given to the psychological principles which motivate people to comply with sound health practices or those which prompt individuals to take unnecessary risks that jeopardize their health. Simple information transfer is not enough. Lectures on health alone, seldom change behavior, and general education appropriate for patients with a disease (such as diabetes) is not always a helpful topic for general health education in a workplace setting (unless specifically targeted to a patient group). The health education component within a workplace health promotion program must be designed to fit the characteristics of the workplace population (age, sex, class, education, health status, language, cultural sensitivity, etc.), the most important health problems in the community as perceived by the workers, the most significant health problems actually present in the community, and the goals to be attained in changing health-related behavior. It is best to get feedback from employees before introducing a topic. For example, if the worksite is composed mostly of women, women's health topics such as screening for breast cancer should normally be featured, but some families and ethnic groups may be reluctant to talk about cancer, or about women's bodies unless the group is limited to women.

Box 30.3 Examples of Rotating Daily Activities

Move it Monday

This Monday, make sure you are active for at least 30–60 minutes. Start a walking club at work, use your lunch break to exercise outside or use free weights at your desk. This is also the day to walk to your co-workers' offices at least a couple of times during the day instead of the usual email or phone call. Once home, get the remainder of your minutes by walking in your neighborhood while also getting to know your neighbors.

Take 15 Tuesday

Let Tuesday be the day that reminds you to take 15 minutes for yourself every day. Sit back in your chair, close your eyes and think of or listen to something soothing. Take a few deep breaths in and out slowly. Concentrate on being very calm and content. Don't worry about the world around you. Just relax. And encourage others, too.

Wednesday Weed-Out

This is the day when you "weed out" any unhealthy food items and other unhealthy habits from your routine. This means no soft drinks (diet or otherwise), no unhealthy snacks or fast food, no smoking (if you do) all day. Encourage co-workers and even family to do the same. See someone in the company walking with a soda on a Wednesday? Throw a yellow flag, or just smile.

Take the Stairs Thursday

This day is "take the stairs day" for all those healthy and able. By taking the stairs, you are adding a simple calorie-burning activity to your daily routine, which will provide a great health return over time. Try to get into the habit of also taking the stairs on other days of the week if you can. The elevator may be more convenient but, remember, hard work pays off. No sign-up or membership fees required.

Fruit and Salad Friday or Far Away Friday

Why not make Friday your fruit and salad day? A day when you only have those colorful fruits and green vegetables. Start the day with a high-fiber cereal with fruit for breakfast; have veggie soup or salad for lunch; and then a vegetarian dish for dinner. Or make Friday the day you park your car further away than usual to get the extra steps in on your way to work. Maybe you can even do both on Fridays!

Tobacco Cessation

One of the most cost-effective wellness initiatives is to help workers stop smoking and quit using other tobacco products. Methods range from individual counseling to group sessions, special aversion methods, pharmacotherapy, nicotine replacement, and creating smoke-free work environments.

A designated task force can be very helpful for policy development and to oversee the process of a worksite becoming tobacco-free. The task force should include top management and workers, and include nonsmokers, smokers, and former smokers. The task force can start by surveying employees about their knowledge and concerns so issues can be addressed before the policy goes into effect.

A clear, simple policy is the most effective and should include enforcement that is consistent with other personnel policies and disciplinary procedures. A goal of a tobacco-free worksite needs to be announced well in advance of implementation, ideally a year before, and come through a letter from the chief executive officer (who should never be seen smoking). Communications can be distributed to educate workers about the reasons for the policy by using resources like paycheck inserts, posters, or company newsletters. Similarly, leadership should continue to inform associates, contractors, vendors, and guests of the policy to be implemented and the exact date it will go into effect. Contact information about other available programs should also be provided through signage, emails, and newsletters. Providing smoking cessation assistance to smokers who try to quit as a result of the policy will increase acceptance of the policy. It is also the best way to maximize the potential health benefits and cost savings of the tobacco-free policy.

Other smoking cessation opportunities may include:

- Smoking cessation educational action plans, online or paper-based.
- Live smoking cessation education classes at the worksite offered several times during the year; these can be done in collaboration with the American Lung Association's Freedom From Smoking program.
- Assessment of the company's health plan options and incentives or discounts offered for smoking cessation products.
- Evaluate and implement, as needed, other programs such as Smokefree.gov (smoke-free text messaging program, step-by-step quit guide, Healthy Monday Challenge, etc.) and National Quitline Number (1-800-QUITNOW).

The task force can also work with staff to post "no smoking" signs, remove ashtrays and tobacco vending machines, and remove smoking waste receptacles as the company gets closer to the chosen Tobacco Free Worksite date. Senior management and wellness leaders need to host a kick-off event on the day the policy starts.

Physical Activity

Physical fitness is an important part of most health promotion programs. It focuses on aerobic exercise, muscle strength, endurance, and joint flexibility. Strategies include individual and group programs that can be modified for gender, age, and physiological capability. Simple physical activity programs can be instituted at the worksite without the need for much oversight or additional expense. These may include promoting walking clubs or encouraging stair use. Creating an environment conducive to physical health where individuals can network and organically grow various programs is essential. For example, by encouraging individuals to learn of one another's health interests through company websites or newsletters may lead them to join others with similar interests for group sports. Linking some of the activities to charity events, such as a heart walk or run, may also prove popular and encourage employees to participate.

Enrolling company-sponsored teams at various physical activity events may promote competition and serve as a great team building exercise. Companies often hold an official annual outdoor picnic with a sports theme and get employees involved. Participation in fitness activities and sports programs provides a regularly scheduled opportunity for conditioning and the sense of belonging to a group, improving the likelihood of success. However, the primary focus for workplace fitness programs should not be oriented to athletes, because this excludes many other workers who can benefit from participation. Persons of normal strength and coordination should be able to set reasonable goals and attain them in any setting. Fitness programs should be fun and should build morale among employees, not rivalry.

Formal exercise programs need direct or indirect supervision by qualified fitness counselors. Most of these programs require participants to have a medical clearance before entry. The medical screen can be done by questionnaire by a fitness counselor but any candidate who has a medical problem should undergo a detailed review by a physician. These programs should accommodate individuals with physical disabilities. Successful physical fitness programs range from state-of-the-art company-owned fitness facilities or private to public clubs where memberships are subsidized or given discounted rates. All fitness activities should incorporate regular tests for measuring progress and to provide encouragement. Some companies require validation of exercise through mobile devices, especially when the company provides substantial health care premium rebates or makes significant contributions to health savings accounts.

Nutrition

This component may entail individual or group classes for nutrition or weight counseling. Special attention is usually placed on the importance of healthy diets to reduce risks for cardiovascular disease, diabetes, and obesity. It is generally preferable to have a qualified nutritionist to provide the counseling and teaching. However, certified wellness coaches and nurses can provide dietary advice that is supplemented with pamphlets, bulletins, or web-based resources from recognized authorities in nutrition. Healthy options should be offered in vending machines and cafeterias. If it is not possible to replace all items with healthier ones, the food choices should be labeled so that the employee has the opportunity to make a knowledgeable selection. A kitchen at the worksite with refrigerators and a microwave will also encourage employees to bring healthier lunches to work as opposed to fast food. Likewise, healthy meals and snacks should be offered at various company special events.

Stress Management

This component focuses on providing support for employees to cope with ordinary day-to-day stress and occasional unusual stressful events. It should not attempt to provide individual counseling or psychotherapy in depth, as this is more appropriately dealt with by an employee assistance program. Care must be exercised in choosing qualified resource persons in this area. Certified psychologists or social workers with specialized training tend to be the best qualified and most credible in this role. All too often, however, persons with questionable credentials present themselves as experts.

Short one-or-two-hour group sessions can be very effective. These sessions should be cheerful and informative. They can be enhanced by distribution of individual questionnaires to determine the levels of stress the participant is experiencing. Web-based questionnaires are also being used to indicate the presence of significant stress or depression and then direct individuals to appropriate resources. Longer sessions of one to three days duration are useful but require considerable commitment of time and resources.

If the employer is unable to provide these more elaborate options, 15–20 minutes of daily meditation may prove very beneficial. This can be supplemented or replaced with simple things such as disconnecting oneself from the day to day routines—phones, emails, interruptions, etc.—for just 15–20 minutes around the middle of the day. Similarly, a "quiet room" can be designated at the worksite where anyone can go to take advantage of a few minutes of rest and solitude, especially for individuals prone to migraines. Rest and meditation can provide real, comprehensive benefits which create a favorable work atmosphere in the company.

Preventive Medicine

Americans receive only about half of the preventive services recommended by agencies such as the US Preventive Services Task Force—a finding that highlights the need to incorporate prevention services into worksite health promotion programs. Employer-based preventive services are typically limited to screening for common medical disorders, lifestyle risk factors, and intervention activities which supplement but do not substitute for personal health care. There is usually a strong emphasis on reducing cholesterol levels and cardiovascular fitness training. The emphasis is on primary prevention, to reduce disease incidence in the working population, and secondary prevention, the early detection of disease and referral for care. Reminders to complete other screenings, such as getting a colonoscopy or a mammogram, are also an integral part of health promotion. Reducing risk factors for future health problems is more easily accomplished in an integrated health promotion program. In such programs group spirit, constant encouragement and feedback, and support network make compliance easier to achieve than on an individual basis.

As part of a health promotions program, some employers sponsor voluntary health evaluations for employees through on-site clinics. These examinations should not be confused with fitness for duty evaluations and any clinical opinion formed by the examining physician must not affect the employment status of the participating worker. They are best performed by physicians who are experienced in preventive medicine. The outcome of this examination is strictly confidential. No fitness-to-work judgment is made. The content of the examination should be based on the age, lifestyle, present and past health status, and family history, as well as the working conditions and requirements of the job. The frequency of the examination is based on clinical judgment relating to the age, outcome, and desire of the employee. Company policy sets the maximum frequency and the cost of the examination.

Safety, CPR and First Aid Training

This component dovetails nicely with employee safety training programs. Employees can be taught CPR, use of automated external defibrillator devices (AEDs), and at least basic first aid in order to create a "first line of defense" at home and in the community. When employees have heart attacks while at work, other workers are usually highly motivated to learn CPR for many weeks and this provides an opportunity for training. Integrating CPR into the wellness program is also a good way of getting employees leveraging efforts to drive a positive change of culture within the organization because it fosters a sense of "all for one" and "watching one another's back."

Ergonomics

Educating employees on ergonomics is an essential component of occupational health. Ergonomics is the science of fitting workplace conditions and job demands to the capabilities of the working population. Effective and successful "fits" promote high productivity, avoidance of illness and injury risks, and increased satisfaction at home and in the workforce. This requires assessing work-related factors that may pose a risk of musculoskeletal disorders and making recommendations to alleviate them. Ergonomic programs can be integrated with health promotion or programs intended to address other workplace hazards.

Incentives

Employers have sometimes made participation in health promotion programs attractive through the use of small gift cards and other rewards. However, low participation rates and the continued increases in health care costs have gradually led employers to link participation in these programs to stronger and more substantial rewards, such as health insurance discounts and, in some cases, even health insurance eligibility. Participation in health promotion programs may not be obligatory, but as incentives have grown participation has become a financial necessity for many employees. With small cash rewards and gift cards, wellness programs had achieved participation rates from 10 to 20 percent of the population, but with the introduction of the health insurance premium incentives, many employers are seeing participation rates between 50 and 90 percent. As the outcomes of these programs continue to improve, their popularity is unlikely to diminish anytime soon. Other than insurance premiums, some organizations may also link participation to contributions to the employee's Health Savings Account, eligibility for tuition reimbursement, or even discounts to gyms and fitness coaches.

Human beings respond to short-term rewards more strongly than the anticipation of long-term benefits. A small incentive to participate, even of nominal value such as a T-shirt, motivates people disproportionately to its cost and creates a bond that improves adherence to the program and ultimate success. That is why the provision of incentives for motivation should not be considered "bribes" for doing what the employee ought to be doing anyway. They are motivational reinforcements that act on the hard-wired human brain to overcome resistance or indifference to participate.

Not all incentives need to be monetary. In fact, recognizing individual effort is central to creating a culture of wellness. An annual awards ceremony where individuals and teams are acknowledged can be great motivation for everyone. Certificates and small tokens of appreciation at such events can go a long way toward encouraging everyone—participants and non-participants—to realize the importance of health promotion. Senior executives should host such events and make them an integral part of a successful organization.

Evaluation

Evaluation of the impact of worksite health promotion programs is an essential part of their management. Evaluation supports future planning and adaptation, financial investment, employee relations, and health insurance planning. Some of the important parameters to quantify include participation rates, overall satisfaction, changes in behavior, and biometric measures (such as weight, body mass index or BMI, skin caliper measurements).

Even when participation rates are high, it is always important to assess employee satisfaction with the program regularly and to implement visibly as many of the recommendations as possible. Employees need to feel that their opinion is respected and that they have choices. Lack of autonomy erodes the morale of the organization in the long run. Programs that are unpopular or poorly attended should be phased out or replaced with more responsive programs.

The ultimate goals of a health promotion program are to improve the employee's health status and enjoyment of life, reduce health care costs through reductions in health risks, and improve productivity. Research shows that productivity is improved, sometimes dramatically, when the workforce becomes healthier. Absence decreases and employees are more productive in their jobs.

Studies have shown that when health risks are reduced, reductions in health care costs follow. Dee Eddington at the University of Michigan has been a pioneer in developing a robust, simplified methodology for such studies. Evaluating the impact the program has had on health risk reduction can be very simple. Just counting the number of high risks an employee has predicts future health status and productivity. Both for that individual and for the group as a whole. First, the individual health risks for various measures to be evaluated need to be defined. These include alcohol use, blood pressure, BMI, cholesterol, fasting blood sugar, physical activity level, and nutrition habits. For example, for blood sugar, high risk is defined as fasting blood sugar that is ≥ 126 mg/dL (7.0mmol/liter) and if an individual moves from a fasting blood glucose level of 126 or above to less than 126 (which is still significantly elevated), it means the person has had one high risk reduction. Similarly, these can be evaluated in terms of the net decrease over time for all the risks measured. In other words, the percentage of those who reported the particular individual health risk in the baseline year who did not have the risk in the follow-up year. Typically a total of 15 risk factors are selected and once high risk cutoff for each is defined, as in the example of fasting blood sugar, the number of high risks are counted for each individual to also help categorize them overall as low (0–2 high risks), medium (3–4 high risks) or high risk (5 or more high risks).

A typical company might have 64 percent of employees at low-risk status, 26 percent at medium-risk status, and 10 percent at high-risk status. A "Markov Chain" analysis is a mathematical technique to examine longitudinal data from the same individuals and is an essential part of the evaluation of any sophisticated health promotion program, but description of this method is beyond the scope of this chapter. Such an analysis will address the status of individuals who remain in a specific risk group and also help in reviewing the risk transitions of others.

Return on Investment Calculations

While there is no industry standard to calculate the return on investment (ROI) on a health promotion program, there are three sources of ROI that one can use in assessing the ROI of such programs (see also Chapter 18):

- Health care costs contained (averted costs through health risk reduction).
- Productivity savings (absence/presenteeism costs lower through health risk reduction).
- Health care costs savings (medical/pharmacy claims lower through health risk reduction).

The first category includes savings that can be attributed to such things as identifying a pre-diabetic (e.g. a person with "metabolic syndrome") and coaching him or her on how to prevent development of adverse outcomes (diabetes or heart disease) and the costly claims associated with such chronic conditions. Such items would not show up on a claims-based savings analysis, yet could be included in an assessment of an ROI from wellness.

The last category includes cost savings that will be seen on a claims analysis. While the first two categories can be leading indicators included in calculating savings early on in the program, a claims-based analysis will show reduction in health care costs as a lagging indicator and should be measured in years or even decades. (See Chapter 17 for a discussion of indicators.)

Experts agree that it takes a minimum of three years before one can begin to see the initial stabilized health care cost savings through a claims-based analysis. Several changes need to take place before an impact on claims is seen: behavior changes, biometric changes, the behavior change consolidated and sustained, health risk changes, and health care cost changes. Prior to this, claims may actually increase because more individuals may be taking advantage of screenings and having additional visits to the physicians for follow-up on medical conditions that were not previously recognized. These individuals may also need medications or surgical interventions for the newly diagnosed conditions. However, observing increased costs in the first few years is actually evidence that the health promotion program is effective in detecting disease early and preventing future complications, both of which are far less costly than unmanaged disease.

Outsourcing Health Promotion

It is often more practical for employers to contract for health promotion services rather than staff them in-house. This creates an opportunity for occupational health services and for consultants to become vendors of such services. There are also practical advantages to contract services, as some employees may be more willing to participate and to share personal health information when they are dealing with an independent, outside entity and not their employer.

Some vendors may also offer additional tools and resources not otherwise available. For example, some wellness companies use the latest in technologies, such as Global Positioning Systems through tracking devices placed on the shoes or cell phones to have members document their walking or jogging. Smart phones are a further means to directly communicate with the individual, and many wellness companies may even offer a smart phone app to further engage the member through reminders, trackers, or a calorie counter.

An internal team needs to evaluate outside vendors and select the one that is a best fit. Box 30.4 lists important considerations when selecting the company to deliver health promotion services. These items can be used by an employer or in-house occupational health service in evaluating a candidate for contract services or it can be used as a checklist by occupational health services to determine when they are ready to provide such services.

The employer and the contractor must mutually agree to specific metrics for assessing the success of the program. These may include participation and engagement rates, definition of risks determining how reductions assessed, and defining performance guarantees. It will be necessary to refine these measurement methodologies over time if needed, and to document all stipulated business requirements specified in the contract. If the employer also expects and wants to explore additional economic impacts, then absence rates, turnover rates, health insurance costs, accident rates, and other measures of employee productivity should be made available, and well documented before the program begins. It may advantageous to contract with an outside research agency to conduct an independent analysis of the program's impact.

Box 30.4 Criteria for the Evaluation of Contract Health Promotion Services

1. General
    1.1. Compliant with HIPAA and GINA regulations for data privacy and security online.
    1.2. Accreditation through a national agency such as the National Committee for Quality Assurance (NCQA) or URAC (formerly the Utilization Review Accreditation Commission, now known by its initials).
    1.3. Provide a robust health website accessible to all employees, with coaching available to moderate and high-risk individuals.
    1.4. Health consultations provided by qualified and trained health educators who use scientifically-proven behavior change models.
    1.5. Experience with clients of similar size with more than a few years servicing such accounts and willing to put fees at risk.
2. Health Risk Assessment (HRA)
    2.1. Online HRA assessment (many proprietary questionnaires available; contractor should have deep experience with at least one that has been validated in the published literature and demonstrate the analytical capability to interpret individual and group results).
    2.2. Tobacco usage and alcohol consumption.
    2.3. Nutritional status.
    2.4. Exercise and physical activity.
    2.5. Biometric measures including blood pressure, cholesterol, blood glucose, height and weight, body mass index (BMI), skin caliper measurement.
    2.6. Weight management.
    2.7. Health status/quality of life.
    2.8. Stages of readiness for behavior change by risk.
    2.9. Symptoms/health problems
    2.10. Social/emotional support systems.
    2.11. Psycho-social issues.
    2.12. Self-esteem, depression, sleep patterns.
    2.13. Musculoskeletal health.
    2.14. Health history (chronic conditions).
    2.15. Use of prescription and non-prescription drugs/medication.
    2.16. Prevention practices/self-care.
    2.17. Job satisfaction.
    2.18. Perception of one's own health.
    2.19. Productivity measures.
    2.20. Lab testing offered on-site or through an affiliate.
    2.21. Individual's top risks identified and customized educational activities provided, including interactive health tools and resources, with participation in challenges and other activities available and tracked.
    2.22. De-identified electronic aggregate and cohort reporting made available to organization.

3. Support Requirements
   3.1. Offer a dedicated implementation/ client service manager; provide monthly, quarterly, and annual reports.
   3.2. Offer a designated wellness account manager and a reporting/data analyst.
   3.3. Ensure communication specialists and resources are available, such as customizable materials and multiple modes of communication (e.g. paper, web-based, telephonic, posters, management debriefings, interactive voice response or IVR, email, internet, etc.).
   3.4. Conduct employee surveys and focus groups, evaluate satisfaction surveys.
   3.5. Provide the required data to implement an incentive based on the health promotion program.
   3.6. Capability to integrate, aggregate, and manage data from multiple sources including mobile applications, claims (medical, pharmacy, disability, EAP), and laboratories.

Principles of Successful Programs

Health promotion programs in industry can be extremely rewarding for both employees and employers. Adherence to the following critical principles will accelerate movement toward success:

- Employees must want and trust the program.
- Employees must participate in its creation and be able to influence its evolution.
- Employers must believe that the program is making a measurable contribution to the well-being of its workforce, families, and to the economics of the organization.
- The program is effectively integrated with the employee health assistance program (alcohol and drug abuse, and stress-related problems).
- The program is effectively integrated with and makes use of available community resources.
- The program focuses on self-responsibility.
- The program must be suitable for the employee population (age, sex, class, education, health, language) and the type of industry (size, type, location).
- The program must be reevaluated on a regular basis with new ideas and concepts being introduced frequently and old or unpopular ideas as quickly discarded.
- Creating a culture of health will lead to sustainability and lower program costs.

Studies are now confirming what has up until now been only inferred. That is, it is well known that employees who do take charge of their health by eating well, exercising regularly, learning to cope with life stresses, eliminating smoking and drug use, who use alcohol in moderation and who use common sense in the everyday activities, live longer and better. They also have fewer days of illness and fewer injuries. In short, they lead better lives than they would otherwise. It is now clear that the benefits of a well managed worksite health promotion programs go beyond just health and quality of life. They directly affect productivity in the workplace. They also help morale and promote positive attitudes in employees and families. Sponsorship of such programs is a tangible gesture of interest in the well-being of the employee on the part of the employer, helping employees create a bond with fellow employees and with the employer as well.

Despite evidence that health promotion and prevention works, the focus of the health care system continues to be on treatment of short-term, acute health problems rather than on prevention of chronic disease. With the current health care model not designed to meet the wellness needs of people and employers facing a large part of the cost burden of a broken system, employers have a unique opportunity and an urgent need to play a stronger role. By focusing on individual responsibility and behavior change, and providing education and social support, people can and will take charge of their health. By understanding and embracing a health promotion strategy employers have the capability and expertise to meet the unique challenges of improving their bottom line and also creating a stronger, healthier workforce.

Recommended Reading and Resources

Bray I (2012) *Healthy Employees, Healthy Business: Easy Affordable Ways to Promote Workplace Wellness.* Berkeley VA, Nolo Press, 2nd ed.

Burton W, Chen C, Conti D (2005) The association of health risks with on-the-job productivity. *J Occup Environ Med*, 47(8): 769–777.

Chenoweth D (2011) *Worksite Health Promotion.* Champagne IL, Human Kinetics, 3rd ed.

Edington, DW (2009) *Zero Trends: Health as a Serious Economic Strategy.* Health Management Research Center, University of Michigan, Ann Arbor, Michigan.

Green LW, Kreuter K (2004) *Health Promotion Planning: An Educational and Ecological Approach.* Mountain View CA, Mayfield, 3rd ed.

University of Michigan Health Management Research Center. The Bank One Wellness Study. Undated (compilation of reprints). Available from 1027 East Huron Street, Ann Arbor MI, 48104-1688.

University of Michigan Health Management Research Center. The Steelcase Wellness Study. Undated (compilation of reprints). Available from 1027 East Huron Street, Ann Arbor MI, 48104-1688.

University of Michigan Health Management Research Center. The Story of Health Promotion at General Motors Corporation. Undated (compilation of reprints). Available from 1027 East Huron Street, Ann Arbor MI, 48104-1688.

US Preventive Medicine Task Force. Available at: http://www.uspreventiveservicestaskforce.org/. Accessed December 22, 2011.

World Health Organization (1986) *The Ottawa Charter for Health Promotion.* Geneva: World Health Organization.

31 Emergency Management at the Enterprise Level

Tee L. Guidotti

The most prominent disasters of the last decade in or affecting North America have threatened workers on the job, critical industries that provide needed goods and services, the survival of employers, and the lives of public safety personnel. However, the experience of the last decade has shown that the death toll and the economic disruption associated with disasters can be mitigated by planning and preparation. Since 2001, both on-site and community-based occupational health services now have a recognized, broader role to play in emergency management and business continuity. Successful management of the H1N1 pandemic of 2009 demonstrated that this could be done effectively and without exorbitant cost.

Natural disasters such as hurricanes are expected to worsen and to become more frequent with climate change. Industrial incidents such as hazardous materials (hazmat) releases, fire, and explosions are a risk in many critical industries, both in transportation and in unsecured plants. Intentional violence against business enterprises and workers may be a contemporary threat from terrorism but was always present in workplace violence in the form of crime, bullying, and disgruntled employees.

The occupational health service is not and never will be in a position to rescue the entire company in the event of catastrophe but that is not its mission. It adds its value in preparedness and planning, and advance networking with community-based public services. Historically, occupational health services have always been most active in disaster planning. An in-house, corporate or on-site plant-level occupational health service usually already has responsibility within the organization for planning the medical response to emergencies, identifying facilities and resources for dealing with serious injuries and mass casualties, and providing health protection for key personnel if required. This can be the foundation for an expanded role that helps it to do its day-to-day work. This adds value, offsets costs, and increases efficiency and reliability.

At the same time, there are many ways that a community-based, provider-venue occupational health service can contribute. Most of these functions overlap and dovetail with its regular occupational health protection functions and add value for the client.

There are two sides to emergency management at the enterprise level: "emergency management" and "business continuity." "Emergency management" is a systematic approach to cope with the event and its consequences. "Business continuity" is a systematic approach to maintain production or the level of service that allows the enterprise to continue to function, delivering its goods or services.

This chapter will begin with an introduction to the specialized world of emergency management, and then consider the occupational health response to these challenges, first through emergency management and then in support of business continuity. The business case for incorporating emergency management into occupational health services will be reviewed. Last, pandemic planning will be discussed both as an example and as a template for management of "distributed emergencies," unfolding events that do not occur in a single place or time.

As in so many matters of public services, the organization of emergency management is markedly different in Canada. In Canada, population centers are widely separated and most provinces are large geographically compared to American states. For this reason and because of the constitutional division of responsibilities, the lead level of government for disasters is provincial, not federal, and lines of authority are generally much simpler than in the US, although local emergency management services are similarly organized and equipped.

Liaison with Public Agencies

All but the largest self-contained enterprises will rely heavily on local public health and emergency response agencies in a disaster. It is essential that the occupational health service build a relationship with local public health and emergency management authorities in advance of an emergency, sharing concerns and information and planning together. Disaster response requires decisions to be made in real time, sometimes in chaotic circumstances, and requires trust, understanding, and reliability among the players. There is a common saying in emergency management that the time to exchange cards for the first time is not at the disaster scene.

The principal US federal agency for emergency response is the Department of Homeland Security (DHS), with the Federal Emergency Management Administration (FEMA) responding in support of state and local agencies to natural disasters, and the Federal Bureau of Investigation (FBI) responding to intentional events with national security implications, including terrorism.

Current federal policy is that the response to natural disasters is a state and local responsibility and that federal assistance is to support the mission of state and local agencies, not to lead. This doctrine has been sorely tested by political reality, particularly in the collapse of state capacity during the catastrophic hurricanes of 2006 (Katrina and Rita), but it is clear that localities and therefore enterprises must depend on their own resources for at least the first 72 hours in a natural disaster.

On the other hand, an intentional assault involving national security, such as a terrorist attack, immediately triggers a federal response in which federal agencies take the lead. Some enterprises in the private sector are highly vulnerable to such intentional assaults, particularly those that are involved in security or military applications and that are highly visible. However, other enterprises have been targeted by terrorists because their destruction multiplies local damage, causes confusion and panic, and degrades the response: hospitals (a particularly "soft" target), communications (including and especially the internet), security services (particularly civilian police), and transportation facilities (such as airports).

In those cases in which goods and services are essential to the community, the nation, and to the economy, these enterprises are technically called "critical infrastructure" and employers may fall under federal contingency planning. DHS has stimulated formation of a number of sector-specific coordinating councils and information sharing and analysis centers (ISACs) in order to support partnerships and a collective response to emergency management. (At the time of this writing, the health care and public health sector organizations had not addressed occupational health, and none of the other sector coordinating councils had placed emphasis on occupational health services in their plans for workforce protection.)

An important concept within emergency management is the "incident command system" (ICS). Occupational health services are unlikely to be integrated into the ICS but a working knowledge of how they work may be useful in an emergency for liaison with public agencies. Basically, the ICS is a standardized system for managing emergencies, capable of integrating trained people quickly, and easily scalable from one person to an integrated network involving different agencies and response teams. There is one person in charge, usually either the first to respond or the person with the most relevant experience, not the person with highest rank. This "incident commander" has decision-making authority for the operational response overall, managing a response structure divided into four functions: operations (the response to the emergency in the field); planning and intelligence (which receives information and determines what needs to be done); logistics (deploying assets, tracking inventory, and ordering back-up or supplies, as needed); and administration and finance (keeping track of personnel assignments, costs, and expenses that will require reimbursement). The incident commander is supported by staff, who take care of four key functions: safety (of the responders), public information, communications (within the response structure), and liaison with other agencies and external stakeholders. The terminology and organization do not vary because standardization is key to making the system work. The National Response Framework, administered by the DHS, is essentially an ICS for the US, with agencies playing the key roles in the system rather than individuals.

Principles of Emergency Management

"Emergency management," not to be confused with emergency medicine (the specialty) or emergency services (police, fire, emergency medical services, and hazmat), is a systematic approach at the managerial level to preparing for and coping with an emergency, which may be a real disaster or a threatened catastrophic event. "Disaster" is defined, paraphrasing the World Health Organization, as a sudden adverse event of sufficient magnitude that it exceeds the community's available capacity to respond and requires external assistance. Thus there are two sides to the equation: how bad the event is or could be and how much capacity the responder has available to deal with it. Emergency services serving a small rural community may have to mobilize a disaster plan for a two-car collision. A large city may be able to cope with casualties from a train derailment without experiencing a strain on resources.

A cardinal principle of emergency management is the wisdom of planning flexibly, with common assets for all plausible risks rather than planning narrowly for a particular threat. This "all threats approach" not only makes best use of deployable assets but makes disaster plans and drills more relevant to rapidly changing, real-life events.

Emergency managers recognize four phases in the emergency cycle in relation to the event:

* *Mitigation*, often *Prevention/Mitigation*, is the pre-event phase of active avoidance of risk, through planning and strengthening resistance or resilience. An enterprise-level example might be the separation of fuel tanks; construction of earthquake resistant pipelines; or installing diesel generators in company facilities to provide electricity in case of power failure. In general, mitigation seeks to prevent the event from becoming a disaster and to limit the magnitude of consequences. The occupational health service contributes to mitigation and prevention through planning and by establishing close working relationships with public health and emergency management agencies in advance of any event.
* *Preparedness* is the pre-event phase of planning for the disaster itself and minimizing its consequences through planned response. Unfortunately, disaster plans are often not kept current and are only rarely tested in drills, so they may fail. Other examples

of preparedness would be installation of self-contained breathing apparatus in key locations; deploying water, food, and medical supplies in advance where they are likely to be needed; or maintaining a state of readiness with a well-drilled emergency response unit, such as a mine-rescue team. The occupational health service contributes to preparedness by, among other functions, fitness-for-duty evaluations for emergency services personnel. Preparedness can be combined with operational risk assessment in support of the enterprise's occupational health responsibilities and regulatory requirements (see Chapter 21).

• *Response* is the event or early post-event phase of dealing with the disaster as it develops. This may take the form of fighting the fire, assessing chemical exposures, advising people in the path of a gas plume to shelter in place, deploying personal protective equipment, search and rescue, evacuating personnel, and so forth. During the event, the occupational health service's own personnel and assets are usually insufficient to deal directly with anything more than a small emergency. The principal value of the occupational health service during response is to protect the health of first responders, to advise on issues (such as chemical threats) within its competency, and to be a liaison between the enterprise and the public health authorities and local medical community.

• *Recovery* begins when the immediate threat is over, and so is the post-event phase. It may take the form of clearing debris, bringing in needed supplies that are not locally available, purchasing relief supplies from local vendors (which is the preferred approach because it gets money circulating in the community), establishing health care facilities, repairing damage, and introducing public health inspections (because a particular threat during recovery from many disasters is food poisoning and waterborne diarrhea). The recovery phase continues until basic services are restored and the community is functioning again. During recovery, the occupational health service may certify workers who have been off duty or injured as fit to return to the workplace, may advise on the risk of reentry to potentially contaminated facilities, and may identify dangerous conditions that persist after the emergency. Ideally, mitigation then follows as lessons learned are applied.

The role of occupational health services is principally pre-event (mitigation and preparedness) and post-event (recovery). Identification and evaluation of hazards, in order to assess and to manage risk in the workplace, is the foundation of modern occupational health and safety, and the field therefore provides relevant templates and tools for assessing and managing risk.

Drills, both "table-top" and in realistic simulations, are essential to emergency preparedness and the quality of response and whenever possible should be joint with public safety and emergency management agencies. These drills play out plausible scenarios so that participants will fully understand what is expected of them, anticipate their emotional response to a crisis, experience unexpected and unpredictable developments, and spot serious gaps in planning and preparedness. All disaster plans must accommodate changing circumstances, complicating situations, and second events. Although no emergency proceeds exactly as predicted, drills using realistic scenarios help to condition the thinking of responders as well as to practice implementation of the plan.

An uncanny side benefit of emergency management planning is that, like occupational safety and ergonomics, it often leads to identification of efficiencies and unanticipated benefits. The "post-modern" era of emergency management may be said to have begun with preparations for "Y2K" (a rather contrived acronym for "Year 2000"). The assumption was that the turn of the 21st century would present a risk of widespread disruption due to a supposed programming limitation in computer clocks that was projected to cause essential timing and pacing functions to fail, with catastrophic results for computerized systems. The exercise of reprogramming or replacement to become "Y2K compliant" was possibly the most massive emergency preparation and mitigation effort in history in terms of scope and global reach. As it turned out, nothing much happened. However, in the course of this work thousands of malfunctioning and obsolete items of equipment were identified and replaced or repaired.

Mission of the Occupational Health Service

The mission of any occupational health service in emergency management is to protect the health of the enterprise's workforce as the critical infrastructure necessary to assure survival and continuity of all economic sectors. The goals of an occupational health service in emergency management are to:

*   Integrate the capabilities of the occupational health system into the enterprise's emergency management preparedness and response effort.
*   Integrate the capabilities of the enterprise into the community's emergency management preparedness and response effort.
*   Health surveillance and monitoring.
*   Enhance preparedness of the occupational health community to protect workers and their families.
*   Maintain business continuity.

The occupational health service is in a strategic position to assist employers in emergency management and in maintaining business continuity. Occupational health professionals have special training in chemical, biological, physical, and psychological hazards in the workplace that translate readily to emergency management in certain situations. By being an important player in protecting the enterprise and its workers, the occupational health service demonstrates its value to the enterprise and makes another strong argument for investment in its services. A role in emergency management also provides the enterprise with a good reason to support and expand the scope of the occupational health service.

Occupational health can play its strongest role in preparedness, especially in partnership with operating units, and mitigation, both of which emphasize analysis and planning. Its role in response is limited by its small size but may include advising management on workforce protection during the period of an emergency and especially monitoring the health and advising on the health risks for emergency response personnel, such as fire and security. During recovery, the role of occupational health would include its usual functions, incident investigation, and risk assessment on emerging hazards experienced due to recovery operations.

There are many practical ways in which an occupational health service can be helpful in a serious crisis, some of them listed in Box 31.1. The response to certain emergencies depends on effective occupational health service planning, such as pandemic management.

Business Continuity

Business continuity (also called "continuity of operations") may take many forms and range to high levels of sophistication. During a major natural disaster, the very survival of the enterprise may be at risk. During a terrorist attack, the survival of people may be on the line. Most emergencies will involve much lower stakes, however.

Box 31.1 The Occupational Health Service and Emergency Management

- Attending to the health of key personnel in a catastrophic event.
- Continuity of business following a catastrophic event.
- Instant connectivity to resources for assistance in a health-related emergency.
- Surveillance of the workforce and the early detection of an outbreak.
- Vaccination programs and other protective measures.
- Fitness for duty, respirator fit testing, and health monitoring of first responders.
- Triage, handling the many "worried well" who seek care in an emergency.
- Fitness-for-duty evaluations of security staff and other first responders.
- Managing personal protective equipment training and fit testing.
- Monitoring employee absence as an indicator of health impact.
- Continuity of business following a catastrophic event.
- Instant connectivity to resources for assistance in a health-related emergency.
- Surveillance of the workforce and the early detection of an outbreak.
- Integration of emergency response with public health agencies.
- Surge capacity in the event of a local event requiring mobilization of all available medical resources.
- Determining acceptable return to work or re-entry of a facility that has been contaminated or damaged.
- Assisting executive personnel with medical problems (e.g. diabetes) during an emergency.
- Survival of key personnel in a catastrophic event.
- Fatality and forensic investigation.

Box 31.2 provides a list of priorities for business continuity that apply to most enterprises. It can be seen as a guide to management concerns.

Box 31.3 is one approach to continuity of operations (COOP, in the jargon). It outlines a logical approach to developing what used to be called a "disaster plan" and now is more commonly referred to as a COOP or emergency management plan. The occupational health

Box 31.2 Conceptual Priorities in Emergency Management at the Enterprise Level (in order)

1. Business viability (survival).
2. Business continuity.
3. Business recovery.
4. Regulatory compliance.
5. Loss prevention.
6. Liability prevention (unfunded).
7. Efficiency, productivity.
8. Reputation.
9. Brand image.
10. Cost containment.

Box 31.3 Steps in Developing a Plan for Continuity of Operations

1. Senior management should be briefed, should declare unequivocal support for the planning effort, and should adopt a policy that risks to continuity of operations should be actively managed within the enterprise. Identify the objectives as:
   1.1. To restore critical services or products as quickly as possible.
   1.2. To protect the workforce and their families from harm.
   1.3. To protect the community of which the enterprise is a part.
   1.4. To resume operations as quickly as possible.
2. The core mission of the enterprise should be reviewed with consideration of its social role in providing a needed product or service. What is essential to the business viability of the enterprise? What is critical about its products or services to the community and to the nation? If the enterprise were to abruptly cease operations, what would happen?
3. Stakeholders who would be affected by the inability of the enterprise to continue operations should be identified and their potential options for getting what they need through alternative suppliers. A communications plan should be formulated for informing or reassuring these stakeholders in the event of a potentially disruptive emergency.
4. Identify the essential processes that are required to maintain core operations, those directly related to the mission of the enterprise.
5. Identify the key positions required to operate these essential processes and establish a database of which employees are currently occupying these positions, current employees who have done these jobs in the recent past but have now been reassigned, and recent retirees in the area who had experience in these positions and were evaluated as showing good job performance. This roster may be invaluable to meet short-term staffing needs in an emergency. The occupational health service should be aware of their health issues or impairments, if any.
6. Formulate a set of realistic scenarios that represent a variety of plausible threats to the enterprise. These should include, but not be limited to: natural disaster (such as earthquake or flood), intentional disruption (terrorism, vandalism, extortion, cyber), fire and explosion, disruptive disaster in an adjacent or nearby property, pandemic influenza, and other scenarios consistent with the location, industrial processes, threats, and vulnerability of the enterprise.
7. Develop contingency plans for each plausible scenario, the simpler the better, and identify commonalities and common resource requirements.
8. Managers should be required to develop contingency plans for their area of responsibility.
9. Identify the assets that are required by the contingency plans, accounting for redundancies and duplications. Use this as the basis for a budget estimate and prioritize for future procurement.
10. Disseminate the plan by every feasible means: online, in hard-copy at key locations (to be accessible in event of an information technology (IT) problem), through training.
11. Drill the scenarios in realistic exercises, varying the scenario but emphasizing common contingency plans wherever appropriate.

12. Update the database of key personnel, revise the plan with every significant change in operations, and expand the plan when new facilities and technology are introduced. This should be done on an ongoing basis, as changes occur, rather than bringing the plan up to date every few years.
13. Conduct debriefings after every major disruptive event or near miss, document what happened, review lessons learned, and incorporate issues raised in future training. Use these disruptive events or near-misses to highlight relevant parts of the COOP plan.
14. Document everything meticulously.

service is not usually the lead department in developing such a plan, but if the opportunity presents itself for the service to take a leadership role, it should be seized. Providing leadership in emergency management is one way for the occupational health service to demonstrate its work and to position itself as central to the mission of the enterprise, rather than as merely a support function. In the past, occupational medicine and occupational health services have always been perceived as support functions, facilitating management priorities but not a core business priority. In the new era of threats to survival and business continuity, the occupational health service may play a role in the survival of the enterprise and its people.

Business continuity can therefore be conceived of as a partnership within the corporate leadership team, with specific roles to play during the emergency management cycle of preparedness, response, recovery, and mitigation:

- Senior management coordinates, especially in the stages of preparedness, recovery, and mitigation.
- Security, health/safety/environment, and other designated technical functions take the lead during response, under direction of senior management.
- Occupational health, and health/safety/environment overall, together with human resources, take the lead in workforce protection.
- Information technology (IT) takes the lead in essential services and communications.
- Finance and the affected business units take the lead in recovery.
- Engineering and facilities management, together with health/safety/environment take the lead in mitigation for physical safety and process engineering to reduce vulnerability.
- Health/safety/environment, together with human resources and IT, take the lead in resilience, redundancy, and work organization (such as work from home during a pandemic).

Business continuity is important to the community as well as to the employer and the workforce throughout the response and recovery phases. Recovery from an emergency requires measures to protect the infrastructure of the country that keeps necessary goods and services available during a crisis and that supports the economy so that recovery can follow. This infrastructure includes: vital resources, such as food, water, and medical care; transportation services; communications; energy supplies; public services, such as police and fire protection; public health; financial services, such as banking, credit, and payroll; manufacturing capacity; construction; and government. Interruptions in these services

Box 31.4 Elements of a COOP Information Package

This standard COOP information package should be accessible online and in hard copy at all times to all company officials, both on- and off-site, for an enterprise at high risk.

- Company phonebook.
- Company board of directors and advisory group communications directory.
- Company facility addresses, general contact, email, and fax numbers.
- Company facility personnel and safeguard and security unit contact list.
- Company management and staff working and travel schedules.
- Company plan for delegation of authority and succession.
- Company off-site contact for disbursement authority for operating accounts and emergency fiscal information.
- Company procurement and transaction log forms.

threaten the fabric of society as well as cause injury to those directly affected, because such disruptions deprive the affected community of badly needed resources in the short term and the ability to rebuild and recover in the long term.

A COOP information package (Box 31.4), available on- or off-site and both online (protected) and off the internet, is essential for the leadership in any enterprise at high risk, so that operations can continue with minimal interruption.

The Business Case

Figure 31.1 presents the elements of a generic value pyramid with an emphasis on the relationships among occupational health service, emergency management, and business continuity. The left-hand face of the pyramid deals with management of external threats. Business sustainability is addressed on the right-hand face of the pyramid, in the management of the financial and economic health of the company; this is the appropriate concern of the leadership and where most managers live. The internal development of the organization, and therefore issues involving the assessment and management of all threats to the company, are addressed on the side of the pyramid the reader cannot see. They are virtually hidden as they usually are in real life.

Table 31.1 presents essential questions that must be asked during emergency planning. If the event does not threaten the enterprise but affects the surrounding community, an opportunity exists for the company and occupational health service to lend assistance but liability issues should be worked out in advance. If the event may cause serious disruption to business and operations, planning must focus on ways to mitigate vulnerability and for effective response. If the event is of large scale and threatens the viability of the enterprise, hard questions may have to be asked regarding the capacity of the enterprise to survive. If the company is isolated, it needs to identify what assets it can rely on until aid is forthcoming to the community from state and federal agencies. Even a large enterprise may not be able to endure if the cost of an emergency exceeds its assets.

Emergency management, poorly managed, can be very expensive. Preparedness may require a substantial expenditure of funds on dedicated assets, such as hazmat gear, that will

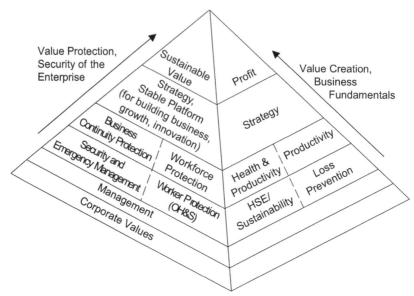

Figure 31.1 Value creation pyramid, adapted from Alcan, showing elements of security and their relationship to business continuity, worker protection, and the creation and protection of wealth

Table 31.1 Risk Matrix for Emergency Management

	Nonessential To Enterprise	*Disruption of Essential Activities**	*Critical to Survival of Enterprise**
Disaster	Can assistance be offered to community or partners? (Address liability issues.)	Can the enterprise survive this event? Does the potential loss exceed assets? Is the enterprise critical to the community?	
Area-wide Disruption			
Major Event		How to minimize the effects of the event? Why is the enterprise so vulnerable?	
Minor Event	Why bother?		

* Refers to events that disrupt a product or service line that is essential for business or that causes damage or loss that threatens the survival of the organization in other ways. This matrix is an adaptation of the risk matrix in Chapter 21.

only be used once or not at all. Emergency management planning and drills detract from normal business activities. Thus, senior managers must balance risk and present cost in most emergency management decisions.

Investing in the occupational health service to play an expanded role in emergency management, however, allows the enterprise to recover some of its investment in improved operating capacity and efficiency for a normal business function, because it supports occupational health protection and workforce productivity. The investment leverages off the already sunk cost of the occupational health services budget. Creating a parallel, special-purpose unit within a company is not a good idea, as it incurs additional expense and operating inefficiencies and its single-minded focus on a rare or unlikely event (albeit one with high consequence) makes it inflexible and may even degrade occupational health and safety because of competition for resources. Perhaps most important, the occupational health service is tested daily with minor health emergencies and a constant stream of challenges.

This operational testing makes response much more reliable in a true emergency than would be the case in a purpose-built organization newly set up within the enterprise.

Emergency management proves to be an excellent investment when an event actually occurs. A critical part of the infrastructure of any enterprise is the people who work in that enterprise, particularly those with experience and those who occupy key production jobs. Workforce protection is therefore a critical part of infrastructure protection, and it is incumbent upon all organizations, public and private, to put in place a series of protocols and procedures to ensure an orderly and cost-effective response through well-founded emergency management and disaster preparedness. Qualified occupational health care providers already have special training on chemical, biological, physical, and psychological hazards in the workplace that translate readily to emergency management.

To perform these duties effectively requires that time be dedicated for preparedness activities, that an occupational health service be structured for the mission and that providers be trained. However, it is costly and inefficient even for large corporations to dedicate a full-time staff and a support structure for the management of an event that may never materialize. This is precisely why adaptation of the existing occupational health service makes sense for employers, especially those in critical or hazardous industries. The investment is not "lost" if an event never occurs, because it still supports the mission of workforce protection of the occupational health service. The same assets and systems support and enhance the traditional occupational health services that employees require.

The theoretical basis for enterprise-level emergency management is based on the model called the "Value Creation Pyramid," pioneered by Alcan and further developed for occupational health and safety by Jean-Pierre Robin at Noranda. The model suggests that any organization that creates wealth and adds value cannot rely on routine operations and public services for protection, and must rest on a foundation that includes special functions designed to assure its security in order to be sustainable. That security may take the form of managing financial risk, protecting the reputation (or brand) of the company, ensuring good relations with stakeholders, preventing catastrophic events, and, at an extreme, measures to ensure the very survival of the enterprise through protecting its leaders, key employees with technical skills, workforce, and assets and with planning for business continuity. An employer may not knowingly face that degree of threat at the moment but it is not wise, whether the threats are physical or fiscal, to make the assumption that it never will.

Pandemic Planning

Most disaster planning is oriented toward discreet emergencies that unfold over days or weeks. Pandemic planning and management differs in principle from other emergency management challenges because the events take place over weeks to months and may recur. Pandemic planning is therefore a paradigm of management for "distributed emergencies," in which the threat occurs in different places at different times and evolves over longer time periods.

Pandemic planning has assumed prominence because of its immediacy in the aftermath of SARS and the H1N1 influenza epidemic and concern over the prospects of a catastrophic H5N1 ("avian influenza") epidemic in the future. Pandemic management is broadly useful, beyond any specific strain of influenza, because it can be activated in any similar emergency, is adaptable in some situations involving bioterrorism, and its individual measures can be used for individual cases and for minor illness outbreaks. Pandemic management in the case of the SARS outbreak of 2003 and the H1N1 influenza pandemic of 2009 has also provided models for occupational health services for the management of distributed emergencies in business and the protection of the workforce.

The primary challenge in pandemic planning, as in other distributed emergencies, is maintaining a sufficient workforce. It is not practical to expect to be able to prevent employees from being affected, because they will be exposed in the community. However, if transmission can be slowed within the workforce, fewer people will be out sick at any one time, making it much easier to continue operations. Likewise, if key people, such as project managers, senior executives, engineers, and essential technical staff, can be kept on the job as long as possible, the enterprise has a better chance of getting through the distributed emergency with minimal disruption.

The key resources for occupational health professionals who are supporting pandemic influenza plans for employers are the federal agencies responsible for population health management: the Centers for Disease Control and Prevention (CDC) in the US, and the Public Health Agency of Canada. They coordinate closely with one another and with the World Health Organization (WHO). The WHO and CDC should not be considered independent sources of information, since the WHO relies heavily on the CDC.

A general plan for management of pandemic infectious disease, specifically influenza, has the following basic elements:

- *"Stay at home" policy.* Employees who become ill should stay at home. This should be a general policy but should be mandatory and vigorously enforced during a pandemic.
- *Hygiene.* Frequent hand washing and the use of antibacterial hand wash interrupts transmission of influenza and cold viruses. Covering the mouth with one's arm and coughing or sneezing into the antecubital fossa (the "vampire cough," as promoted by CDC) rather than hands should be encouraged in the workplace at all times, becoming the new social norm, and should become mandatory during a pandemic. Research shows that textiles are efficient at trapping liquid aerosols from a cough or sneeze and have much less transmission potential than skin.
- *Changing health behaviors.* A pandemic may provide an opportunity to change behaviors in ways that promote health and ultimately make health gains if they can be sustained as part of the enterprise culture beyond the emergency. Many customs accepted in daily life are counterproductive with respect to health. One of them is shaking hands, which is an efficient way of transmitting viral pathogens. A pandemic provides an opportunity for introducing socially acceptable substitutes for shaking hands (such as the Indian "namaste" gesture (palms together, fingers up), touching elbows, or the American "fist bump") which can be done in a light-hearted and even humorous way to make the change in custom more acceptable.
- *Social isolation.* Keeping a skeleton team on duty during a disaster is generally possible only in a local disaster, not a distributed disaster such as a pandemic. However, at least half a dozen communities in the US missed the 1917 pandemic influenza outbreak entirely because they were socially isolated and could restrict access. Enterprises can limit access to headquarters to designated key personnel and essential vendors. However, social isolation cannot be sustained for long.
- *Social distancing of individuals.* This strategy rests on remote work and telecommuting. Supervisors should have contingency plans for implementing this strategy for critical functions wherever possible. Efforts should be made to reduce the frequency of face-to-face contact among employees in order to slow transmission, such as video conferencing, distance learning, telecommuting, cessation of face-to-face meetings when business can

be conducted electronically, and work at home. CDC has developed a severity index for pandemic infections and intends to advise increasing social isolation and distancing with increasing severity index. However, this recommendation will be intended for the general public and schools.

- *Social distancing of workplaces.* Any enterprise that is not strictly virtual offers direct transmission opportunities among its employees because of their patterns of interaction. It will be better protected by interrupting transmission pathways early, especially those between branches or nodes of the operation, to prevent facilitating transmission. Eventually, employees will face the same risk as the public in general but social distancing should delay and attenuate peak absence and cause less disruption. If social distancing works well overall, the pandemic is likely to develop in "slow motion" in the enterprise compared to the community, making it easier to manage.
- *Prioritization.* Nonessential activities requiring face-to-face meeting may be curtailed. Some services may have to be suspended or curtailed. Wherever possible, services that workers need to access should be moved online or redesigned to be contact-free.
- *Increased vigilance and security.* Operating with a skeleton crew on site and with social distancing will make the organization less efficient and may reduce access to IT personnel. The enterprise may therefore be more vulnerable to disruption from hacking and cybersecurity breaches during the emergency. Steps should be taken to ensure that security is maintained and even enhanced, including protecting confidential medical records.
- *Travel restrictions.* Nonessential travel involving regions where the outbreak affects the general public or employees in the organization, particularly from a branch or node of the business that is affected to one that is unaffected, should be temporarily prohibited. On the other hand, travel restrictions should make sense. During the SARS multifocal epidemic, some organizations prohibited travel to all of Canada, although the outbreak there was limited to one hospital serving one area of one city, Toronto.
- *Surveillance.* Any such outbreak will be tracked closely by local public health agencies and by CDC. In the past, CDC has not always seen providing timely information to employers as a priority and has tended to treat the occupational health community as members of the general public. Collateral information sensitive to business purposes can be essential in fine-tuning the response to the pandemic, as demonstrated during the SARS outbreak when a small number of companies networked with their divisions in Asia and a prominent regional airline to monitor conditions on the ground for themselves.
- *Personal protection.* In a pandemic, there will be a huge demand for N95 respirators, which is the personal protection of choice for individuals who report to the workplace, are on the job in public, who communicate with face-to-face contact, or are several days out from an illness that might have been influenza. Stockpiles must be protected and controlled by occupational health personnel or supervisors because employees will inevitably want to take some home in order to protect their families.
- *Adaptation and interpretation.* Understandably, most of CDC's communications on occupational health risk and mitigation are directed at health care institutions and workers. Hospitals have special requirements and procedures for N95 respirators that may not apply to other enterprises. The occupational health service may need to adapt and interpret the risk for other sectors, always keeping in mind liability issues. For example, there is no obvious reason why a worker outside of a health care institution could not reuse an N95 respirator or take it on or off many times during the day, as

long as it is clean, does not become saturated with moisture, and there is not a high risk of contamination on the surface. This practice would not be acceptable in a hospital. However, if such practices were later suspected of spreading H5N1 in the community the assertion would be difficult to disprove and could lead to liability issues.

- *Home care and triage.* Persons showing symptoms of influenza should be encouraged to stay at home if their symptoms are low-grade. If they require a higher level of care, current plans call for establishing designated intermediate care centers in schools and churches, and only admitting people to hospital if they are severely ill. This strategy may require a liberal policy of allowing employees flexibility to take care of dependents while working from home, perhaps expediting leave procedures. If the pandemic lasts a long time, this may exceed mandates under the Family and Medical Leave Act and the capacity of employees to take time off without pay (see Chapter 24).
- *Vaccine development.* Vaccines are developed as soon as the antigenic determinants are known but normally take months to produce in quantity. New vaccine antigen production techniques look very promising, however.
- *Immunization.* Employers should arrange or cooperate in encouraging mass immunizations for employees against both seasonal influenza and special strains, as they become available. Immunization rests on several strategies. The primary strategy for pandemic influenza control is that as soon as a specific vaccine is available, it will be administered as widely as possible, with priority given to certain groups (such as health care workers) for the earliest batches. A secondary strategy is to encourage immunization against seasonal influenza in order to remove a burden to the health care system and minimize confusion in diagnosis. A third strategy, more applicable to other infectious diseases, is the so-called "ring" strategy, in which probable contacts of a known case are immunized to prevent secondary transmission. (For some diseases, such as anthrax, which happens not to be transmissible person to person, immunization is also an effective treatment, if performed promptly after exposure.) How immunization is used will therefore depend on the pathogen and the epidemic curve of the pandemic.
- *Antiviral medication.* The role of these agents is limited because supplies are finite, resistance is common in many strains of influenza, and treatment inhibits the development of immunity, so that once treatment ends patients remain at risk for recurrent viral infection. Policy and protocol on antiviral medication will therefore have to wait until the characteristics of an outbreak are known.
- *Crisis communication.* The employer should be prepared to maintain close communications with all employees on a daily basis in the course of the pandemic, including those who are telecommuting. This is important not only to disseminate information but to monitor employee work and support engagement with the enterprise, since some employees are likely to feel alienated and may lose motivation.
- *Psychological support.* The presence of a pandemic in the community and in the workplace will place unprecedented stress on the workforce. Employee assistance program services should support the workforce with telephone and online counseling (see Chapter 28).

Recommended Reading and Resources

American Medical Association. *Disaster and Public Health Preparedness.* Monthly journal.

Ciottone GR, ed. (2006) *Disaster Medicine.* Philadelphia, Elsevier.

Guidotti TL (2010) *The Praeger Handbook of Occupational and Environmental Medicine.* Santa Barbara CA, Praeger. See Chapter 22, on "Emergency Management."

Guidotti TL (2011) What is the role of emergency management in occupational medicine? *J Occup Environ Med*, 53(7): 822–823. Occupational Medicine Forum, ed. Schwerha JJ.

Haddow G, Bullock J, Coppola DP (2011) *Introduction to Emergency Management*. Burlington MA, Butterworth-Heinemann.

Hogan DE, Burstein JL (2002) *Disaster Medicine*. Philadelphia, Lippincott Williams & Wilkins.

McEntire DA, Lindsay JR (2012) One neighborhood, two families: a comparison of intergovernmental emergency management relationships. *Journal of Emergency Management*, 10(2): 93–107. (Provides a useful overview of emergency management in Canada.)

Upfal M, Krieger GR, Phillips S, Guidotti TL, Weissman D, eds (2003) Terrorism: biological, chemical and nuclear. *Clinics in Occupational and Environmental Medicine*. Orlando FL, Elsevier Science, May. Entire issue of this bound journal devoted to topic of terrorism, with an emphasis on occupational health.

32 Medicolegal Services

Tee L. Guidotti

Medical testimony is used to inform dispute resolution on matters of health. This is an ancient and venerable function of health professionals. Expert witnesses (often referred to simply as "experts") are usually retained by lawyers to help in understanding the technical aspects of the case, in forming a theory about what happened, in preparing an opinion regarding what caused the injury, and in articulating the opinion clearly so that it can be understood by a lay judge or jury. Often a medical expert is also asked to determine the degree of injury or impairment (see Chapter 26) and may conduct an independent medical evaluation (IME, see Chapter 25). Several experts may be involved, each focusing on an aspect of the case.

Occupational health professionals provide opinions in disputed workers' compensation cases, tort cases (usually third party lawsuits against manufacturers of allegedly unsafe products, since employers are protected by the workers' compensation exclusion), and in civil litigation involving alleged discrimination or unfair practices under the Americans with Disabilities Act (ADA) or Family and Medical Leave Act (FMLA). Other situations, such as criminal prosecution or medical malpractice, are rare for experts in occupational health and will not be discussed here because they follow somewhat different rules.

The law, in general, respects the opinion of physicians, nurses, and other expert witnesses. However, in the real world, serving as an expert in a civil case is tough, demanding, and difficult. In the past, the opinion of health professionals, without reference to the evidence, carried much greater weight than it does today. Now, much greater justification and demonstration of evidence is required to support an opinion.

Serving as an expert witness, as opposed to testifying as a treating professional or witness to a fact, is not something that most occupational health practitioners can or should do on a regular basis without extensive preparation and years of experience. Opinions that are not tightly reasoned will not withstand scrutiny and the results can harm the client and can be embarrassing for the expert.

Although physicians are subject to the requirements of the legal system when they serve as expert witnesses, the law recognizes professional standards and the norms of medicine and, increasingly, epidemiology. Medical and other professional societies often develop codes of ethics for the deportment and honesty of their members who serve as expert witnesses but these codes are designed to prevent the most egregious breaches and abuses, not to set normative rules.

This chapter will not address the application of scientific evidence to the resolution of disputes involving health, because it is beyond the scope of this book. (The "Recommended Reading" list features books that will better prepare the new expert intellectually than any short chapter could do. *Science on the Witness Stand* was written specifically for occupational health professionals.) Rather, it emphasizes the process, the skill set of an expert, and how the civil litigation system works. Criminal cases have their own dynamics and will not be discussed.

Role of the Expert Witness

All occupational health professionals are called upon to provide medicolegal services of some kind, usually by attesting to a medical fact, conducting an IME, or writing a letter of opinion for a workers' compensation case. The physician (because almost all expert witnesses on medical matters are physicians) practicing occupational medicine also becomes involved in civil litigation (resolving a dispute between two parties), adjudication of workers' compensation claims, and the decisions of pension and other authorities. Most civil litigation in which an occupational health professional is likely to be involved involves "personal injury," in which the plaintiff is claiming damages from the defendant for a "tort," a wrongful act, whether by commission or omission, that causes damage or loss. The other systems and venues, such as workers' compensation appeals, grew out of tort litigation with the intention of simplifying the process and reducing cost, and are called "alternative dispute resolution" methods. Workers' compensation (see Chapter 2) was the first alternative dispute resolution approach adopted in North America but there are now many such venues. They follow many of the same rules as court cases but usually with somewhat relaxed rules of evidence and procedure.

On a practical level, the legal system lacks the capacity to evaluate the validity of knowledge independently and therefore relies heavily on expert opinion. Until 1994, there were no broad, generally agreed-upon rules for the application of medical, nursing, public health, and for that matter any scientific knowledge, except in the rules of evidence and precedent. This was particularly evident in tort litigation, where liability for causing injury is under consideration, and often rests on theories of disease etiology and the circumstances surrounding exposure to a hazard. The Federal Judicial Center, in Washington DC, has since produced the *Reference Manual on Scientific Evidence*, which provides guidance to judges and lawyers.

Serving as an expert witness comes with certain exceptional obligations and privileges. For example, the expert is exempted from the usual rule that second-hand knowledge, what is commonly called "hearsay," is not admissible in court, because the expert is allowed to quote from the literature and to "opine" (deliver an opinion) on the medical practices of others to establish a standard of practice. The culture of scientific investigation and the legal privileges given expert witness are reflected in British and Commonwealth (including Canadian) law and in American law and procedure, notably in the (US) Federal Rules of Evidence (Article IV), which gives special consideration to epidemiology.

The "Theory" of the Case

A critical function of the expert is to make sense of the evidence by formulating an explanation for what happened. The explanation is called the "theory" of the case. It must be based on facts, be robust in argument, and integrate sound technical and medical knowledge, often from different disciplines. (The intrinsic interdisciplinary nature of occupational medicine gives physicians in this field an advantage.) Exactly how to do that is beyond the scope of this chapter and the cognitive skills and discipline required to sort out a complicated case may require years of experience as well as education.

In the past, the expert's word was taken more or less at face value. However, junk science and the spectacle of dueling experts provoked a backlash. The Frye Rule (from a federal district court ruling in *Frye v. United States*, 1923), which is still the basis for the rules of evidence in many states, elevated acceptance of the expert's opinion to a collective level by requiring that the methods used by the expert should have gained general acceptance in the professional field as a whole before the court can accept the testimony. Frye has been superseded in federal courts and most states by the Daubert Rule, which was the result of a Supreme Court decision and is discussed in detail below. Daubert requires the court to serve as a gatekeeper on the validity of scientific evidence and requires each step in the approach to the opinion to be justified by the expert.

Theories most likely to be given weight in court are those that are simple, easy to explain, and based on unbiased evidence analyzed by methods that can be understood by the average person. A personal or idiosyncratic interpretation of the facts contributes little to the case and may undermine the expert's credibility. However, in a courtroom, even a reasonable theory developed to fit the particulars of a highly unusual case can be ridiculed or made to appear idiosyncratic, even bizarre, by the lawyer on the "other" side. The key, therefore, is to support the theory of the case with solid evidence, simply explained, with as few confusing alternative explanations or complications as possible.

There is always a temptation for the inexperienced expert to "show off" by suggesting that the case is somehow so complicated that only he or she understands it, or to invoke a detailed chain of events to explain what happened, or to trump the "other side" with a new fact and recently published finding. These temptations should be avoided. Very few cases hinge on one particular scientific finding and when they do, the most recent finding may not yet have been replicated, interpreted by the scientific community, or integrated into the body of scientific knowledge; it might even be reversed in the next publication. It is almost always the body of evidence that matters, not any individual study, in scientific evidence.

A simple theory of the case with as few steps as possible is always desirable, as well as being much easier to communicate to a judge or jury. It is also more likely to be true, by the principle of Occam's razor. An apparently rational but overly elaborate theory of a case requires too many contingent steps, each of which has to be justified and is vulnerable to attack.

Most issues requiring expert explanation are obscure to the court and to the lay public but very familiar, even mundane to the expert. Technical knowledge is important but deep specialization is usually irrelevant except for the most unusual and highly technical cases. A good mastery and nuanced understanding of the field is usually more valuable than technical brilliance. Discipline is also important in mental terms, because it is too easy to come to a premature conclusion about a case and then see only the details in the record that confirm that preconception. The effective expert should keep an open mind while reviewing the case (not only to generate a valid opinion but to anticipate rebuttal challenges), focus on the issues that really matter, consider other points of view and address them in his or her opinion, conduct a thorough literature review rather than cherry-picking articles that support his or her opinion or reading only abstracts, and cooperate with the lawyer who has retained the expert, whatever he or she may think of the lawyer and the client. (If the expert does not trust the lawyer or the client, he or she should get out of the case before being declared to the court as a witness.) Deference to legal counsel is also important because, very often, the lawyer may actually be arguing the case on another point and the expert's role may be less critical than the expert thinks it is.

There is nothing unethical about holding one opinion with respect to the legal interpretation of a set of findings and another with respect to the scientific interpretation, because the standards of certainty are hugely different. One may legitimately consider a matter to be very likely but not scientifically proven (such as asbestos as a cause of colon cancer). Often, the scientific evidence for an association is strong but not conclusive. In such cases, it is entirely reasonable and responsible, although frequently uncomfortable, for an expert witness to maintain on the witness stand that there is or is not an association, on the basis of an interpretation of "the weight of evidence," but to maintain in a scientific forum that the association is not proven because it has not been proven beyond a reasonable doubt. What counts in the end in a legal case is the weight of what evidence exists.

Expert Witness Practice

Most expert services begin with a request to review the medical record, review the relevant scientific literature, and to prepare a letter of opinion. This may be followed by deposition (during the phase of pre-trial preparation called "discovery"), and later by testimony in court, although the great majority of cases are settled before they go to trial.

Almost all lawyers consistently represent one side or the other, plaintiff or defense, and these days usually specialize in one type of case, particularly within the general area of personal injury. Experts may, and for their credibility should, be associated with both sides in different cases that show variety. However, circumstances of expertise and the referral network among lawyers often favor one side or the other. Sometimes lawyers from the defense in a very big case will try to retain experts who usually work on the plaintiff side, in order to tie them up and prevent them from serving as plaintiff experts in the same case.

A telephone call usually comes from the lawyer on one side or the other asking about the expert's availability and interest in assisting with a case (or claim, in disputed workers' compensation cases). Experts will normally be asked for a current curriculum vitae and a list of recent cases in which the expert participated, usually for the previous ten years, as these will be submitted into evidence when the expert is declared as a witness. Once declared to the court, an expert witness usually cannot be replaced and so there is an implied commitment once one agrees to serve as an expert to see the case through for the duration.

Merit Review

The expert should first offer to review the merits of the case. This may not require a detailed record review, as long as the essential facts are available. An oral opinion is given to the lawyer as to whether their case makes sense on the face of it. This initial evaluation, called a "merit review," is not about the expert's sympathies, but about whether the case is well grounded. Many lawyers will drop the case at this point if the expert tells them that the case does not hold water; others will shop around for another expert, which is not unethical. On the other hand, if the case is considered at this preliminary stage to be meritorious, the expert will normally be asked to proceed to a full record review and preparation of a written opinion.

The opinion in a preliminary merit review must be oral. No opinion letter should be written at this point, because the consultation is still preliminary. The complete record has not been reviewed and so the expert's opinion cannot be final and may be wrong. Besides, another expert may have a different point of view, a different theory of the case, and possibly a better analysis. A premature written opinion may be in error, incomplete, or off point but because it is subject to subpoena, a discordant preliminary opinion would have to be produced during discovery and will certainly be used to discredit the final opinion of that or another expert. It therefore is presumptuous and unacceptable to write an opinion letter in spite of the request of the lawyer not to do so. Some naive experts insist on doing this in order to force their own opinion into the record. This is inappropriate and contrary to the adversarial system of justice, in which both sides are expected to put forward their best case. To do so is therefore viewed as a hostile act on the part of the expert, not to mention a supreme act of egotism.

Reviewing Medical Records

Medical records review in a legal case is usually more extensive than is required for an IME (see Chapter 25, guidance from which also applies to medicolegal opinions) but the same principles apply.

The time it takes to review a medical record bears little relationship to its size, once the record is about an inch thick or more. Most medical records have many duplicate documents in them, especially laboratory tests and hospital discharge summaries. Records of subsequent medical treatment or management of complications following the initial diagnosis of an occupational disease are usually irrelevant in assessing causation. An exception might be that a newer record might mention a disputed smoking history or a family history suggesting a predisposition to a disease.

Every expert has his or her own routine in reviewing a record. The novice expert usually begins by reviewing the record page by page, making notes as he or she goes along, and then integrates the material before writing the case summary in the opinion letter. With experience, this can be streamlined by beginning with the documents that provide the most complete explication of the case (usually hospital discharge summaries, referral letters, and emergency department notes) and then formulating an idea of what the case is about and a preliminary theory of what happened. Following the "Pareto principle," 80 percent of the information is likely to be in just 20 percent of the records. By going where the most information is, the experienced expert can write a preliminary working draft with the basics and then refine, correct, and in some cases revise it in real time while reviewing the rest of the record. The medical record can then be reviewed systematically for contrary facts as if it were a test of a scientific theory, with the expert actively seeking to poke holes in his or her own theory of the case, whether working for the defense or the plaintiff.

Whichever approach the expert uses, he or she should always remember that any notes, electronic or handwritten, and any drafts of a letter of opinion that are prepared along the way are subject to subpoena. Small differences, expressed uncertainties (such as marginal notes to check something or question marks or exclamation marks), second thoughts, and just lines to make it easy to find some passage, will be exploited to create doubt in court, even though they reflect a perfectly legitimate process of questioning and evaluating evidence. Therefore, working notes and drafts should be kept to a minimum and dispensed with altogether if possible. As a practical matter, for experts without photographic memories, this means that cases are usually most easily reviewed in long marathon sittings while, if possible, preparing the opinion letter as one goes along instead of making multiple drafts.

The opinion letter must be professional, concise, and structured for easy access to critical information. One popular format for opinions regarding causation is outlined in Box 32.1. In a simple case, not all items may be needed and each item may only require a paragraph or so. In most cases, the letter is divided into sections so that the reader can find important material easily. Opinions on level of impairment or other issues will take other forms.

Box 32.1 Organization of the Opinion Letter in a Medicolegal Case

1. Expert's qualifications.
2. List of documents reviewed.
3. Case summary (highly detailed, not unlike the history of the present illness that a medical student might write).
4. IME results (if applicable, see Chapter 25).
5. Exposure history (including identification of significant hazards).
6. General causation (scientific evidence for causation).
7. Specific causation (evidence for causation in this particular case).
8. Opinion (elaborated in detail and justified).
9. Conclusions (summarizing the opinion, expressing the degree of certainty the expert has in the opinion "to a reasonable degree of medical certainty").
10. "References Relied Upon" (a list of key references from the literature on which the opinion is based).

Testimony may be by deposition or on the witness stand at a trial. The expert should receive a subpoena or court order to testify because this places him or her under the court's protection as someone compelled to testify and therefore independent at that moment from any obligation to or arrangement with the client. Generally, the subpoena will stipulate certain files, records, or billing information the expert is expected to bring. Only what is asked for should be brought.

Deposition is a procedure for taking testimony from the expert and from witnesses under oath. Most depositions are recorded in audio only or taken down using a stenotype machine by a court reporter and the product is a transcript. The transcript does not show gaps or pauses, and so the expert should never feel rushed or under pressure to provide an immediate answer. A thoughtful answer is better than an impulsive response. A videotaped deposition is more like testimony at trial, where patterns of speech and body language are important to perception. (It is unclear who besides the opposing counsel would ever sit through a video instead of just reading a transcript, so its value probably has more to do with detecting hesitation and unease on the part of the witness for later exploitation in court.) The court reporter is often unfamiliar with the terminologies of medicine, chemistry, and science that are used in occupational and environmental medicine and it is both entirely proper and very helpful for the expert witness to provide him or her with a list of words and names, correctly spelled.

After the transcript is produced, the witness has the opportunity to submit corrections to errors in an addendum to the transcript. (The transcript itself is not changed and often contains abundant errors.) The experienced expert will read the transcript carefully and take advantage of this opportunity. Although it is unlikely that a single erroneous passage will play a major role in the later proceedings, making the correction heads off the temptation for the opposing counsel to play games with it and makes clarification easier if the matter comes up again in court.

The expert's level of compensation will usually be raised at the end in cross-examination, with the intent of making the expert's testimony appear to be financially motivated. The best response is to simply state the facts and not to react defensively. Juries know that good experts are expensive.

Witnesscraft

An expert witness requires specific skills, as for any professional service. These skills come with practice and experience:

- The ability to speak in clear and understandable language about technical matters. (An expert's opinion does not matter if he or she cannot communicate it.)
- Technical knowledge. (Above all, the expert has a duty to be correct, to the best of his or her ability.)
- Discipline. (The effective expert prepares thoroughly for the case, regardless of distractions.)
- The ability to anticipate counterarguments and address them before they are presented by the "other" side. (This is where scientific training, with its emphasis on alternative hypotheses, is invaluable.)
- Deference. (A good expert follows the lead of the lawyer and does not try to pull the case in a certain direction.)

Novice expert witnesses often become absorbed with issues of deportment, proper dress, and "tricks of the trade" in giving oral testimony at trial. Too much emphasis is placed on these aspects of being an expert. Basically, the expert should simply present him- or herself in a manner appropriate to the professional role he or she plays, erring on the side of conservatism. It is certainly allowable to show flashes of individuality and to have a personality. However, the test of whether clothing and style are appropriate should not be what makes the expert look more credible. It should be whether the expert's appearance and deportment draws attention away from the proceedings, distracting the court from the serious business at hand, or creates a negative impression that undermines the expert's credibility.

A male physician or nurse, for example, is expected to appear in court dressed in a conservative business-style suit and a tie. These are not unreasonable expectations and so when an expert does not do so, the message in the back of the mind of judge and jury alike is "why"? A physician who showed up in jeans, even in Oregon, would not be perceived as showing respect for the court. (However, a mechanic or laborer might be given a pass.) A physician who showed up in court in whites with a stethoscope around his or her neck would be seen as acting the part and would be completely unbelievable. A physician or nurse who took the stand in an elegant, expensive, and fashionable or flamboyant suit would probably antagonize a jury but an investment banker who did the same would not get quite the same reaction. A health professional who showed up in a ridiculously loud tie or jacket or showing a provocative décolletage would be perceived as a blowhard or to be showing off, trying to draw attention to him- or herself. Conservative dress, therefore, is not about wearing a uniform and showing conformity but about keeping the attention of the people in the courtroom who matter on what is actually important.

Anything about the professional's appearance, speech, or mannerisms that is highly unusual (wheelchairs and prostheses are exceptions), that appears affected (such as some speech mannerisms or flamboyant facial hair), or that reflects a visibly controversial or alternative lifestyle commitment (such as a prominent earring, pink hair, or a tattoo) is an obstacle to communication. Affectations project an unclear message that the judge and jury don't need to think about, because they will not encounter the expert again and his or her lifestyle is irrelevant to the case at hand. The mental energy required to get beyond an expert's unusual appearance is energy that is taken away from thinking about the case and concentrating on what the expert is saying. The case is not about the expert and if the expert draws attention to him- or herself instead of the opinion, he or she will be doing a disservice to the client.

After gaining a little experience, experts all too often try to play lawyer. Some try to read the jury or judge as they testify, as if they were the lawyer for the side that brought them into the case. It cannot be said too emphatically: the expert is not the lawyer. Even if he or she has a law degree, the expert is not the lawyer in the case at hand.

Almost all experts form strong opinions about what is true in the case and some become very attached to the side they are supporting. Some consciously try to nudge the court to reach the "right" decision, which is not correct. The role of the expert is to provide a valid framework for thinking about the technical issues in the case within their scope of practice and to translate technical meaning into language a judge and jury can understand. The judge or the jury decide.

Experts may also chafe under the rules in court and wish to be "more scientific" in their testimony or (more often in the case of a treating physician) to show sympathy for the plaintiff. The legal system has its rules and they are not arbitrary. They are designed to resolve the matter decisively on the basis of current knowledge and allow the parties to move on, with justice done when it can be. The expert fits within those rules; the expert does not bend the court to the rules of science and medicine.

The first part of a deposition or testimony on the stand is normally to qualify the witness as an expert. Training, experience, and even publications may be reviewed in detail, especially if there is an opening for the "other side" to discredit the witness. It is strongly to the expert's advantage to hold formal credentials (degrees, certifications, diplomas, fellowships, proof of having passed a qualifying test) in every field in which he or she purports to be an expert, medical or nonmedical, health-related or not. For physicians, it is important for credibility to be actively practicing medicine, even if the case is not about a particular clinical issue. Any awkward, embarrassing, problematical, or contentious issues (such as a gap in practice or a malpractice lawsuit) should be raised by the lawyer who brought the expert into the case on direct examination and preferably fully explained before the substantive testimony even starts, in order to make it more difficult for opposing counsel to exaggerate its significance.

The expert needs to have a thick skin. Every time one testifies, one's credibility and reputation are placed on the line. If the expert consistently testifies on behalf of a plaintiff (or claimant) or defendant, he or she will be called partisan at best or a hack or a stooge. If the expert testifies for both at different times, coming to an opinion based on the facts of the case, he or she will be called a hired gun whose opinion can be bought by either side. This calumny comes with the territory, but it is one reason why many serious, thoughtful professionals who would otherwise have much to contribute do not want to have anything to do with litigation. The challenge and test of credibility inherent in serving as an expert witness also attracts a good many personality types who should not be doing it.

There are certain guidelines learned from experience that an expert would be wise to follow in giving testimony. These are summarized in Box 32.2.

Business Management

Lawyers who retain experts expect to be asked to sign a retainer agreement. The retainer itself is an up-front payment that is applied to the account later as services are billed. The retainer agreement should be prepared in advance by the expert and should provide a fee schedule for the various services (usually billed hourly, with a daily rate for cases that run for

Box 32.2 Guidance for Expert Witnesses

- *Avoid jargon.* Professional language has a role in professional communication but not in a deposition or in the courtroom. Use common, every day language to the extent possible. If you must use technical terms, define them and explain their significance. If you cannot explain a complicated issue in your field to an average person in less than five minutes, you should not be an expert witness.
- *Watch the tone of your verbal language.* Do not speak like a professor giving a lecture, if you can help it, and do not talk down to the judge or jury. Keep the level and vocabulary more or less conversational. Your sole purpose is to explain, not to impress.
- *Watch your body language.* Your body language should be relaxed and confident, not tense or defensive. Suppress idiosyncratic habits, like shaking your leg (a common habit), and gestures like fiddling with the microphone cord. Watch your eye contact. It should be on the person asking you the question or the judge or jury, not staring off into space or at the plaintiff. Basically, try to look like a normal person.
- *Avoid distractions and affectations.* Clothes, speech patterns, mannerisms, excessive jewelry, tattoos, shocking hair color, prominent piercings, and other distractions draw attention to the expert and away from the expert's opinion. This is not about personal choice and lifestyle. It is about communicating a message and allowing people to hear it undistracted.
- *Be explicit and as conclusive as you can be.* This is not a scientific exercise and the standard of certainty is not scientific certainty. The hedges that characterize scientific language are inappropriate in a venue in which the standard of certainty is already established as "more likely than not." Drop the distracting qualifiers, such as "essentially," "not significantly different," and "may suggest that," because they are impediments to understanding, and inadvertently convey uncertainty and diffidence to a jury. Simply state at the beginning of your testimony that you are offering your opinion based on the weight of evidence, taking into account uncertainties.
- *Be explicit.* Never assume that the judge or jury can reason from your foundation to a conclusion by themselves if you have not spelled out the logic and the conclusion for them. You are there precisely because you are the expert and they are not.
- *Answer only the question that is asked and do not volunteer further information.* Do not use a question as a springboard to give a lecture. Remember that it is the job of the lawyer on the side that brought you into the case to clarify unclear statements in redirect.

a full day or more). It should include the expert's policy regarding the expert's travel expenses (reimbursed in full, with a charge for time spent travelling) and how much compensation will be paid to the expert if and when (as is often the case) a deposition is cancelled or a trial is postponed or the case is settled on short notice. The usual cutoff for such changes is cancellation less than 48 hours in advance. Most cases settle, in part because most cases that do go to court are decided for the defense.

Medicolegal services are prone to misunderstanding of terms and to collection problems. This is especially true on the plaintiff side, because the law firm is usually working for a contingency fee for individual cases, may be facing long odds of success, and may be financially strained. Unless and until they win the judgment, the expenses of the case are paid by the law firm itself, which for major cases has normally taken out a line of credit at a bank. If the plaintiff does not win, the law firm loses all the money they have invested in the case, as well as the interest on the debt. On the other hand, large class action lawsuits are increasingly often financed by investors, who put up capital in anticipation of winning a large judgment, not unlike picking stocks. The firm, on behalf of its own lawyers and the financial backers, then takes a fraction of the judgment from the plaintiff if they win. For a plaintiff firm, it is therefore important to have several legal actions going at any one time so that an occasional big win will offset the more frequent losses.

On the defense side, there may be confusion over who is directly responsible for the invoice: the law firm, the client, or an insurance company. It is extremely important to know who, exactly, is responsible for payment and how to communicate with them: law firms will normally channel all communications to the payer through themselves and they may or may not be motivated to collect the expert's fee from a recalcitrant insurance company or a client who has lost the case.

For cases of short duration, a final invoice is usually sufficient. Frequent, preferably monthly, invoices during periods when there is activity in a case are much preferred in a long-running case to infrequent (quarterly or semiannual) invoices or invoicing everything at the end of the case. Most clients would prefer to receive regular, small invoices rather than single large invoices, even if the total amount is the same or slightly higher, which it should be because of processing expense. Single large invoices raise audit questions, break annual budgets, and straddle fiscal years, all of which cause additional issues and expense to the firm.

Failure to pay an expert's invoice may occur for many reasons, not the least of which is that the actual payer may not have received the invoice, there may be an error in the invoice, or the services or hours given in the invoice may be disputed. It is imperative to deal with such matters quickly. Accounts receivables that last past 60 days have a poor chance of being collected.

There are legal means, such as liens and lawsuits, to coerce payment in the case of deadbeat clients but they should only be used as a last resort. For the expert, such measures are complicated, unpleasant, and will certainly alienate clients. The best way to ensure collection is to prevent problems in the first place by charging a large retainer, invoicing frequently, and obtaining written agreement (email is fine) whenever the scope of work changes (for example, when additional records are received that were not in the original batch, when the number of billable hours will clearly exceed the range previously agreed upon, and when a rebuttal or response to the other side's expert is requested).

The most difficult part of the business side of being an expert may be remembering to keep track of hours. A timesheet or computer-based billing clock is ideal from the accounting perspective but impractical. One simple way to record hours is to enter blocks of time spent on a case in the expert's calendar (for example on Outlook) as if they were past appointments. Then, using the calendar to prompt memory, record the total time spent on each case every day at 5:00 or the close of business. It is important to remember to carry over work done after the close of business to the following day, because many and perhaps most experts do their best work on opinions after hours, free of distractions.

Recommended Reading and Resources

American College of Physicians (1990) Guidelines for the physician expert witness. *Ann Intern Med*, 113(10): 789.
Cohen FL (2004) The expert witness in legal perspective. *J Leg Med*, 25(2): 185–209.

Federal Judicial Center (2011) *Reference Manual on Scientific Evidence.* Washington DC, 3rd ed.

Guidotti TL, Rose SJ (2001) *Science on the Witness Stand: The Evaluation of Scientific Evidence in Law, Adjudication, and Policy.* Beverly Farms MA, OEM Press. Written primarily for physicians and other health professionals in occupational and environmental medicine.

Jasanoff S (1995) *Science at the Bar: Law, Science and Technology in America.* Cambridge MA, Harvard University Press, Twentieth Century Fund.

Lukcso D, Green-McKenzie J (2009) What are some of the essential elements physicians should consider when in the role of expert witness? *J Occup Environ Med,* 51: 1350–1352.

Lukcso D, Green-McKenzie J (2010) What are some terms commonly encountered by the physician expert witness? *J Occup Environ Med,* 52: 109–110.

Meyer C., ed. (1999) *Expert Witnessing: Explaining and Understanding Science.* Boca Raton FL, CRC Press.

Muscat JE, Huncharek MS (1989) Causation and disease: biomedical science in toxic tort litigation. *J Occup Med,* 31(12): 997–1002.

Appendix 1: An Occupational Health Audit

This audit instrument is not comprehensive and does not address specific technical issues such as particular chemical hazards and safety measures. It does provide a framework for evaluating the performance of an employer and for the occupational health professional who is called upon to participate in a visit to the workplace, or "walk through," in an incident investigation, or in a performance audit.

Occupational health and safety (OHS) audits can come in many forms. In general, many organizations recognize five specific types of audits. These audit types, their definitions, the source of auditors, and the suggested audit frequencies are noted below.

Type of Audit	Definition	Auditors	Frequency
Management System Audit	Assessment of management system(s) against recognized standards (e.g. OSHAS 18001, etc.).	External—Accredited Certifiers Internal auditor(s) can be used for pre-audit support	Based on the Standards' requirements.
Audit of OHS Audit Program	An assessment of the OHS Audit Program itself for compliance with the organization's audit process.	Internal or external auditors may be employed but must be external to the part of the business owning the audit system.	Suggested minimum— every three years.
Due Diligence Audits for Acquisitions and Divestitures	Evaluation of OHS-related performance and an assessment of risks to identify potential and actual issues, including costs, and business impacts and liabilities prior to completion of the transaction.	Internal and/or external auditors can be employed. Must have the technical skills to understand and assess the processes and activities of the entity being audited.	Prior to the completion of potential acquisition or divestiture.
Specific Audit	Audit focused on one or several specific issues.	Internal and/or external auditors can be employed providing they have the appropriate skill sets.	As required.
Comprehensive Audit	Assesses compliance to regulatory, site-specific, and organizational requirements as well as best practices and overall effectiveness of the Management System.	Internal Audit Team plus external auditors as necessary for specialized or technical expertise, or as additional general auditors.	Audit frequency may be based on risk levels established through the baseline comprehensive audit and in rsponse to performance on previous audits.

There are many approaches to scaling audit findings. The sample audit format noted in the following pages uses a relatively simple but effective format: "inadequate," "needs improvement," and "satisfactory." Other approaches can be more specific such as the one with four levels of findings that is described below.

- *Level 1 findings.* These findings require immediate action and include findings that: (1) are immediately or foreseeably dangerous to life and health (IDLH) or could cause significant or extensive damage; (2) reflect failures of compliance with legislation or organizational policies; (3) are key risks, which could result in serious injuries, death, or significant longer term health impacts to employees or others, or are legal charges against company personnel; and/or (4) relate to issues which have a reasonable chance of damaging the organization's reputation.
- *Level 2 findings.* Highly significant findings which do not fall into the definition of category 1, but should be given high priority to resolving these findings (e.g. within three to six months).
- *Level 3 findings.* These findings have lower significance and resolution priority, but still must be addressed and closed.
- *Level 4 findings.* Findings that do not require action but reflect recommendations or best practice references which will assist the site on the road to excellence.

The model for an occupational health audit noted below is intended to be a tool that *assists the reader to understand the audit process* and can be used during a visit to any industrial facility. It is *not* intended to be comprehensive and/or all-inclusive. Such an audit approach for health and safety would be far more intensive and encompass many additional topics not covered here. Nevertheless, with the appropriate modifications, this format can be adapted for use in working units in many different types of organizations. This audit is presented as a questionnaire divided into sections, each with a series of questions and associated measures. The measures (as noted previously) have been kept simple and qualitative. No two areas of a workplace are in the same situation and no two employers are the same. Where a rating is less than satisfactory, corrective action must be initiated. Similarly, the format of audits can vary greatly from one company to another (for internal audits) and from one auditing organization to another (for external, contracted, auditing services).

The original version appeared for the first time in the first edition of this book. It was used internally in a Canadian oil pipeline company called NOVA by Dr. John Cowell, who was an author of the book in its first edition. This version was adapted, with many changes and additions, by Marion Stecklow and by Ian Arnold.

Description	Inadequate	Needs Improvement	Satisfactory
1.0 Occupational Health and Safety Policy			
1.1 The policy enjoys wide acceptance and publicity throughout the organization.			
1.1.1 A written and signed policy statement affirms the employer's commitment to protecting the health and safety of all persons affected by their operations.			
1.1.2 Officers and senior management of the company endorse, and publically support, the policy.			
1.1.3 All legislated occupational health and safety standards are considered to be the minimum standards acceptable and will be exceeded where possible.			
1.1.4 The policy is accessible, posted, distributed, and communicated to all employers throughout the organization, in an appropriate language.			
1.1.5 The policy is regularly reviewed and updated to reflect changes in legislated and company requirements.			
1.1.6 Each aspect of health, safety, and hygiene is covered in the policy including psychological health and safety.			
1.2 The policy is compatible and consistent with corporate policy in other areas and meets regulatory requirements as applicable.			
2.0 Occupational Health and Safety Administration			
2.1 There is a clearly defined approach to managing health and safety that includes the following:			
2.1.1 Roles and responsibilities are clearly defined for all levels of employees in the organization including health and safety professionals.			
2.1.2 Defined expectation for action to resolve health and safety issues.			
2.1.3 Established preference for proactive, preventive programs.			
2.1.4 Understanding among all levels of management and by safety professionals of the priorities of the program and the expectations placed on them for its successful implementation.			
2.1.5 Qualified resource personnel are available in the following disciplines as determined by the organization's needs:			
2.1.5.1 safety			
2.1.5.2 occupational hygiene			
2.1.5.3 occupational medicine			
2.1.5.4 occupational health nursing.			
2.2 The following aspects are clearly defined:			
2.2.1 safe work practices			
2.2.2 workplace standards			
2.2.3 personal protective equipment standards.			
2.3 There is a written procedure requiring proper incident/accident investigation that clearly defines the role and duties of all personnel involved.			

Description	Inadequate	Needs Improvement	Satisfactory
2.4 There is a written, clearly established procedure for reporting and recording data on all incidents and accidents, conforming at a minimum to Occupational Safety and Health Administration (OSHA) requirements or other regulatory compliance			
2.5 There is a well established program to communicate current health and safety issues to employees and employers that includes the following:			
2.5.1 Regular health and safety meetings of management, supervisors, and local health and safety specialists.			
2.5.2 Regular health and safety meetings that involve and engage all employees.			
2.5.3 Regular health and safety inspections.			
2.5.4 Written communications of incident/accident investigation reports to all personnel with responsibilities that may be affected.			
2.5.5 Films, bulletins, posters, and other posted information in appropriate language, and simple illustrations to maintain health and safety awareness.			
2.5.6 Communication to employees in appropriate language and the use of graphics for known or potential hazards associated with the workplace, and their possible effects.			
2.6 Each area within the workplace has a coordinated annual health and safety program that includes:			
2.6.1 Clearly defined goals established by operating management in consultation with company health and safety personnel.			
2.6.2 An identified plan to achieve the goals.			
2.6.3 Consistent and thorough reviews involving management and health and safety specialists to examine performance and to adjust the above plan as necessary.			
2.6.4 Written objectives for each health and safety specialist specifying how their activities support the goals established by the operating components of the employer.			
2.7 A written plan is in place that demonstrates the ability to respond to all levels of emergency incidents, including:			
2.7.1 Identification of potential emergencies.			
2.7.2 Identification of personnel assigned to handle an emergency and their responsibilities in the event of an incident.			
2.7.3 Identification and organization of resources available to manage emergencies.			
2.7.4 Documented practice sessions to ensure readiness in the event of an incident.			
2.8 Regular health and safety inspections are performed and documented by:			
2.8.1 supervisors			
2.8.2 health and safety specialists.			
2.9 Local health, safety and work procedures are reviewed regularly to ensure:			
2.9.1 Compliance with current internal and legislated standards.			
2.9.2 Suitability for use in the workplace.			

Description	Inadequate	Needs Improvement	Satisfactory
2.9.3 Availability and familiarity in the workplace.			
2.10 Management and the local health and safety specialists are involved in the review.			
2.11 All action items are identified, documented, and resolved in a timely manner.			
3.0 Site Management			
Site managers are required to:			
3.1 Consider occupational health and safety as a normal part of operations that must be planned for, organized, controlled, and measured.			
3.2 Understand their responsibilities related to health and safety.			
3.3 Ensure that their employees know their responsibilities related to health and safety, and hold them accountable			
3.4 Ensure that procedures/instructions are established and followed regarding:			
3.4.1 Health and safety practices			
3.4.2 Job/work practices			
3.4.3 Enforcement of health, safety, and work regulations			
3.4.4 Accident investigation			
3.4.5 Workplace hazard identification and risk assessment and control			
3.4.6 Exposure to health hazards, both physical and psychological			
3.5 Ensure that all employees are properly trained to perform their specific job tasks safely			
3.6 Receive training and demonstrate competence in:			
3.6.1 Management's responsibility for occupational health and safety, as expressed in company policy and legislation			
3.6.2 Basic principles of hazard recognition and accident prevention.			
3.6.3 Basic principles of occupational hygiene			
3.6.4 Basic principles of psychological health and safety			
3.7 Actively participate in the health and safety program by:			
3.7.1 Holding regular recorded meetings to discuss health and safety issues and performance involving:			
3.7.1.1 their manager/supervisor			
3.7.1.2 occupational health personnel			
3.7.1.3 safety personnel			
3.7.1.4 industrial hygiene personnel			
3.7.1.5 worker representatives where applicable			
3.7.2 Participate in safety tours.			
3.7.3 Provide routine reports on health and safety issues and their resolution.			

Description	Inadequate	Needs Improvement	Satisfactory
3.7.4 Ensure that adequate resources are in place to support the health and safety activities.			
3.7.5 Review all accident, injury, and occupational illness reports and ensure that proper corrective action is implemented.			
4.0 Foremen/Supervisors			
The foremen/supervisors are responsible for:			
4.1 Maintaining records of the health and safety performance of the workers in their area.			
4.2 Including health and safety as a regular part of their daily activities, and encouraging a positive, safe attitude on the part of employees.			
4.3 Ensuring that their employees are trained in and follow health and safety practices associated with their particular job. Only competent and trained employees or employees under the direct supervision of a competent employee are permitted to perform a hazardous task.			
4.4 Maintaining the necessary training in the areas of:			
4.4.1 Supervisory responsibilities related to health and safety			
4.4.2 Accident prevention techniques			
4.4.3 Hazard recognition risk assessment and risk control			
4.4.4 Occupational hygiene			
4.4.5 Accident investigation			
4.4.6 First aid and cardiopulmonary resuscitation			
4.4.7 Local emergency procedures.			
4.5 Ensuring that the written procedures, in appropriate language, apply to any job involving work of a hazardous nature are available and reviewed with the employees involved.			
4.6 Performing regular health and safety inspections in their area, and recording the results and any corrective action required.			
4.7 Working with the local health and safety specialist to ensure that proper, safe work practices and procedures are established for the area.			
4.8 Ensuring that the facilities for which they are responsible are maintained in a safe and healthy condition.			
5.0 Joint Employee–Management Health and Safety Committee (sometimes known as the Joint Health and Safety Committee)			
5.1 A committee exists in accordance with:			
5.1.1 employee–management agreement			
5.1.2 legislation			
5.1.3 other (specify)			
5.2 The committee meets regularly and follows an agenda.			
5.3 There is representation from the following:			
5.3.1 senior management			

Description	Inadequate	Needs Improvement	Satisfactory
5.3.2 operations			
5.3.3 facilities management.			
5.3.4 employees.			
5.4 The committee performs regularly scheduled health and safety inspections in the area.			
5.5 A training program is maintained to ensure that the members have sufficient knowledge of health and safety matters to function effectively.			
5.6 The committee issues minutes of the meetings on a regular basis.			
5.7 The minutes are action- oriented, identifying tasks to be done.			
5.8 There is a positive and timely response to the action items by operational personnel.			
5.9 The committee is perceived as effective by both the employees and management.			
5.10 The committee reviews all incident/accident reports.			
6.0 Training Program			
6.1 A standard training format has been established to provide the health and safety training required for the preparation of:			
6.1.1 supervisors			
6.1.2 employees.			
6.2 A standard training program is in place to ensure that all operators are properly trained or supervised before they operate any of the facility's mechanical/electrical equipment or operational/manufacturing equipment.			
6.3 Employees' assigned responsibilities are directly in compliance with the training that has been successfully completed.			
6.4 All new employees are given a health and safety orientation covering the following:			
6.4.1 job hazards			
6.4.2 health hazards, including psychological health hazards, and related risks			
6.4.3 use of protective equipment			
6.4.4 proper work procedures			
6.4.5 work restrictions			
6.4.6 health and safety regulations			
6.4.7 hazard reporting			
6.4.8 first aid resources.			
6.5 All new employees are closely supervised until they are capable of working without risk of injury.			
6.6 Are all employees aware of:			
6.6.1 Potential and existing hazards and the risks from these hazards that may pose a threat to their health and safety?			
6.6.2 Proper work procedures?			

Description	*Inadequate*	*Needs Improvement*	*Satisfactory*
6.6.3 Proper use and limitations of protective equipment?			
6.6.4 Health and safety regulations?			
6.6.5 Special skills necessary to perform their job safely?			
6.7 Sufficient numbers of people are qualified in:			
6.7.1 first aid			
6.7.2 cardiopulmonary resuscitation			
6.7.3 fire fighting			
6.7.4 use of respiratory protection			
6 .7.5 special hazard awareness			
6.7.6 special hazard detection			
6.7.7 hazardous chemical control and use			
6.7.8 incident/accident investigation			
6.7.9 other (specify)			
6.8 All the training programs offered meet current company and legislated standards.			
6.9 The training program includes:			
6.9.1 Permanent records of all health, safety, and job training courses completed by each employee.			
6.9.2 Training documentation includes the title of the training session, the instructors name and qualification, session duration, date, employee printed name and signature.			
6.9.3 A periodic review to ensure that the required level of expertise is maintained.			
7.0 Incident/Accident Handling			
7.1 All incidents/accidents are suitably investigated to determine the following:			
7.1.1 A clear understanding of what occurred and all factors contributing to the incident.			
7.1.2 The direct and indirect causes of the accident.			
7.1.3 The basic causes (root cause) that allowed the incident/accident to occur at all.			
7.1.4 The proper short- and long-term corrective action(s).			
7.2 There is a written procedure for recording and reporting the incident/accident and communicating findings to:			
7.2.1 the required employer representative			
7.2.2 required government authorities			
7.2.3 supervisors			
7.2.4 employee representatives.			
7.3 The investigation involves all appropriate levels of management, supervisors, health and safety professionals, and employee representatives (as applicable).			

Description	Inadequate	Needs Improvement	Satisfactory
7.4 There is a clearly defined procedure to ensure that options for corrective actions are reviewed by management and appropriate action is taken to resolve the problems identified, and to ensure appropriate and timely follow-up.			
7.5 All types of incidents/accidents are covered, including the following:			
7.5.1 personal injury (physical and psychological)			
7.5.2 occupational illness			
7.5.3 property damage			
7.5.4 vehicle accidents			
7.5.5 near miss (incidents/accidents that are narrowly avoided).			
7.5.6 transportation incidents.			
7.6 The following incidents are discussed with all employees:			
7.6.1 personal injury (physical and psychological)			
7.6.2 occupationally related illnesses			
7.6.3 property damage			
7.6.4 vehicle accidents			
7.6.5 transportation incidents.			
8.0 Occupational Health and Safety Specialist			
8.1 At least one employee is assigned to management with responsibility for coordinating health and safety programs.			
8.2 The duties, responsibilities, and relationships of the health and safety specialist(s) are clearly described and known to workers.			
8.3 The people assigned to health and safety duties are adequate in number and skills to fulfill their responsibilities in all areas, including the following:			
8.3.1 occupational health			
8.3.2 safety			
8.3.3 occupational hygiene			
8.3.4 emergency response			
8.3.5 transportation of hazardous materials.			
8.4 Technical and management specialist(s) are provided with adequate opportunities to maintain and to improve their qualifications by attending seminars and courses.			
8.5 Adequate facilities and equipment are provided to support the responsibilities of the specialist(s) including the following:			
8.5.1 appropriate clinical health facilities, including equipment and supplies.			
8.5.2 office and records storage			
8.5.3 meeting room facilities			
8.5.4 audiovisual materials			
8.5.5 specialized equipment (including emergency supplies)			

Description	Inadequate	Needs Improvement	Satisfactory
8.5.6 biohazard containment equipment			
8.5.7 defibrillator and intubation equipment			
8.5.8 meets or exceeds regulatory requirements for accessibility for disabled persons			
8.5.9 capacity for storage of controlled drugs.			
8.6 The facilities and equipment are regularly maintained.			
8.7 The specialist(s) is required to submit reports to management at a frequency that is relevant to the organizational needs about their activities and outcomes.			
8.8 The specialists are required to prepare an annual plan, in cooperation with management, to coordinate the sustainability of their programs.			
9.0 Facilities and Equipment			
9.1 A visual inspection of the facilities finds that it is free of significant problems in:			
9.1.1 housekeeping			
9.1.2 adequate work areas and access paths			
9.1.3 material and chemical storage			
9.1.4 ventilation—temperature/noise levels			
9.1.5 provision of guardrails and handrails			
9.1.6 machine tools, equipment guards, and protective devices			
9.1.7 roadways and walkways			
9.1.8 lighting			
9.1.9 facilities and equipment maintenance.			
9.2 Access to areas with significant health and safety hazards/risks is restricted to employees who have had an appropriate health assessment and appropriate and documented training, and have a reason to be in the area.			
9.3 Waste material is properly collected and disposed of.			
9.4 The fire protection systems are adequate in the following ways:			
9.4.1 suited to the facility and equipment therein			
9.4.2 properly located			
9.4.3 properly maintained (with maintenance recorded).			
9.5 All hazardous confined spaces are properly identified and controlled.			
9.6 Adequate, accessible first aid facilities are provided.			
9.7 A suitable program is in place to ensure proper maintenance in the following areas:			
9.7.1 Regular maintenance checks of the condition of all equipment. Negative findings are reported and resolved in a timely manner.			
9.7.2 All work is performed only by competent and trained personnel.			

Description	Inadequate	Needs Improvement	Satisfactory
9.7.3 Proper locking and tagging procedures are used to isolate all hazardous energy sources during maintenance work.			
9.7.4 Written maintenance records are kept in accordance with policy and legislated regulations.			
9.7.5 Critical failures, or processes that have the potential for significant risks in the event of failure, are identified and corrected.			
9.8 When facilities are modified or expanded, procedures are in place to ensure that:			
9.8.1 All plans are reviewed by a qualified health and safety specialist.			
9.8.2 Government authorities are notified as required by the employer's policy and by law.			
9.8.3 All construction work is observed and managed in accordance with the employer's policy, legal regulations, and the following:			
9.8.3.1 Health and safety policies of the contractor.			
9.8.3.2 Adherence by the contractor to the employer's policies, legal regulations, and accepted practices.			
9.8.3.3 Construction and material quality standards.			
9.8.3.4 Standing with the workers' compensation carrier.			
9.9 A process analysis (or the equivalent) has been completed to identify possible hazardous areas that could endanger workers.			
10. Safety Programs and Procedures			
10.1 Published guidelines on safe work practices are available to all employees in appropriate language.			
10.2 Management reviews and regulates personnel who perform work that requires specialized knowledge, training, or licensing.			
10.3 There is a work control system to identify hazards, and assess and control risk through a system of safe work permits.			
10.4 Mobile equipment is qualified as safe when purchased, is properly maintained, and is operated only by competent, authorized operators.			
10.5 A program is in place to ensure that hoisting and lifting equipment is in a safe condition when purchased, is properly maintained, and is operated only by competent, authorized operators.			
10.6 All inspection and maintenance work done on mobile and lifting equipment is documented.			
10.7 Vehicle operations require the following:			
10.7.1 Vehicles used on company business are maintained in safe condition and are operated in a safe manner and in accordance with all laws.			
10.7.2 Only properly licensed employees may operate a motor vehicle on company business.			
10.7.3 Vehicles requiring a licensed operator other than a holder of a Class 5 license (or equivalent) are operated only by a properly licensed operator.			

Description	Inadequate	Needs Improvement	Satisfactory
10.7.4 Seat belts and/or other restraining devices should be mandatory.			
10.7.5 All company vehicles must be driven with lights on.			
10.7.6 Consideration should be given to implementing driver training courses when hazards may exist that could pose special risks to the employee or others.			
10.8 A complete written procedure exists for locking, tagging, and blocking equipment that ensures that the equipment is in a state of "zero energy" (i.e. will not roll, snap, spring, or discharge) before and during the time it is worked on.			
10.9 Written standards are provided that cover the storage and use of flammable materials and include the following:			
10.9.1 proper ventilation			
10.9.2 proper storage cabinets or rooms			
10.9.3 suitable fire extinguishing equipment, which is checked regularly and is readily available			
10.9.4 separation of potentially reactive materials			
10.9.5 proper grounding of containers			
10.9.6 limits on the quantities of flammable materials kept in work areas			
10.9.7 control of ignition sources close to flammable materials in work and storage areas.			
10.10 Maintenance employees and others, as needed, are trained in proper procedures of performing elevated work, including the following:			
10.10.1 proper use of ladders and scaffolds			
10.10.2 proper use of personal protective equipment.			
10.11 Work on electrical equipment is controlled to ensure that:			
10.11.1 only qualified competent personnel perform the work			
10.11.2 proper locking and tagging procedures are followed.			
10.12 All excavation and trenching work is controlled to ensure that:			
10.12.1 Excavations are properly prepared prior to entry by any personnel.			
10.12.2 Buried hazards and cables are identified and safely exposed by hand digging.			
10.12.3 Trenches are properly shored according to sound work practices and legislation.			
10.13 Written procedures are followed to ensure that the opening of pipes, sumps, valves, tanks, and cisterns during maintenance is properly controlled and done only by competent personnel.			
11. Occupational Hygiene Program			
11.1 A program is in place to identify all existing and potential chemical, physical, and biological hazards, including the following:			
11.1.1 Identification of hazards associated with raw materials and their location.			

Description	Inadequate	Needs Improvement	Satisfactory
11.1.2 Identification of hazards associated with process chemicals and additives, and their location.			
11.1.3 Identification of process by-products and their locations.			
11.1.4 Identification of equipment and activities that can give rise to such physical hazards as heat, noise, and radiation.			
11.1.5 Assessment of the potential exposure in the event of a process failure, or a system breakdown.			
11.1.6 Assessment of all new processes, equipment, and process chemicals to deter the potential hazard.			
11.2 A program has been established to identify all chemical products used or stored at the facility that includes the following elements:			
11.2.1 A complete written inventory of all chemicals and their location.			
11.2.2 A standardized format for Safety Data Sheets (SDS) that meets all legislated requirements.			
11.2.3 A review of the accuracy and completeness of all safety date sheets performed by qualified personnel.			
11.2.4 A process for updating the chemical inventory list on a regular planned basis.			
11.2.5 Sufficient distribution of SDS to ensure that all employees have access to them.			
11.2.6 An ongoing evaluation of new chemical products during their initial research and later industrial development to identify any health and safety concerns before the products are used within the company.			
11.2.7 An ongoing evaluation of new chemical products throughout the process by which they are developed for industrial and commercial use that aims at identifying all health and safety concerns.			
11.3 A program is in place to identify hazards associated with products. This program includes the following elements:			
11.3.1 Identification of all components of the products and a review of their potential hazard.			
11.3.2 Identification of potential product contaminants that could be hazardous or that could increase the hazard of the product.			
11.3.3 Preparation and provision of accurate SDS to customers.			
11.3.4 Documentation, including the date of issue, for the distribution to customers of SDS for the product.			
11.3.5 Testing of equipment for physical hazards (noise, vibration, heat, radiation).			
11.4 A program is in place to ensure that any known or potential carcinogens and other hazardous substances, including bloodborne pathogens, have been identified and controlled.			
11.5 A program is in place to evaluate exposure to health hazards and includes the following elements:			

Description	*Inadequate*	*Needs Improvement*	*Satisfactory*
11.5.1 Regular monitoring of potential employee exposures under operational conditions and the potential for exposure to blood-borne pathogens (BBPs)			
11.5.2 Testing and analysis of the workplace by qualified specialists.			
11.5.3 Comparison of all readings to recognized standards in order to evaluate the need for control.			
11.5.4 Recognized monitoring and analytical methods.			
11.5.5 A suitable procedure for verification of and follow-up of problems.			
11.5.6 Equipment calibration and maintenance.			
11.6 A hazard control program is in place that includes the following:			
11.6.1 Engineering, administration, and personal protective controls, as appropriate.			
11.6.2 A control strategy that considers the following responses, in order of preference:			
11.6.2.1 elimination and/or replacement of the hazardous substance			
11.6.2.2 engineering controls to minimize or eliminate the exposure potential			
11.6.2.3 administrative controls to protect employees from exposure			
11.6.2.4 use of suitable personal protective equipment to protect employees from overexposure.			
11.7 A follow-up program is in place to ensure that the controls that have been implemented are effective and maintained.			
11.8 A training program is in place to ensure that employees are made aware of all health hazards and the proper procedures associated with protecting workers from exposure. This program includes an SDS retrieval and interpretation exercise to assist in dealing with all hazardous materials and including the potential for exposure to BBP.			
11.9 A hearing conservation program is in place to control exposure to harmful noise levels that includes the following:			
11.9.1 noise measurements			
11.9.2 employee hearing tests (baseline and periodic)			
11.9.3 employee training			
11.9.4 suitable controls.			
11.10 A complete program is in place to control entry into confined spaces, in accordance with the employer's policy and legislated standards.			
11.11 The required "Codes of Practice" are all in place.			
12. Transportation of Hazardous Materials			
12.1 The requirements of legislation are considered to be the minimum standard and are to be improved upon if possible.			
12.2 The facility is registered as a shipper/manufacturer of hazardous materials, as required by law.			
12.3 An emergency response plan has been filed with government authorities.			
12.4 There is a complete listing of all regulated goods used at the facility.			

Description	Inadequate	Needs Improvement	Satisfactory
12.5 There is a training program in place in accordance with legislated requirements.			
12.6 There is a program in place to monitor changes in legislation.			
12.7 Regulated wastes generated by the facility are identified and monitored.			
12.8 Copies of all bills of lading are stored in one place and available for review.			
12.9 Copies of all federal and state or provincial inspection reports are easily available for review.			
12.10 This facility has participated in an audit on the handling of hazardous materials.			
12.11 A program is in place to ensure proper placarding (signage on the vehicle) of vehicles transporting hazardous materials.			
13. Personal Protective Equipment			
13.1 A written program is in place to control the selection, use, and maintenance of personal protective equipment.			
13.2 The selection of personal protective equipment available to workers at the worksite takes into consideration the following:			
13.2.1 nature of the specific hazards			
13.2.2 employee fitting and fit testing for use o frespirators (as applicable)			
13.2.3 employee training.			
13.3 The selection available includes all necessary personal protective equipment to protect employees adequately from all hazards in the workplace (foot, head, face, eye, skin, respiratory, hearing, fall protection, etc.) and gives them a choice wherever possible.			
13.4 Personal protective equipment is made available to all employees in accordance with the employer's policy and legislated standards for employee protection.			
13.5 The supervisors, in consultation with health and safety personnel, specify which type of personal protective equipment is required by their workers on all jobs.			
13.6 Prior to the specification or purchase of any personal protective equipment, a qualified occupational health or safety professional reviews and approves the purchase order so as to ensure that the final selection of equipment is in accordance with recognized standards and operational requirements.			
13.7 Supervisors actively promote and require the use of personal protective equipment by their workers, and set an example by using the appropriate equipment themselves.			
13.8 Supervisors make sure that all workers understand the need for proper use of the personal protective equipment and the limitations on their effectiveness. Appropriate disciplinary actions for failure to use required personal protective equipment are in place and understood by all employees.			

Description	Inadequate	Needs Improvement	Satisfactory
14. Occupational Health Service Policy and Procedures			
14.1 The occupational health personnel have direct access to designated management personnel at the workplace.			
14.2 Regular staff meetings are held and documented. (Identify the frequency and the date of the last meeting.)			
14.3 Occupational health personnel members have job descriptions that are current.			
14.4 Occupational health personnel members work from annual goals/ objectives. (Identify the person responsible for setting goals.)			
14.5 Occupational health personnel members are given the opportunity to attend professional courses, conferences, and seminars.			
14.6 A detailed policy and procedure manual is reviewed and signed annually, and is readily available.			
14.7 The manual reflects corporate policy regarding occupational health and safety and includes a clear description of the organization's approach to the confidentiality of medical records.			
14.8 The manual includes statements on the following:			
14.8.1 individual personnel responsibilities, including job descriptions			
14.8.2 control and dispensing of medication			
14.8.3 use of special equipment			
14.8.4 authorization for medical procedures, including signed standing orders, reviewed and documented annually			
14.8.5 liaison with health resources in the community			
14.8.6 services on weekends and after normal hours			
14.8.7 communications with hygiene and safety departments, where applicable			
14.8.8 communications with employer management			
14.8.9 transportation of sick and injured			
14.8.10 emergency care policy and procedures, including appropriate documentation			
14.8.11 sickness absence follow-up			
14.8.12 disability management procedures			
14.8.13 work appointments' procedures			
14.8.14 record-keeping procedures			
14.8.15 retention time for records			
14.8.16 occupational health staff meetings			
14.8.17 laboratory procedures			
14.8 18 objectives and procedures for health programs			
14.8.19 in-house safety procedures			
14.8.20 procedures concerning investigations of incidents/accidents.			

Description	Inadequate	Needs Improvement	Satisfactory
14.9 The manual includes the following:			
14.9.1 disaster plan outlining the appropriate response of the occupational health services			
14.9.2 use of record and requisition forms			
14.9.3 contracts for hospital and emergency services.			
14.10 The manual is reviewed regularly by all parties responsible. (Specify date of last review.)			
14.11 The occupational health service meets regulatory requirements in the following areas:			
14.11.1 hearing conservation			
14.11.2 examination of vehicle operators			
14.11.3 workers' compensation reports			
14.11.4 substance abuse testing			
14.11.5 examinations relating to all legislated substances and hazards.			
14.12 The most significant illness and injury problems arising in the workplace (specify) have been identified and discussed with:			
14.12.1 the physician and/or the occupational health nurse			
14.12.2 the occupational health manager			
14.12.3 employer management			
14.12.4 employee representatives.			
14.13 The most frequent occupational injuries and illnesses in the workplace have been addressed by effective programs or controls.			
14.14 The principal health and safety hazards presented by this workplace are known to all service personnel and are frequently discussed.			
14.15 The occupational health personnel have a mechanism in place for becoming aware of and knowledgeable about changes in hazards and conditions in the workplace. These include:			
14.15.1 Safety Data Sheets or their equivalent			
14.15.2 site visits (regularly and as needed)			
14.15.3 review of clinical records (regularly and as needed)			
14.15.4 worker complaints			
14.15.5 union complaints			
14.15.6 industrial hygiene notifications			
14.15.7 management consultations			
14.15.8 special studies conducted on the workplace			
14.15.9 other (list).			
14.16 The physician, certified occupational health nurse, and appropriate occupational health personnel have become familiar with the processes, materials, and products found in the workplace.			

Description	Inadequate	Needs Improvement	Satisfactory
14.17 The physician and appropriate occupational health personnel make regular and frequent site visits.			
15. Health Service Programs and Activities			
Evaluations of services provided have demonstrated satisfactory performance of the following:			
15.1 Acute injury and illness management.			
15.2 Fitness-to-work evaluations:			
15.2.1 preplacement health assessment			
15.2.2 return-to-work evaluation			
15.2.3 job transfer health assessment			
15.2.4 continuing education			
15.2.5 changes in health conditions			
15.2.6 changes in working conditions			
15.2.7 performance-initiated health assessment			
15.2.8 voluntary periodic health evaluation			
15.2.9 substance abuse testing.			
15.3 Health surveillance.			
15.4 Health monitoring.			
15.5 Assessments of fitness to wear respirators.			
15.6 Audiograms.			
15.7 Immunizations.			
15.8 Ongoing therapy, monitoring of chronic health conditions.			
15.9 Psychological health and safety programs:			
15.9.1 employee assistance			
15.9.2 stress reduction			
15.9.3 substance abuse counseling			
15.9.4 other psychological health and safety program components (specify)			
15.10 Low back care and prevention of back injury.			
15.11 Smoking cessation.			
15.12 Physical fitness.			
15.13 Dietary consultation and nutrition.			
15.14 Workplace rehabilitation.			
15.15 Site health surveys and health hazard evaluations.			
15.16 Health and safety committee.			
15.17 Worker health training.			
15.18 Management health training.			

Description	Inadequate	Needs Improvement	Satisfactory
15.19 Collection of illness/trauma data.			
15.20 Analysis of illness/trauma data.			
15.21 Reporting of results of analysis to employer management.			
15.22 Incident/accident investigation.			
15.23 First aid/cardiopulmonary resuscitation (CPR) training.			
16. Health Service Resources Facility			
The location, main components, and age of the occupational health service facilities are appropriate to the service's use and function.			
16.1 The facilities are accessible to workers with adequate parking available.			
16.2 The facilities are accessible to the handicapped.			
16.3 The facilities ensure the privacy of workers who come for care and are in compliance with Department of Transportation and/or employer requirements for substance abuse testing.			
16.4 The facilities are quiet.			
16.5 The facilities are well maintained and clean.			
16.6 Equipment is properly maintained and, if applicable, calibrated,			
including the following:			
16.6.1 diagnostic and treatment equipment			
16.6.2 training equipment			
16.6.3 administrative and office equipment.			
16.7 Information resources are available and include the			
following:			
16.7.1 medical and nursing texts			
16.7.2 occupational health newsletters			
16 7.3 occupational health journals			
16.7.4 occupational health regulations			
16.7.5 SDS			
16.7.6 first aid manuals			
16.7.7 internet and electronic data capabilities.			
17. Record-Keeping and Documentation (Electronic and Paper)			
17.1 Access to confidential records is controlled in a satisfactory manner.			
17.2 Occupational history records are maintained for each worker.			
17.3 Hazard exposure records are maintained for each worker.			
17.4 Consultation and treatment records are maintained for each worker.			
17.5 Periodic health evaluation records are maintained for each worker.			
17.6 Medical records are prepared and maintained to keep separate confidential documents from non-confidential documents.			

Description	Inadequate	Needs Improvement	Satisfactory
17.7 A satisfactory flagging system is in operation for special cases and for scheduled evaluations.			
17.8 Biological monitoring records are maintained.			
17.9 Immunization records are maintained.			
17.10 Authorization for release of information documents are appropriate, available, and used as needed.			
17.11 Fitness-for-work certificates are used and include documentation/ communication to:			
17.11.1 employee			
17.11.2 employer (management and supervisor)			
17.11.3 workers' compensation (where applicable)			
17.11.4 occupational health.			
17.12 Site-survey reports are maintained.			
17.13 A daily log (visit record) is kept.			
17.14 Minutes of meetings are retained.			
17.15 A record of equipment maintenance and calibration is kept.			
17.16 Records of the purchasing and maintenance of equipment, supplies and inventory are maintained.			
17.17 Drug dispensing records are kept.			
17.18 Records are maintained of equipment loans, such as crutches, canes, splints.			
17.19 Substance abuse testing records are maintained in a confidential manner, isolated from the medical record.			
17.20 Employer's workers' compensation insurance information or other appropriate insurance and billing information is available and current.			
18. Additional Items Specific to the Enterprise			

Appendix 2: A Reference Bookshelf for an Occupational Health Service

American College of Occupational and Environmental Medicine (2004) *Occupational Medicine Practice Guidelines*. Chicago IL, ACOEM, 3rd ed. in hard copy, one-year access to APG-1 online version included in purchase. APG-1 is revised frequently and is also available as a free-standing application.

ACOEM Health and Productivity Toolkit. Chicago IL, American College of Occupational and Environmental Medicine. Online resource available by subscription. See www.acoem.org.

American Medical Association (2010) *AMA Guides to the Evaluation of Disease and Injury Causation*. Chicago IL, 6th ed. is current edition. Different states may require different versions. See Chapter 26.

Guidotti TL (2010) *The Praeger Handbook of Occupational and Environmental Medicine*. Santa Barbara CA, Praeger ABC-Clio, 3 volumes. Written by the editor of this work; the most recent comprehensive textbook of occupational medicine. Does not address clinical aspects of injury care.

Guidotti TL, Rose SG (2001) *Science on the Witness Stand: Evaluating Scientific Evidence in Law, Adjudication, and Policy*. Beverly Farms MA, OEM Press.

Hartenbaum N, Hegman K, Wood E (2010) *The DOT Medical Examination: A Guide to Commercial Driver's Medical Certification*. Beverly Farms MA, OEM Press, 5th ed.

Hathaway GJ, Proctor NH (2004) *Proctor and Hughes' Chemical Hazards of the Workplace*. New York, Van Nordstrand, 5th ed.

International Commission on Occupational Health: Code of Ethics. Available at: http://www.icohweb.org/site_new/ico_core_documents.asp#. Accessed May 16, 2011.

Mitchell, F (2002) *Instant Medical Surveillance*. Beverly Farms MA, OEM Press.

Moser R Jr. (2008) *Effective Management of Health and Safety Programs: A Practical Guide*. Beverly Farms MA, OEM Press, 3rd ed. An alternative to the present book, providing a different point of view.

Palmer KT, Cox RAF, Brown I (2007) *Fitness for Work: The Medical Aspects*. London and New York, Oxford University Press, 4th ed.

Rogers B (2003) *Occupational and Environmental Health Nursing: Concepts and Practice*. Philadelphia PA, Saunders, 2nd ed.

Rogers B, Randolph S, Mastroiani K (2008) *Occupational Health Nursing Guidelines for Primary Clinical Conditions*. Beverly Farms MA, OEM Press, 4th ed.

Rom WN (2007) *Environmental and Occupational Medicine*. Philadelphia PA, Lippincott Williams & Wilkins 4th ed. The most recent comprehensive but not clinical textbook of occupational medicine, an alternative to the *Praeger Handbook of OEM*. Does not address clinical aspects of injury care.

Rosenstock L, Cullen MR, Brodkin CA, Redlich CA (2005) *Textbook of Clinical Occupational and Environmental Medicine*. Philadelphia PA, Elsevier. Clinically oriented, but does not address clinical aspects of injury care.

Swotinsky R, Smith DR (2010) *The Medical Review Officer's Manual: MROCC's Guide to Drug Testing*. Beverly Farms MA, OEM Press, 4th ed.

Talmadge JB, Melhorn JM (2007) *A Physician's Guide to Return to Work*. Chicago IL, American Medical Association, 6th ed.

Periodicals

Journal of Occupational and Environmental Medicine
Workplace Health & Safety: Promoting Environments Conducive to Well-Being and Productivity (formerly the *American Association of Occupational Health Nurses Journal* (AAOHN Journal))
Other journals, depending on location and emphasis in practice.

Online

Occupational and Environmental Medicine List (Occ-Env-Med-L), the indispensable social media vehicle for occupational health professionals, moderated since 1993 by Dr. Gary Greenberg. Occ-Env-Med-L reaches approximately 4,000 recipients in 75 countries. http,//occhealthnews.net/occ-env-.htm.

There are many online groups in occupational health, particularly in LinkedIn.

Index